Equine Neurology

Editor

STEPHEN M. REED

VETERINARY CLINICS OF NORTH AMERICA: EQUINE PRACTICE

www.vetequine.theclinics.com

Consulting Editor
RAMIRO E. TORIBIO

August 2022 • Volume 38 • Number 2

ELSEVIER

1600 John F. Kennedy Boulevard • Suite 1800 • Philadelphia, Pennsylvania, 19103-2899

http://www.vetequine.theclinics.com

VETERINARY CLINICS OF NORTH AMERICA: EQUINE PRACTICE Volume 38, Number 2
August 2022 ISSN 0749-0739, ISBN-13: 978-0-323-81341-9

Editor: Taylor Hayes
Developmental Editor: Ann Gielou Posedio

Veterinary Clinics of North America: Equine Practice (ISSN 0749-0739) is published in April, August, and December by Elsevier Inc., 360 Park Avenue South, New York, NY 10010-1710. Business and Editorial Offices: 1600 John F. Kennedy Blvd., Suite 1800, Philadelphia, PA 19103-2899. Subscription prices are $299.00 per year (domestic individuals), $777.00 per year (domestic institutions), $100.00 per year (domestic students/residents), $341.00 per year (Canadian individuals), $789.00 per year (Canadian institutions), $372.00 per year (international individuals), $789.00 per year (international institutions), $100.00 per year (Canadian students/residents), and $180.00 per year (international students/residents). To receive student/resident rate, orders must be accompanied by name of affiliated institution, date of term, and the signature of program/residency coordinator on institution letterhead. Orders will be billed at individual rate until proof of status is received. Foreign air speed delivery is included in all *Clinics* subscription prices. All prices are subject to change without notice. **POSTMASTER:** Send address changes to *Veterinary Clinics of North America: Equine Practice*, 3251 Riverport Lane, Maryland Heights, MO 63043. Customer Service (orders, claims, online, change of address): Elsevier Health Sciences Division, Subscription **Customer Service, 3251 Riverport Lane, Maryland Heights, MO 63043. Tel: 1-800-654-2452 (U.S. and Canada); 314-447-8871 (outside U.S. and Canada). Fax: 314-447-8029. E-mail: journalscustomerservice-usa@elsevier.com (for print support);** E-mail: **journalsonlinesupport-usa@elsevier.com (for online support).**

Reprints. For copies of 100 or more of articles in this publication, please contact the Commercial Reprints Department, Elsevier Inc., 360 Park Avenue South, New York, NY 10010-1710. Tel.: 212-633-3874; Fax: 212-633-3820; E-mail: reprints@elsevier.com.

Veterinary Clinics of North America: Equine Practice is covered in *MEDLINE/PubMed (Index Medicus), Excerpta Medica, Current Contents/Agriculture, Biology and Environmental Sciences,* and *ISI.*

Contributors

CONSULTING EDITOR

RAMIRO E. TORIBIO, DVM, MS, PhD
Diplomate, American College of Veterinary Internal Medicine; Professor and Trueman Endowed Chair of Equine Medicine and Surgery, College of Veterinary Medicine, The Ohio State University, Columbus, Ohio, USA

EDITOR

STEPHEN M. REED, DVM
Diplomate, American College of Veterinary Internal Medicine; Equine Internal Medicine, Rood and Riddle Equine Hospital, Adjunct Professor, Gluck Equine Research Center, University of Kentucky, Lexington, Kentucky, USA; Emeritus Professor, Veterinary Clinical Sciences, The Ohio State University, Columbus, Ohio, USA

AUTHORS

MONICA ALEMAN, MVZ Cert, PhD
Diplomate, American College of Veterinary Internal Medicine (Large Animal Internal Medicine, Neurology); Professor, Terry Holliday Equine and Comparative Neurology Endowed Presidential Chair, SVM: Department of Medicine and Epidemiology, University of California, Davis, Davis, California, USA

CARRIE J. FINNO, DVM, PhD
Diplomate, American College of Veterinary Internal Medicine (Large Animal Internal Medicine); Department of Veterinary Population Health and Reproduction, School of Veterinary Medicine, University of California, Davis, Davis, California, USA

MARTIN O. FURR, DVM, PhD, MA Ed
Diplomate, American College of Veterinary Internal Medicine; Department of Physiological Sciences, College of Veterinary Medicine, Oklahoma State University, Stillwater, Oklahoma, USA

KATHERINE S. GARRETT, DVM
Diplomate, American College of Veterinary Surgeons (Large Animal); Rood and Riddle Equine Hospital, Lexington, Kentucky, USA

WILLIAM F. GILSENAN, VMD
Diplomate, American College of Veterinary Internal Medicine (Large Animal Internal Medicine); Rood and Riddle Equine Hospital, Lexington, Kentucky, USA

LUTZ S. GOEHRING, DVM, MS, PhD
Veterinary Science Department, Institute of Infectious Diseases and Zoonoses, Ludwig-Maximilians University, Munich, Germany; Department of Veterinary Science, The

Maxwell H. Gluck Equine Research Center, College of Agriculture, University of Kentucky, Lexington, Kentucky, USA

BARRIE GRANT, DVM, MS, MRCVS
Diplomate, American College of Veterinary Surgeons; Bonsall, California, USA

CAROLINE HAHN, DVM, MSc, PhD, MRCVS
Diplomate, European College of Equine Internal Medicine; Diplomate, European College of Veterinary Neurology; Senior Lecturer in Veterinary Clinical Neurosciences, Royal (Dick) School of Veterinary Sciences, The University of Edinburgh, Roslin, United Kingdom

DANIEL K. HOWE, PhD
Professor, Department of Veterinary Science, M.H. Gluck Equine Research Center, University of Kentucky, Lexington, Kentucky, USA

GISELA SOBOLL HUSSEY, DVM, PhD
Department of Pathobiology and Diagnostic Investigation, College of Veterinary Medicine, Michigan State University, East Lansing, Michigan, USA

JENNIFER G. JANES, DVM, PhD
Diplomate, American College of Veterinary Pathologists; Associate Professor, Department of Veterinary Science, University of Kentucky Veterinary Diagnostic Laboratory, Lexington, Kentucky, USA

AMY L. JOHNSON, DVM
Diplomate, American College of Veterinary Internal Medicine (Large Animal Internal Medicine, Neurology); Department of Clinical Studies, University of Pennsylvania School of Veterinary Medicine - New Bolton Center, Kennett Square, Pennsylvania, USA

SHERRY A. JOHNSON, DVM, MS
Diplomate, American College of Veterinary Sports Medicine and Rehabilitation; PhD Candidate, Department of Clinical Sciences, Orthopaedic Research Center at the C. Wayne McIlwraith Translational Medicine Institute, College of Veterinary Medicine and Biomedical Sciences, Colorado State University, Fort Collins, Colorado, USA

SANNE LOTTE JOURNÉE, DVM
Equine Diagnostics, Wijns, the Netherlands; Research Group of Comparative Physiology, Department of Translational Physiology, Infectiology and Public Health, Faculty of Veterinary Medicine, Ghent University, Merelbeke, Belgium

HENRICUS LOUIS JOURNÉE, MD, PhD
Department of Neurosurgery, University of Groningen, University Medical Center Groningen, Groningen, the Netherlands; Department of Orthopedics, University of Utrecht, University Medical Center Utrecht, Utrecht, the Netherlands

ROBERT J. MACKAY, BVSc (Dist), PhD
Professor Emeritus of Large Animal Medicine, Department of Large Animal Clinical Sciences, College of Veterinary Medicine, University of Florida, Gainesville, Florida, USA

YVETTE S. NOUT-LOMAS, DVM, PhD
Diplomate, American College of Veterinary Internal Medicine; Diplomate, American College of Veterinary Emergency and Critical Care; Associate Professor Equine Internal Medicine, Department of Clinical Sciences, Colorado State University, Fort Collins, Colorado, USA

NICOLA PUSTERLA, DVM, PhD
Department of Medicine and Epidemiology, School of Veterinary Medicine, University of California, Davis, Davis, California, USA

REBECCA E. RUBY, MSc, BVSc
Diplomate, American College of Veterinary Pathologists; Diplomate, American College of Veterinary Internal Medicine-Large Animal Internal Medicine; Assistant Professor, Department of Veterinary Science, University of Kentucky Veterinary Diagnostic Laboratory, Lexington, Kentucky, USA

JACOB M. SWINK, DVM, MS
Diplomate, American College of Veterinary Internal Medicine (Large Animal Internal Medicine); Brown Equine Hospital, Somerset, Pennsylvania, USA

RAMIRO E. TORIBIO, DVM, MS, PhD
Diplomate, American College of Veterinary Internal Medicine; Professor and Trueman Endowed Chair of Equine Medicine and Surgery, College of Veterinary Medicine, The Ohio State University, Columbus, Ohio, USA

STEPHANIE J. VALBERG, DVM, PhD
Diplomate, American College of Veterinary Internal Medicine (Large Animal); Diplomate, American College of Veterinary Sports Medicine and Rehabilitation; Professor, MaryAnne McPhail Dressage Chair in Equine Sports Medicine, Michigan State University, Large Animal Clinical Sciences, College of Veterinary Medicine, East Lansing, Michigan, USA

BRETT WOODIE, DVM, MS
Diplomate, American College of Veterinary Surgeons; Surgery, Rood and Riddle Equine Hospital, Lexington, Kentucky, USA

Contents

> The neurological examination is undertaken to determine whether any deficit is due to a lesion in the nervous system and, if so, where within the nervous system any possible lesion or lesions are located. The examination of horses has challenges not encountered when doing the equivalent examination in dogs and cats, principally that spinal reflexes and postural reactions are impossible/difficult to assess in most animals. The anatomy book can be consulted later but at the end of the neurological examination the clinician then should be able to determine broadly which area of the neuromuscular systems is affected.

> Diagnostic imaging is often an important part of the diagnostic approach to neurologic disease. Advanced imaging techniques such as myelography, computed tomography (CT), and magnetic resonance imaging (MRI) provide more information than radiography and ultrasonography but are more limited in their availability. The clinician should be cognizant of the findings of the clinical examination when interpreting diagnostic imaging findings.

> Depending on the localization of the lesion, spinal cord ataxia is the most common type of ataxia in horses. Most prevalent diagnoses include cervical vertebral stenotic myelopathy (CVSM), equine protozoal myeloencephalitis (EPM), trauma and equine degenerative myeloencephalopathy (EDM). Other causes of ataxia and weakness are associated with infectious causes, trauma and neoplasia. A neurologic examination is indispensable to identify the type of ataxia. In addition, clinical neurophysiology offers tools to locate functional abnormalities in the central and peripheral nervous system. Clinical EMG assessment looks at the lower motoneuron function (LMN) and is used to differentiate between neuropathy in peripheral nerves, which belong to LMNs and myopathy. As LMNs reside in the spinal cord, it is possible to grossly localize lesions in the myelum by muscle examination. Transcranial (tc) stimulation techniques are gaining importance in all areas of medicine to assess the motor function of the spinal cord along the motor tracts to the LMNs. Applications in diagnostics, intraoperative neurophysiological monitoring (IONM), and evaluation of effects of treatment are still evolving in human

medicine and offer new challenges in equine medicine. Tc stimulation techniques comprise transcranial magnetic stimulation (TMS) and transcranial electrical stimulation (TES). TMS was first applied in horses in 1996 by Mayhew and colleagues and followed by TES. The methods are exchangeable for clinical diagnostic assessment but show a few differences. An outline is given on the principles, current clinical diagnostic applications and challenging possibilities of muscle evoked potentials (MEP) from transcranial stimulation in horses.

Carrie J. Finno and Amy L. Johnson

Neuroaxonal degenerative disease in the horse is termed equine neuroaxonal dystrophy (eNAD), when pathologic lesions are localized to the brainstem and equine degenerative myeloencephalopathy (EDM) and degenerative changes extend throughout the spinal cord. Both pathologic conditions result in identical clinical disease, most commonly characterized by the insidious onset of ataxia during early development. However, later onset of clinical signs and additional clinical features, such as behavior changes, is also observed. A definitive diagnosis of eNAD/EDM requires histologic evaluation of the caudal medulla and cervicothoracic spinal cord. Strong evidence has suggested that eNAD/EDM is an inherited disorder and there seems to be a role for vitamin E acting as an environmental modifier to determine the overall severity of the phenotype of horses affected with eNAD/EDM.

Brett Woodie, Amy L. Johnson, and Barrie Grant

Cervical vertebral stenotic myelopathy is a common cause of ataxia in horses secondary to spinal cord compression. Early articles describing this problem indicate genetic predisposition as a known risk factor. Further studies have shown the problem is a developmental abnormality which might have genetic predisposition and environmental influences.

Robert J. MacKay and Daniel K. Howe

Advances in the understanding of equine protozoal myeloencephalitis (EPM) are reviewed. It is now apparent that EPM can be caused by either of 2 related protozoan parasites, Sarcocystis neurona and Neospora hughesi, although S neurona is the most common etiologic pathogen. Horses are commonly infected, but clinical disease occurs only infrequently; the factors influencing disease occurrence are not well understood. Epidemiologic studies have identified risk factors for the development of EPM, including the presence of opossums and prior stressful health-related events. Attempts to reproduce EPM experimentally have reliably induced antibody responses in challenged horses, but have not consistently produced neurologic disease. Diagnosis of EPM has improved by detecting intrathecal antibody production against the parasite. Sulfadiazine/pyrimethamine (ReBalance) and the triazine

their presence. The goal of this article is to provide an overview on patho-physiologic and clinical aspects of nonarboviral equine encephalitides, specifically on lyssaviruses (rabies) and bornaviruses (Borna disease).

Although equine herpesvirus myeloencephalopathy (EHM) is a relatively uncommon manifestation of equine herpesvirus-1 (EHV-1) infection, it can cause devastating losses during outbreaks. Antemortem diagnosis of EHM relies mainly on the molecular detection of EHV-1 in nasal secretions and blood. Management of horses affected by EHM is aimed at supportive nursing and nutritional care, at reducing central nervous system inflammation and preventing thromboembolic sequelae. Horses exhibiting sudden and severe neurologic signs consistent with a diagnosis of EHM pose a definite risk to the surrounding horse population. Consequently, early intervention to prevent the spread of infection is required.

Mechanisms of traumatic nervous system injury to a degree are similar, but differences exist in etiology, pathophysiology, and treatment of brain, spinal cord, and peripheral nerve injury. The most common clinical abnormalities seen in the horse are abnormal level of consciousness, abnormal behavior, seizures, cranial nerve deficits, vestibular disease, tetra- and paraparesis or paraplegia, cauda equina syndrome, specific gait deficits, and muscle atrophy. Treatments are directed toward reducing inflammation and swelling, halting secondary injury, and promoting mechanisms of neuroregeneration and plasticity. Prognosis depends on the severity of primary injury and the neuroanatomic location and extent of nervous tissue damage.

Rehabilitation of the neurologic horse represents a unique challenge for the equine practitioner. Improving postural stability and balance control through improving the strength of the spinal stabilizer muscle multifidus remains one of the most promising rehabilitative targets. This muscle can be targeted through the use of physiotherapeutic exercises, various forms of perturbation, and even whole-body vibration. Neuroanatomic localization and diagnosis specificity enable the practitioner to determine suitability for such rehabilitative tasks, and with the advent of evolving strategies and commercially available equipment, the bandwidth for professionally guided programs is continuously being developed and is expected to improve traditional outcomes.

The vestibular system (VS) is the primary specialized sensory system responsible for maintaining balance (equilibrium) and orientation of the eyes, neck, trunk, and limbs during rest and movement. Two important reflexes are responsible for maintaining balance: vestibulo-ocular and vestibulospinal reflexes. These reflexes involve peripheral and central components of the VS. Whether central or peripheral disease, most of the disorders of the VS result in ipsilateral neurologic deficits. A few uncommon exceptions present with contralateral signs to the site of the lesion. This article provides a brief review of functional anatomy, vestibular disease, clinical signs, and examples of disorders affecting the VS.

 Video content accompanies this article at http://www.vetequine. theclinics.com.

Movement disorders are defined as involuntary movements that are not due to a painful stimulus or associated with changes in consciousness or proprioception. Diagnosis involves ruling out any lameness and neurologic disease and characterizing the gait during walking backward and forward and trotting. Shivers causes abnormal hindlimb hypertonicity during walking backward and, when advanced, a few strides walking forward. Stringhalt causes consistent hyperflexion during walking forward and trotting and variable difficulty when walking backward. Classification and potential causes are discussed as well as other enigmatic movement disorders in horses are presented. Cerebellar abiotrophy is reviewed.

The variety of neurologic diseases which affect horses makes pathologic examination of the nervous system a complex and lengthy process. An understanding of the common causes of neurologic disease, antemortem neurolocalization, and supplementation of the necropsy examination with ancillary testing will help to diagnose a large number of causes of neurologic disease. A general understanding of neuropathology and collaborative relationship with your local pathologists will aid in the definitive diagnosis of neurologic diseases.

VETERINARY CLINICS OF
NORTH AMERICA: EQUINE PRACTICE

SERIES OF RELATED INTEREST

Veterinary Clinics of North America: Food Animal Practice
https://www.vetfood.theclinics.com/

THE CLINICS ARE NOW AVAILABLE ONLINE!
Access your subscription at:
www.theclinics.com

Preface

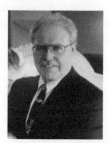

Stephen M. Reed, DVM
Editor

The recognition and understanding of equine neurologic diseases have been a challenge for equine veterinarians. The advent of new, more sophisticated diagnostic techniques has allowed equine practitioners to more accurately diagnose disorders of the nervous system. In addition, better understanding of how the nervous system responds to trauma, infection, and other types of injury, such as oxidative damage, has led to more rapid and effective treatments for congenital, developmental, infectious, and inherited diseases of the central and peripheral nervous systems.

The goals of this *Veterinary Clinics of North America: Equine Practice* issue are to provide a comprehensive review of equine neurologic diseases, to introduce the use of new diagnostic testing for neurologic diseases, and to emphasize the benefits provided by use of technologies such as computed tomography, MRI, and transcranial electrical and magnetic stimulation to evaluate the central nervous system. Equally important are the advances in interpretation of diagnostic testing on blood, spinal fluid muscle, and nerve tissues.

In this issue of the *Veterinary Clinics of North America: Equine Practice*, known diseases, such as equine degenerative myeloencephalopathy (EDM), equine herpesvirus-1 myeloencephalopathy (EHM), and viral infections of the nervous system, as well as the use of electrodiagnostic techniques, have been given expanded coverage. Of particular interest is the apparent recognition of EDM in quarter horses and warmblood horses over the past 8 to 10 years.

The emphasis of this issue is on anatomic diagnosis—the basis for successful clinical practice. Each article provides detailed information about the cause of the clinical condition, the signs associated with damage to a particular anatomic location, and thorough discussion on essential diagnostic tests needed to accurately diagnose and treat the condition.

Separation of some neurologic conditions from musculoskeletal problems is sometimes difficult, which is the reason one article on performance of the neurologic examination emphasizes the importance of proper neuroanatomic localization. I hope this *Veterinary Clinics of North America: Equine Practice* is on the shelf of all equine

Vet Clin Equine 38 (2022) xiii–xiv
https://doi.org/10.1016/j.cveq.2022.06.001
0749-0739/22/© 2022 Published by Elsevier Inc.

hospitals and is carried in the ambulatory vehicles of many practitioners to be used in their daily examination of horses in their practice.

The authors are recognized as experts in the articles they authored, and I commend and thank each of them for their contributions and their attention to detail. As a result of their hard work, all readers will have a better understanding of the many neurologic problems encountered on a daily or weekly basis in our practices.

Stephen M. Reed, DVM
Equine Internal Medicine
Rood and Riddle Equine Hospital
Lexington, KY, USA

Veterinary Clinical Sciences
The Ohio State University
Columbus, OH, USA

Gluck Equine Research Center
University of Kentucky
2150 Georgetown Road
Lexington, KY 40511, USA

E-mail address:
sreed@roodandriddle.com

Neurological Examination of Horses

Caroline Hahn, DVM, MSc, PhD, DipECEIM, DipECVM, MRCVS

KEYWORDS

- Neurological examination • Equine • Horses • Ataxia • Paresis

KEY POINTS

- The neurologic examination in equids is a modified version of the examination in small animals; spinal reflexes and postural reactions are difficult to assess in most animals.
- Methodical examination of the head, neck and trunk, perineum, and gait and posture allows for an effective assessment of the nervous system.
- Tight circling of ataxic patients is useful to disclose ataxia and paresis of limbs, and pulling on the tail while the horse is moving is the most useful test for upper motor neuron paresis.
- The severity of ataxia and paresis should be evaluated (mild, moderate, severe for paresis, 0 to 4+ for ataxia). Compressive lesions classically result in clinical signs that appear more severe in the pelvic limbs and a two-grade difference in spinal cord ataxia is possible with a lesion in the cervical spinal cord.
- Autonomous zones for individual sensory branches of the major spinal nerves to the limbs of horses have been established; there is no autonomous zone for the radial nerve.

BACKGROUND

The neurological examination is undertaken to determine whether any deficit is due to a lesion in the nervous system and, if so, where within the nervous system any possible lesion or lesions are located. The examination of horses has challenges not encountered when doing the equivalent examination in dogs and cats, principally that spinal reflexes and postural reactions are impossible/difficult to assess in most animals. Nevertheless, assessment of the function of the nervous system is possible given sufficient care and observations.[1] A detailed knowledge of neuroanatomy is not essential as long as all the deficits are noted. The anatomy book can be consulted later[2] but at the end of the neurological examination the clinician then should be able to determine broadly which area of the nervous system is affected:

- Cerebrum
- Brain stem
- Cerebellum

Royal (Dick) School of Veterinary Sciences, The University of Edinburgh, Room 160 Middle Wing, Easter Bush, Roslin EH25 9RG, United Kingdom
E-mail address: Caroline.Hahn@ed.ac.uk

Vet Clin Equine 38 (2022) 155–169
https://doi.org/10.1016/j.cveq.2022.05.001
0749-0739/22/© 2022 Elsevier Inc. All rights reserved.

- Spinal cord (which segment?)
- Peripheral nerve
- Muscles (and neuromuscular junction)

EQUIPMENT

Very little equipment is required to carry out a neurologic examination, but the author is always equipped with a strong light source (most recently a mobile phone light), a pair of forceps, and a video camera! A handler is essential to hold and move the animal; the horse should be led from the same sides as the examiner so that the kicking end can be safely turned away if the patient objects to having his tail pulled or his perineum prodded. In cases with focal muscle atrophy, it may be useful to use ancillary aids such as electromyography, as in horses disuse atrophy can be remarkably difficult to differentiate from neurogenic muscle atrophy.

HISTORY

It is always useful to speak to the owner to find out exactly what they think the problem is and to assess whether the horse's current behavior is normal—is this really the quietest 2-year old colt in the county or does the patient suffer from a degree of depressed mention? If the problem is episodic, for example, head-shaking, are the episodes seasonal? Was the onset sudden or progressive? Keep in mind, however, that animals with, for example, cervical vertebral malformation can present with acute severe sign despite the process being due to a progressive lesion.

STEPS IN THE NEUROLOGIC EXAMINATION

1. Head
2. Neck and trunk
3. Perineum
4. Gait and posture
5. Recumbent animals
6. Autonomous zones

Steps 1 to 4 are always performed, and it behooves the clinician not to take any shortcuts; localizing the lesion, that is, making an "Anatomic Diagnosis,"[3] requires that the entire system has been assessed. The horse that is clearly ataxic in all limbs may not have a cervical vertebral compression after all, something that could have been ascertained had the *medulla oblongata* deficits been noted. Examination of recumbent animals is much like that in small animals except that the equipment is much bigger, for example, using a hammer handle to elicit equine patellar reflexes.

The neurologic examination begins at the head and ends at the tail, emphasizing the anatomical location of any lesion. The examination consists of evaluation of the head and evaluation of the entire body in the stable, and finally, evaluation of gait and posture while the animal is led in-hand. In addition to the results of the neurological examination, any bony and muscular asymmetry, localized sweating, focal muscle atrophy, decreased pain perception, and localized painful responses should be noted.

The following sequence for the equine neurological examination is used by the author:

- Behavior and mentation (forebrain)
- Head posture (cranial nerve [CN] VIII)
- Head muscle mass (motor CN V)

- Nasal septum sensory perception (forebrain, sensory CN V)
- Tongue tone (CN XII)
- Eye movement (CN III, IV, VI, and VIII)
- Symmetry of eye position with head elevation (CN VIII)
- Menace response ("vision": CN II, visual cortex, CN VII, and cerebellum)
- Pupillary light reflex and swinging light test (CN II and parasympathetic III)
- Palpebral response (CN V and VII)
- Local cervical reflex and cervicofacial reflex (cervical dorsal and ventral spinal roots andN VII)
- Cutaneous trunci reflex (dorsal roots, cranial thoracic spinal cord, and C8 spinal cord lateral thoracic nerve)
- Anal sensation and reflex, tail tone (caudal equina)
- Tail pull (upper motor neuron function)
- Gait in straight lines, circling, zigzagging, walking down slope with head elevated (upper and lower motor neurons, general proprioception, cerebellum, vestibular system)

First examine the patient when standing still; signs of bony and muscular asymmetry, localized sweating, focal muscle atrophy, decreased pain perception, and localized painful responses are searched for and documented. Areas of sweating and analgesia and depths and diameters of muscle masses should preferably be accurately measured.

Head

An evaluation of behavior, mentation, head posture and movement, and cranial nerves is undertaken to determine if there is evidence of brain or cranial nerve disease. Begin by observing the patient; is the horse inquisitive and is mental status appropriate (forebrain function)? Does the patient have normal ears movement with a nose that is not pulled to one side (facial nerve, **Fig. 1**)? Is the head posture straight (vestibular nerve)? Are masseter and temporal muscles the same size on both sides (trigeminal nerve)? Can the patient pick up and swallow a polo mint (facial musculature, tongue, and pharynx function)? Motor trigeminal and facial nuclear lesions that result in atrophy of the muscles of mastication or facial paresis are often seen with equine protozoal myeloencephalitis, and it is very important to carefully interpret such subtle asymmetry of the head in horses that have come from countries in which protozoal myeloencephalitis may be suspected.

Significant changes in the horse's behavior will be obvious but you will often notice subtle changes as you examine the animal. Acceptable medical terms for the progressive loss of a patient's sensorium are dullness, lethargy, obtundation, semicoma (stupor), and coma (note that the word "depressed," a term used for humans, is not on this list). The most common site for a focal lesion to cause progressive obtundation or stupor is the thalamus, presumably from the interruption of the ascending reticular activating system at this level.

Sensation of the face (CN V) is best assessed by gently touching the nasal mucosa with a pair of forceps, a horse with normal mentation should object to this. The difference in responses left and right is important, so take time to carefully compare them. Although nasal sensation is mediated though the trigeminal nerve, this test is really used as a crude assessment of forebrain function; detection of slight asymmetry in the behavioral (avoidance) response to a stimulus applied to the nasal septum, that is, hyperalgesia, can take considerable patience but may confirm the presence of asymmetric forebrain disease.

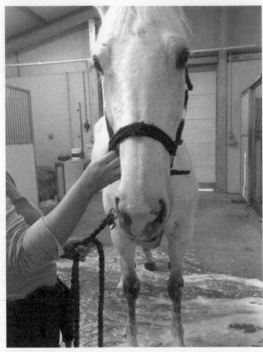

Fig. 1. Horse with a mild, transient left-sided facial nerve neuropraxia following general anesthesia with the head collar on.

The motor innervation of the tongue (CN XII) is examined by grabbing it and assessing its strength; often cases of botulism will present with poor tongue tone. A "dirty" tongue is also a potential sign of botulism or potentially a swallowing problem such as choke. Some horses appear to not mind the tongue being manipulated, so further evidence of a disease process should be established.

The next step in the rostral to caudal examination is the eyes, and both function and movement need to be assessed. While examining the eyes you can appreciate whether they are normally positioned in the orbits. Abnormal eye positions could be due to a retroorbital mass (most commonly) or reflect a lack of innervation of the extraocular muscles or a disorder with the vestibular system. The latter is most common and results in ventral strabismus, which is most evident when the head is lifted (**Fig. 2**). A quick assessment of the motor function of the oculomotor nerve is to test for normal physiologic nystagmus (oculocephalic reflex) by moving the head side to side. The fast movement of physiologic nystagmus is in the same direction as the head movement.

The examination of vision (**Fig. 3**) is crude in horses and is generally limited to appraising the response to a threatening gesture; the horse should close its eyes when a threatening hand is moved toward it; this is a learned response that requires vision (CN II), an intact cerebellum and a functional facial nerve, and may not be apparent in foals until they are a week to 10 days of age. Make sure to test the whole visual field, as retinal lesions may result in visual field abnormalities: nasal retinal fibers decussate at the optic chiasm, whereas temporal retinal fibers do not so that each cerebral hemisphere receives information from contralateral visual field. In the absence of a menace response do not forget to assess the palpebral response (CN V afferent,

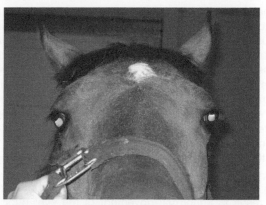

Fig. 2. Horse with a right-sided central vestibular lesion. Note the exaggerated ventral strabismus in the right eye with elevation of the head.

CN VII efferent) and check if the horse is able to close its eye when the palpebra are touched before declaring that the horse is blind; a lesion to the facial nerve is much more common than a lesion to the eye or optic nerve. The strength with which a horse closes its eyes when menaced is so strong that often an audible "click" can be heard, and suspicion of a facial nerve paresis should be raised if this click is heard on one side but not the other.

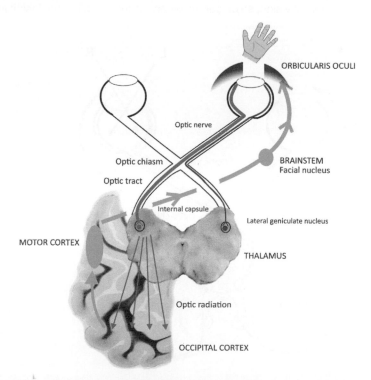

Fig. 3. Optic pathway and transmission of light stimuli to the visual cortex.

To evaluate whether a light impulse reaches the midbrain, use a strong light in a darkened stable to elicit the pupillary light reflex (PLR). Eighty percent of equine optic nerve axons decussate in the optic chiasm (**Fig. 4**), resulting in unequal pupillary responses in the illuminated and unilluminated eye. Both the direct and indirect reflex should be assessed but to overcome the operational difficulty of visualizing the eye on the opposite side of the large horse's head, the "swinging light test" should be used: light is alternately shifted from eye to eye and both pupils should constrict to an equal degree when stimulated. The pupil of the eye with a degree of blindness, however, will have constricted indirectly but will now dilate when the light is swung across to shine on that side, a disconcerting experience!

Depending on the anatomy of the lesion, internal ophthalmoplegia (impairment of pupillary function due to sphincter muscle dysfunction, presence of an atropine-like drug or a lesion in the parasympathetic portion of the oculomotor nerve or its nucleus) may or may not result in abnormal movement of the eye; pupillomotor fibers are located superficially and as a result may be preferentially damaged with no extraocular muscle dysfunction. External ophthalmoplegia (dysfunction of the motor fibers of CN III) is characterized by ptosis, lateral strabismus, and inability to rotate the globe dorsally, ventrally, or medially. Isolated external ophthalmoplegia is rare and generally seen with central lesions.

Localizing lesions in the visual pathway are puzzles to be solved and broadly can be characterized as follows: (1) with optic nerve lesions, both vision and PLR are abnormal, (2) with cortical lesions, vision is affected but PLRs are normal, and (3) with efferent arm lesions, the PLR is abnormal and vision is unaffected. An important caveat here is that PLRs are often maintained even with retinal or optic nerve lesions that result in the loss of vision, so be careful when diagnosing a central lesion in a blind

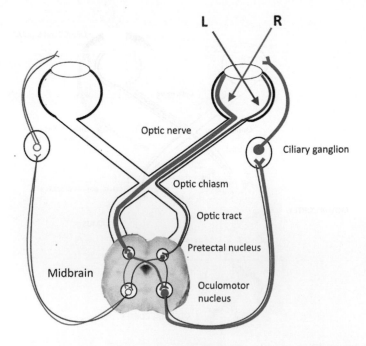

Fig. 4. Anatomy of the pupillary light reflex pathway.

horse with apparently operational PLRs. Interestingly, and for reasons not elucidated, generalized cerebellar dysfunction produces bilateral mydriasis and PLR deficits but of course these would result in obvious additional clinical signs.

One condition unrelated to vision that might be uncovered during an examination of the eyes is Horner syndrome, caused by a lesion to the sympathetic input to the eye (but nothing to do with the facial nerve, a common misconception). Classic ophthalmic signs of Horner syndrome are ptosis, miosis, and enophthalmos with associated protrusion of the nictitating membrane but in horses ptosis is the most consistent clinical sign and may be the only sign observed (**Fig. 5**). Additional clinical signs are usually observed, particularly if the lesion is severe and acute:

1. Lesions in the region of the guttural pouch and cranial cervical ganglion will result in sweating of the face (most prominent at the base of the ear) and the cranial neck down to the level of C2.
2. Lesions further down the neck involving the sympathetic trunk may result in sweating of the face and the neck extending down to the level of C3 to C4
3. Lesions in the thoracic inlet can result in this sweating extending down to the level of the shoulder.
4. Although extremely rare, lesions of the spinal cord involving the descending sympathetic pathway can result in Horner syndrome and sweating of the whole side of the body ipsilateral to the lesion.

Neck and Trunk

After the evaluation for evidence of brain and/or cranial nerve abnormalities is completed, reflexes involving the neck and trunk can be undertaken (**Fig. 6**). Tapping the skin over the *brachiocephalicus* muscle with closed tip of the hemostat from the cranial end of the neck to the back of the shoulder should result in contraction of the *brachiocephalicus* and *cutaneous colli* muscles as well as twitching of the facial muscles at the commissure of the lips. Interruption of reflex components in the cervical nerves or roots (sensory or motor) or local cervical spinal cord segments or facial nerve can affect these reflexes. The response can be reduced at the level of a cervical spinal cord lesion but is normal cranial and caudal to the lesion and should result in a local cervical reflex (a local reflex) and cervicofacial reflex (a compound reflex involving at least cervical dorsal and ventral spinal roots and CN VII).

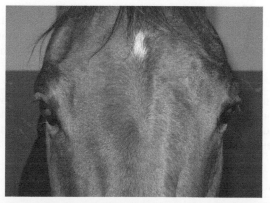

Fig. 5. Horse with guttural pouch mycosis resulting in Horner syndrome in the left eye. Note the enophthalmos, ptosis, and particularly the downward pointing eyelashes.

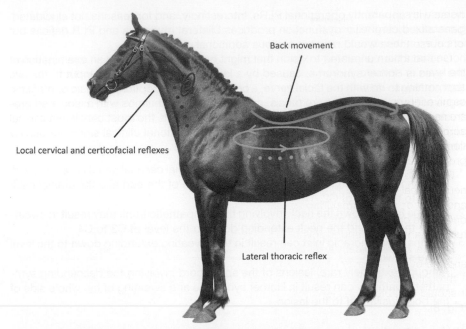

Back movement

Local cervical and certicofacial reflexes

Lateral thoracic reflex

Fig. 6. Examination of local cervical and cervicofacial reflexes.

Next the author examines movement and reflexes of the back. Make sure that the horse is standing squarely, then stroke the closed tip of the hemostat caudally along the skin over the longissimus muscle, from midthorax caudally to the level of the tuber coxa. The expected response is a brisk downward extension of the back and pelvis followed by back flexion when the hemostats are over the croup. If the horse has back pain, there may be obvious resistance to any back movement, but if the horse is ataxic in the pelvic limbs then not uncommonly the horse will have difficulty extending the pelvic limbs to return to a normal position and will wobble the pelvis up and down in an effort to extend the pelvic limbs.

Progressing further caudally, the cutaneous trunci reflex can be elicited by tapping the skin over the middle of the ribcage with the same pair of forceps at short intervals from cranial to the caudal thorax. A normal response is twitching of the skin but unlike the local cervical responses, this is a long reflex, with the pathway running from the point of the stimulus dorsally to the spinal cord via sensory axons, then cranially along the spinal cord to the C8 segment and then caudally along the lateral thoracic nerve; the reflex will be absent if there is a spinal cord lesion anywhere cranial to the stimulus.

Perineum

The final step of the portion of the examination undertaken in the stable is the evaluation of the perineal reflex. Manipulating the tail and stimulating the skin of the perineum should result in closure of the anus and flexion of the tail, and paresis in these responses suggests a lesion in the nerves of the cauda equina or spinal cord sacral segments.

Gait and Posture

At this point the author has the horse led out of the stable to proceed with examination of gait and posture, and considerable time should be taken on this when spinal cord disease is suspected. The basis of gait generation in quadrupeds is the central pattern generator, biological neural circuits that drive rhythmic and stereotyped motor behaviors even in the absence of input from higher brain areas; this has the advantage to the horse that a normal gait can be generated even in the presence of significant lesions to the brain or spinal cord, but the disadvantage is for the clinician who tries to disclose abnormalities. Maneuvers that alter the visual, gravitational, vestibular, and proprioceptive inputs to the nervous system, such as tight circles and maneuvering slopes, are needed to disclose subtle sensory or motor deficits; examination of horses walking across curbs have however not proved to be a useful test of proprioceptive dysfunction, and unlike in dogs, manually placing a limb in an abnormal position has not proved to be helpful (**Fig. 7**).

Given the impossibility of eliciting voluntary responses in our patients, the veterinary neurological examination is perforce limited to examining reflexes; however, in dogs and cats or small ruminants a reasonably comprehensive examination is possible due to the opportunity of examining postural reactions and limb reflexes; these unfortunately are mostly impossible to elicit in horses.

From a neurological perspective the gait is assessed for both paresis and ataxia and the overall severity of any gait abnormality in each of the 4 limbs can be graded 1 through 4 as subtle, mild, moderate, or severe. If the horse is found to be ataxic, it should be able to decide in which region of the spinal cord a lesion is located in (**Fig. 8**).

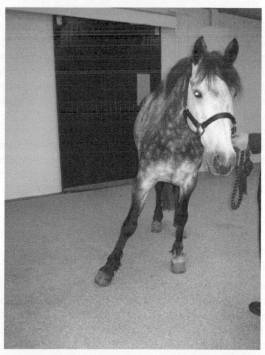

Fig. 7. A normal horse, presumably in an effort to be helpful, will frequently not immediately replace limb that has been placed in an abnormal position, and so this is not a good test for conscious proprioception. Normal horse not replacing a limb placed in an unexpected position.

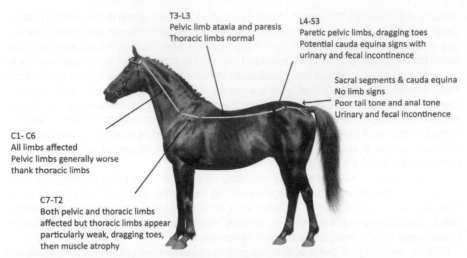

T3-L3
Pelvic limb ataxia and paresis
Thoracic limbs normal

L4-S3
Paretic pelvic limbs, dragging toes
Potential cauda equina signs with
urinary and fecal incontinence

Sacral segments & cauda equina
No limb signs
Poor tail tone and anal tone
Urinary and fecal incontinence

C1- C6
All limbs affected
Pelvic limbs generally worse
thank thoracic limbs

C7-T2
Both pelvic and thoracic limbs
affected but thoracic limbs appear
particularly weak, dragging toes,
then muscle atrophy

Fig. 8. Neuroanatomic localization to the spinal cord segments.

1. *Paresis* is defined as a reduction in motor function,[3] which may predominantly involve flexor or extensor muscle groups and can be caused by lesions in motor neurons in the brain (upper motor neurons, UMN) or in the spinal cord (lower motor neurons, LMN). LMNs are efferent neurons that connect the central nervous system (CNS) with the smooth or skeletal muscle to be innervated. Injury to the neuron causes flaccid paralysis and neurogenic atrophy and electromyography changes of skeletal muscle. UMNs are responsible for the initiation of voluntary movement and the maintenance of tone and posture. In horses UMNs consist of scattered groups of interconnected neurons in the cortex and brainstem, which ultimately synapse with LMNs. Injury to the cell bodies, or more commonly their axons, produces spastic paralysis—absence of voluntary movement with increased tone and increased or primitive reflexes due to the lack of UMN inhibition. Paresis may predominantly involve flexor or extensor muscle groups.

2. *Ataxia* on the other hand is the clinical sign that follows a deficit in proprioception, that is, the sense of position of both where the limbs are relative to the body and the position of the body in space. A lesion in any nervous system structure that is concerned with proprioception, that is, the cerebellum, and in animals to a lesser extent the forebrain, as well as the vestibular system or any of the pathways to those structures such as the spinal cord can result in ataxia. The word ataxia incidentally comes from Greek, with *A* (without) and *TAXIA* (order), and a good description of most ataxic gaits are disordered and inconsistent. Ataxia can be characterized as having components of hypometria or plasticity and hypermetria or high striding.

The neurological examination attempts to accentuate both paresis and ataxia while remembering that the most common neurological gait deficit in horses is caused by spinal cord damage, and the resulting gait is the result of a combination of paresis and ataxia. Nevertheless, the degree of both paresis and ataxia should be evaluated as mild, moderate, or severe for paresis and 0–4 for ataxia. Compressive lesions classically result in clinical signs that appear more severe in the pelvic limbs (probably due to the more peripheral location of the spinocerebellar tracts in the spinal cord), and a 2-grade difference in spinal cord ataxia is possible with a lesion in the cervical spinal cord.

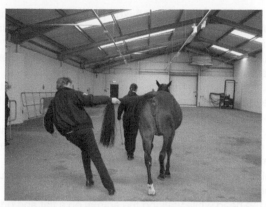

Fig. 9. Evaluating upper motor neuron paresis by pulling on the horse's tail while walking.

This is the sequence used by this author to examine the gait of neurological patients:

- Stand the patient square and pull on the tail; this initiates an extensor (patellar, quadriceps) reflex, and a poor response suggests a lower motor neuron lesion at the level of L_{3-5}, and therefore, the patient will demonstrate weakness while standing still (hypotonia). A patient with paresis due to an UMN lesion, for example, cervical spinal cord disease, will not show paresis when the tail is pulled when standing.
- Have the patient walk back and forth, looking for excessive swinging in the back end and inconsistent movements when turning; it may give you a clue that there is a deficit before starting more complex maneuvers. Horses with lower motor neuron paresis, for example, botulism or equine motor neuron disease, may show consistent but short strides with a low head-carriage.
- Have the handler walk in a straight line and perform a tail pull while walking next to the horse, gently at first and then firmly when the horse has got used to it. Observe the placement of the limbs and whether you can pull the horse toward you—a horse with a cervical lesion and thus damage to UMN axons may be easily pulled to the side when walking, particularly if the lesion is acute (**Fig. 9**).
- In the author's experience ataxia is most consistently revealed by circling the horse (**Fig. 10**)—wide circles, tight circles, serpentines; look for low foot flight

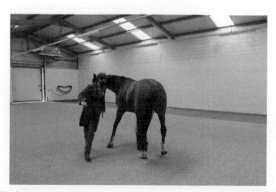

Fig. 10. Assessing limb movement during tight turning, a relatively complex maneuver. This horse had mild (grade 1) ataxia in the thoracic limbs and moderate (grade 3) ataxia in the pelvic limbs.

or dragging of toes (hypometria, flexor paresis), overreaching (hypermetria), excessive circumduction of particularly the outside pelvic limb when turning buckling of limbs.
- Pelvic limb and/or thoracic limb paresis can be further detected by pulling on the halter and tail at the same time while guiding the horse to circle around the handler (**Fig. 11**). This test requires a certain amount of practice to ensure that it is the horse that is doing the circling and not the handler! This is particularly useful if there is asymmetry in the degree of weakness. Normal, alert horses resist such pulling, whereas a paretic animal is easy to pull to the side. Releasing the tail abruptly often exacerbates ataxic movements of the thoracic and especially the pelvic limbs.
- To detect milder degrees of ataxia, additional postural maneuvers may need to be performed, which include the following:
  1. Elevating the head while walking the animal on a flat and on a sloping surface; ataxic horses can find this difficult, and the thoracic limbs often overreach, particularly when the head is elevated while walking down a slope
  2. Turning tightly when stopping abruptly from a trot
  3. Backing

Recumbent Animals

Horses can become recumbent for a variety of reasons and need to be managed carefully due to their size and temperament. Readers are referred to references below for excellent reviews of the management of the recumbent horse.[4–6] An accurate history and consideration of the signalment is likely very helpful, and a thorough physical examination is essential; every attempt should be made to rule out nonneurological causes of recumbency including musculoskeletal, cardiovascular, and metabolic disorders.

As in the standing horse, the goal of the neurologic examination is to establish whether a neurologic lesion exists and if so to localize it. Broad categorizations to the brain, spinal cord, or neuromuscular system should be possible even after an abbreviated examination. The neurological examination of the recumbent horse is perforce limited and has to be modified depending on the situation. Assessment of mentation should be possible bearing in mind that the patient likely will be stressed. Assessment of cranial nerves and vision should be possible, as can local cervical,

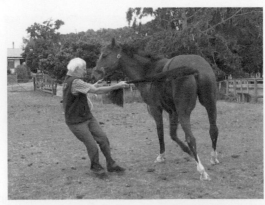

Fig. 11. Pulling on the halter and tail while turning the horse in a circle around the examiner (Dr Joe Mayhew) to test limb extensor muscles.

cervicofacial, and cutaneous trunci reflexes, at least on the accessible side. If the horse can adopt a dog sitting position then an injury caudal to T2 is likely. If the horse is unable to raise the head, particularly with abnormal respiration, then a proximal cervical spinal cord or a diffuse neuromuscular disease such as botulism (make sure to test tongue tone!) should be high on the differential list. Severe, acute unilateral vestibular disease on the down side is also possible; attempt to move the head and examine the eyes for spontaneous nystagmus.

Recumbent horses present a unique opportunity to examine limb reflexes, but examiner safety must be considered. Just as in small animals it is important to attempt to evaluate limb tone, and repeatedly flexing carpal and tarsal joints should be informative. Increased tone is compatible with a spinal cord lesion and a lack of UMN toning down of reflexes, whereas markedly decreased tone suggests neuromuscular disease. The patellar reflex (femoral nerve and L4-5 spinal cord segments) can be elicited with the wooden handle of a hammer, and withdrawal reflexes can be tested by carefully pinching the coronary band with a hemostat. Pelvic limb flexion is mediated by the sciatic nerve and caudal lumbar and sacral segments. Thoracic limb flexion involved all the major nerves of the brachial plexus and the whole cervical intumescence. Withdrawal of the forelimb is achieved via the nerves of the brachial plexus and the C6-T2 spinal cord segments. Tail tone and anal tone can be examined and depending on the period of recumbency bladder tone, size and ability to express urine may be evaluated via a rectal examination. Muscle tone, including that of the eyelid and tongue, should be evaluated carefully, as paresis is a characteristic finding with botulism. If the lesion cannot be localized then it may be worth assisting the horse to stand, which may elucidate whether the horse is suffering from a CNS, neuromuscular, or orthopedic injury.

Autonomous Zones

Equine cases with monoparesis should be evaluated for specific areas of sensitivity (**Fig. 12**). Unlike autonomous zones in dogs, in horses these can be variable from case to case and, significantly, do not have an autonomous zone for the radial nerve.[1] Testing for hypalgesia is best examined with a 2-pinch test; this is performed by holding the skin in a fold, inserting the fold into the jaws of a strong hemostat or needle holder, and after the patient has settled to this, a brief, sharp squeeze is applied to

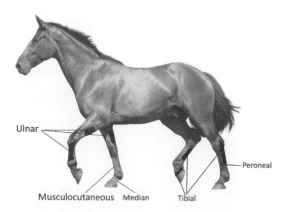

Fig. 12. Autonomous zones for individual sensory branches of the major spinal nerves to the limbs of horses.

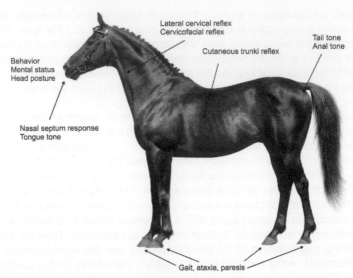

Lateral cervical reflex
Cervicofacial reflex

Tail tone
Anal tone

Cutaneous trunki reflex

Behavior
Mental status
Head posture

Nasal septum response
Tongue tone

Gait, ataxia, paresis

Fig. 13. Summary of the equine neurological examination.

elicit a pain (behavioral) response. Covering the ipsilateral eye may help to establish which nerve or nerves are involved.

EQUINE NEUROLOGICAL EXAMINATION SUMMARY

See **Fig. 13**.

CLINICS CARE POINTS

- Ataxic horses can look remarkably better when excited; it is worth giving the horse time after arrival to the hospital before examining it for mild neurological signs.
- Horses with chronic spinal cord lesions may appear ataxic but have mild paresis on tail pull. Conversely severe upper motor neuron paresis in an ataxic horse suggests an acute lesion.
- Horses can make remarkable adjustments to a vestibular lesion with vision; to accentuate a loss of balance (carefully) examine the patient after applying a blindfold.
- The pupillary light reflex can appear normal even when vision is obviously affected by a retinal or optic nerve lesion.

DISCLOSURE

The author has nothing to disclose.

REFERENCES

1. Mayhew I. Large animal neurology. 2nd edition. Hoboken, New Jersey: Wiley-Blackwell; 2008.
2. Thomson C, Hahn C. Veterinary neuroanatomy: a clinical approach. 1st edition. Philadelphia: Saunders Ltd.; 2012.

3. DeLahunta A, Glass E, Kent M. de Lahunta's veterinary neuroanatomy and clinical neurology. 5th edition. Philadelphia: Saunders; 2021.
4. Davis GE, Bonnie RR. Equine recumbency: defining the problem and establishing the differential diagnosis. Compendium 2004;26(1):67–76.
5. Gardner RB. Evaluation and management of the recumbent adult horse. Vet Clin North Am Equine Pract 2011;27(3):527–43.
6. Nout YS, Reed SM. Management and treatment of the recumbent horse. Equine Vet Educ 2005;17:324–36.

Special Diagnostic Techniques in Equine Neurology (Radiography, Ultrasonography, Computed Tomography, and Magnetic Resonance Imaging)

Katherine S. Garrett, DVM

KEYWORDS

- Radiography • Ultrasonography • Computed tomography
- Magnetic resonance imaging • Myelography • Cervical spine • Brain

KEY POINTS

- Although radiography and ultrasonography are widely available and noninvasive, their diagnostic value is more limited as compared with myelography, computed tomography (CT), and magnetic resonance imaging (MRI).
- Diagnostic imaging findings should be interpreted in light of the clinical signs.

INTRODUCTION

Diagnostic imaging is often an important part of the diagnostic approach to neurologic disease. Although the same modalities are available for equine patients as are used in humans and small animals, there are significant differences in how these modalities can be used in horses due to the large size of horses and the need for general anesthesia for some modalities. Advanced imaging techniques such as myelography, computed tomography (CT), and magnetic resonance imaging (MRI) provide more information than radiography and ultrasonography but are more limited in their availability.

RADIOGRAPHY
Plain Radiography–cervical Spine

Radiography is often the imaging modality first pursued when neurological disease is suspected to originate from the cervical spine region. Although diagnostic quality radiographs can be obtained with portable x-ray generators, image quality in the caudal

Rood and Riddle Equine Hospital, PO Box 12070, Lexington, KY 40580, USA
E-mail address: kgarrett@roodandriddle.com

Vet Clin Equine 38 (2022) 171–188
https://doi.org/10.1016/j.cveq.2022.04.001
0749-0739/22/© 2022 Elsevier Inc. All rights reserved.

cervical spine is generally better with more powerful clinic-based systems. Sedation improves patient compliance as the horse must remain still and some horses are nervous with equipment close to their heads.

Laterolateral views from C1-T1 are included in a standard study of the cervical spine in adult horses. With a larger detector (14 × 17 inches), these can generally be obtained in 3 images. Using a larger detector also assists with vertebra identification on the images, as C2 and C6 can be identified by their distinctive shapes. Radioopaque markers taped to the skin in the images can also help with vertebra identification. Left and right ventrolateral-dorsolateral oblique views at a 45 to 55° angle serve to separate the left and right sides of the vertebrae and highlight the articular processes (**Fig. 1**).[1]

General principles of radiographic image evaluation should be followed for interpretation. Common pathologies in the cervical spine include articular process enlargement, degenerative joint disease, osteochondral fragmentation, vertebral body subluxation, narrowing of the intervertebral space, and fracture (**Figs. 2–4**). The clinician should be aware that there can be variation in the appearance of the transverse processes of C6 and C7 which are generally not associated with clinical signs.[2-4] Additionally, articular process enlargement alone in the caudal neck may not be associated with clinical signs.[5]

For horses with suspected cervical spine pathology, one of the primary differential diagnoses is cervical vertebral stenotic myelopathy (CVSM). Standing laterolateral cervical spine radiographs are generally the first imaging modality pursued in these cases. In addition to the assessment of morphologic changes in the spinal column, measurements of various spinal canal dimensions have been used in an effort to identify potential sites of spinal cord compression. Although the use of minimum sagittal diameter and longitudinal ratios has been described, most clinicians use intravertebral

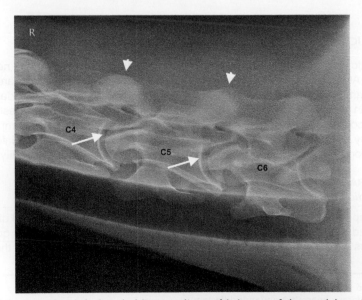

Fig. 1. Right-ventral to left-dorsal oblique radiographic image of the caudal cervical spine. Cranial is to the left of the image. The right cranial and caudal articular processes (*arrowheads*) are superimposed over one another and the joint spaces between the left cranial and caudal articular processes are highlighted (*arrows*).

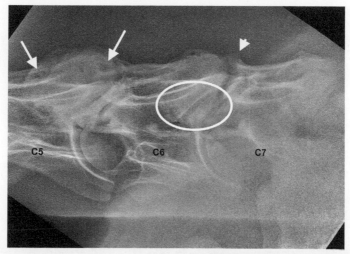

Fig. 2. Laterolateral radiographic image of the caudal cervical spine. Cranial is to the left of the image. At C5-C6, the articular processes are enlarged with areas of lysis and sclerosis (*arrows*). Osteophytes are present on the joint margin at C6-C7 (*arrowhead*) and the subchondral bone is irregular (*circle*).

sagittal ratios (minimum vertebral canal sagittal diameter/maximum height of the cranial aspect of the same vertebral body) and intervertebral sagittal ratios (minimum intervertebral distance/maximum height of the cranial aspect of the caudal vertebral body) to determine potential sites of spinal cord compression (**Fig. 5**).[6–8] For intravertebral ratios, Rush Moore *and colleagues*[7] recommended using a cut off value of 0.52

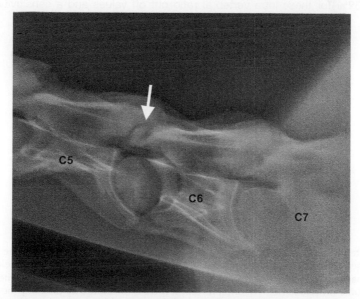

Fig. 3. Laterolateral radiographic image of the caudal cervical spine. Cranial is to the left of the image. An osteochondral fragment is present at C5-6 (*arrow*).

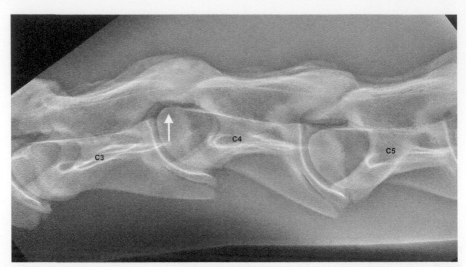

Fig. 4. Laterolateral radiographic image of the mid-cervical spine of a horse with grade 3 to 4 ataxia in all limbs. Cranial is to the left of the image. There is subluxation at C3-C4 leading to spinal canal narrowing (*arrow*). The intravertebral ratio at this site was 0.42 and the intervertebral ratio was 0.33.

for C3-4, C4-5, C5-6, and a cut off value of 0.56 for C6-C7 to determine sites of possible spinal cord compression (**Fig. 6**). For intravertebral ratios, Hahn *and colleagues*[8] recommended using a cut off value of 0.485 for all sites from C3-C7. However, there are limitations to using sagittal ratios as decision criteria. The sensitivity and specificity of these cut-off ratios are not ideal. One study using histology as the criterion standard for spinal cord compression found a sensitivity of 84% and specificity of 32% for these intra-vertebral ratio cut off values and a sensitivity of 20%

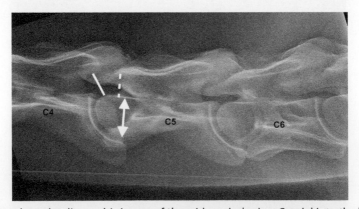

Fig. 5. Laterolateral radiographic image of the mid-cervical spine. Cranial is to the left of the image. The intravertebral sagittal ratio is calculated by dividing the minimum height of the spinal canal (*dotted line*) by the maximum height of the cranial aspect of the same vertebral body (*double arrowed line*). The intervertebral ratio is calculated by dividing the minimum intervertebral distance (*solid line*) by the maximum height of the cranial aspect of the caudal vertebral body (*double arrowed line*).

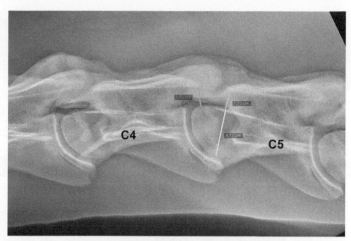

Fig. 6. Laterolateral radiographic image of the mid-cervical spine. Cranial is to the left of the image. The intravertebral ratio at C4-C5 is 1.75 cm (*blue line*)/4.17 cm (*yellow line*) = 0.42 and the intravertebral ratio is 1.75 cm (*orange line*)/4.17 cm (*yellow line*) = 0.42, both of which are below the recommended cut off values that suggest spinal canal narrowing.

and specificity of 100% for this intervertebral ratio cut off value.[9] Additionally, interobserver agreement for these ratios is considered low.[9,10] The clinician should interpret the radiographic findings in light of the horse's clinical signs as well as with the knowledge that these cut-off points for the diagnosis of CVSM on standing laterolateral radiographs have limitations.

Radiographic Myelography–cervical Spine

As a result of the limitations of standing plain radiography, myelography has become the technique of choice for the diagnosis of CVSM. Myelography involves the injection of radio-opaque positive contrast media in the subarachnoid space at the atlanto-occipital space. For radiographic myelography, contrast injection is followed by laterolateral radiographs in neutral, flexed, and extended neck positions. General anesthesia is required and the use of a purpose-built myelogram table to assist with horse and detector positioning can greatly reduce the physical demands on the personnel performing the procedure as well as protect the digital detector. From a technical perspective, kV should be kept low to maximize the contrast of the contrast media and the forelimbs should be pulled caudally to improve image quality in the caudal neck. Strategic placement of pads keeps the vertebral column straight to avoid oblique images.

Myelographic images have been evaluated for extradural spinal cord compression at vertebral articulations using a variety of criteria. The 2 most commonly used are a 50% reduction in the height of the dorsal contrast column as compared with the height of the dorsal contrast column in the cranial vertebra and a 20% reduction in the total dural diameter of the contrast column as compared with the total dural diameter of the contrast column in the cranial vertebra (**Fig. 7**).[6,11–13] Van Biervliet *and colleagues*[11] investigated the sensitivity and specificity of various cut off values for dorsal contrast column reduction and total dural diameter reduction to determine spinal cord compression at individual locations using histology as the criterion standard. The reader is directed to this article for the details, but from C3-C6, the authors

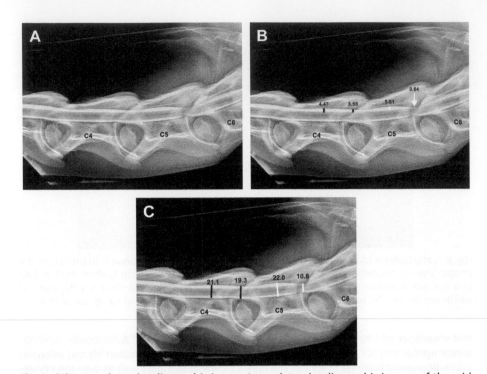

Fig. 7. (*A*) Latero-lateral radiographic image. Laterolateral radiographic images of the mid-cervical spine after subarachnoid contrast administration. Cranial is to the left of the images. (*B*): Dorsal contrast column measurements (in mm). Black lines indicate the measurement sites for C4-C5 and white line and arrow indicate the measurement sites for C5-C6. At C4-5 the dorsal contrast column is narrowed by 21% and at C5-6 it is narrowed by 89%. (*C*): Total dural diameter measurements (in mm). Black lines indicate the measurement sites for C4-C5 and the white lines indicate the measurement sites for C5-C6. At C4-5 the total dural diameter is narrowed by 9% and at C5-6 it is narrowed by 51%.

recommended cut off values of 20% total dural diameter contrast column reduction in the neutral view and a 70% dorsal contrast column reduction in the flexed view to maximize specificity with the knowledge that sensitivity will be low. At C6-7, 100% sensitivity and 90% specificity were achieved with a cut off value of 70% reduction of the dorsal contrast column in the neutral position and a sensitivity and specificity of 100% with a cut off value of a 25% reduction of the total dural diameter in the flexed position. Another study showed a sensitivity of 71% and a specificity of 65% for the 50% dorsal contrast column reduction cutoff using postmortem findings from C2-C7 as the criterion standard.[13] As with sagittal ratio compression criteria, no perfect cut-off value exists and sensitivity and specificity of various values is lower than is ideal, so the clinician is again faced with a complex decision matrix. Additional factors to consider include the implications of false negatives versus false positives in light of the clinical signs, intended use of the horse, and owner wishes.

For both plain radiography and myelography, interpretation is complicated by the fact that obtaining orthogonal views of the cervical spine in an adult horse is not possible. In practical terms, lesions on the lateral aspect of the spinal column are difficult to identify so radiographic myelography may not identify lateral compression of the spinal cord.

Skull

Horses with signs of head trauma can be evaluated with skull radiographs. The most common abnormal finding in this situation is fracture (**Fig. 8**). Horses with vestibular disease should be evaluated for temporohyoid osteoarthropathy, which may include radiography. However, in general, skull radiographs can be difficult to evaluate due to the complexity of the anatomy and superimposition, so if CT is available, it often yields superior diagnostic information.

ULTRASONOGRAPHY

Although the spinal cord and brain are generally inaccessible via ultrasonography due to their location within the skull and spinal cord, ultrasonography does have a role in diagnostic and therapeutic procedures of neurologic disease. General principles of ultrasonography are applicable. The area to be imaged should be clipped if possible, the skin or hair cleaned, and acoustic coupling gel applied. Machine settings such as frequency, focal zone location, and depth should be appropriately adjusted. Sedation often improves patient compliance.

Although examination of the vertebral column is limited to the lateral aspects of the spine, the articular processes can be examined for the signs of osteoarthritis (**Fig. 9**). Perhaps the most common use of ultrasonography in equine neurologic disease is ultrasound-guided injection of the synovial joints of the cervical spine. Various techniques are described but all involve the visualization of the joint space and needle placement within the synovial joint to deposit the therapeutic product (**Fig. 10**).[14–16] Ultrasonography may also be used to collect cerebrospinal fluid from the atlantoaxial space in the standing, sedated horse.[17] More recently, ultrasound-guided approaches to deliver therapeutics to the region of the spinal nerves have been described but as of this writing, there have been few reports of clinical use and outcomes of these techniques.[18,19] Although linear transducers can be used, curvilinear transducers are helpful with their smaller footprint and wedge-shaped image.

Osteomyelitis and septic synovitis affecting the vertebral column is seen in foals and presents in a wide variety of ways. Ultrasonography can identify areas of bony irregularity or synovial effusion and assist with the sampling of abnormal areas (**Fig. 11**).

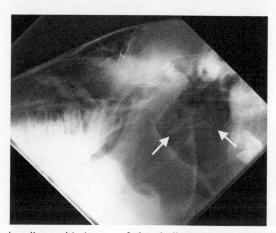

Fig. 8. Laterolateral radiographic image of the skull. Cranial is to the left of the image. There is a fracture of the basisphenoid bone with ventral displacement of the fragment (*arrows*).

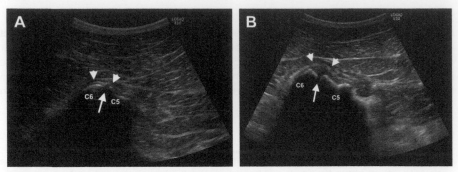

Fig. 9. Ultrasound images from the lateral aspect of the neck at the level of the C5-C6 articular processes. Dorsal is to the right of the images (*A*) is a normal horse and (*B*) is a horse with osteoarthritis indicated by the irregular bony contour (osteophytosis) and synovial effusion. The arrow indicates the joint space and the arrowheads indicate the joint capsule.

MAGNETIC RESONANCE IMAGING

Magnetic resonance imaging is the imaging modality of choice to examine the brain and spinal cord. Current designs limit the areas accessible in the adult horse to the brain and cranial-most portion of the spinal cord. However, in foals that can be positioned within the bore of the magnet, the entire spinal cord, and vertebral column can be imaged. General anesthesia is required and examinations typically take between 30 to 60 minutes to complete. Magnet strength influences both the duration of the examination and the resolution that is able to be achieved.

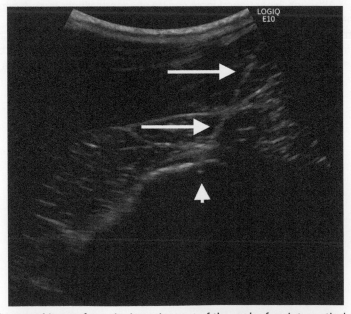

Fig. 10. Ultrasound image from the lateral aspect of the neck of an intra-articular injection of a cervical synovial joint. Dorsal is to the right of the image. The needle (*arrows*) seems as a hyperechoic line extending to the joint space (*arrowhead*).

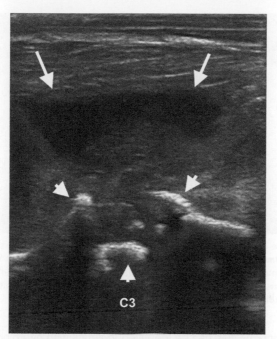

Fig. 11. Ultrasound image from the lateral aspect of the neck at the level of C3 of a foal with neck pain and swelling. Cranial is to the right of the image. There is bony irregularity of the vertebra (*arrowheads*) and an associated hypoechoic, encapsulated area (*arrows*) consistent with an abscess that communicates with the area of bony irregularity.

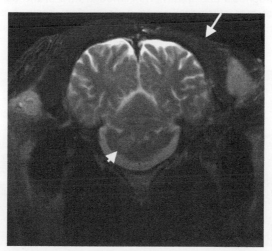

Fig. 12. Transverse T2W MR image of the brain at the level of the rostral cerebellum of a horse with an acute onset of ataxia progressing rapidly to recumbency. Left is to the right of the image. There is a region of T2 hyperintensity in the brainstem (*arrowhead*). Protozoal organisms were found in this area on postmortem examination. Temporal muscle atrophy is also apparent (*arrow*).

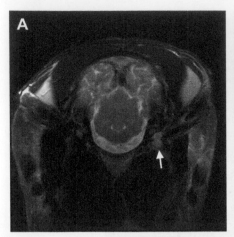
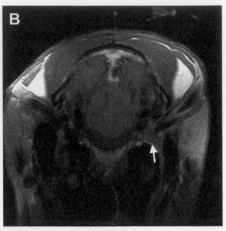

Fig. 13. Transverse T2W (*A*) and T1W postcontrast (*B*) MR images of the skull at the level of the tympanic bullae of a horse with otitis media who presented with a head tilt. Left is to the right of the images. The left tympanic bulla (*arrows*) contains material with heterogeneous signal intensity. The lining of the tympanic bulla undergoes contrast enhancement but the material within it does not.

A variety of abnormalities can be identified in adults with neurologic disease localized to the head, including multifocal inflammation consistent with equine protozoal myeloencephalopathy, otitis, hydrocephalus, intracranial abscessation or hemorrhage, cerebrovascular events, temporohyoid osteoarthropathy, nigropallidal encephalomalacia, brain edema, and neoplasia (**Figs. 12–16**).[20,21] MRI examinations are often normal in horses who present with seizure, narcolepsy, or headshaking as the primary complaint.[20,21] The findings of an MRI examination (even if negative) can help determine prognosis and treatment. Although MRI of the cervical spine of the adult horse is not currently possible on a premortem basis, postmortem studies have shown that it may be useful for the diagnosis of intervertebral disc disease and CVSM.[22,23]

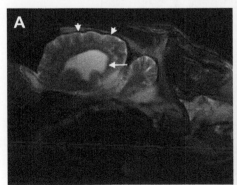
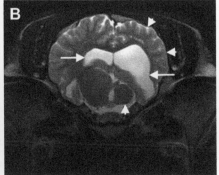

Fig. 14. Paramedian (*A*) and transverse (*B*) T2W MR images of the brain of a 3-year-old horse with hydrocephalus who presented with abnormal behavior and possible vision abnormalities present since birth. Cranial is to the left in image A and left is to the right of image B. The lateral ventricles are dilated (*arrows*) and the brain parenchyma is distorted with decreased volume (*arrowheads*).

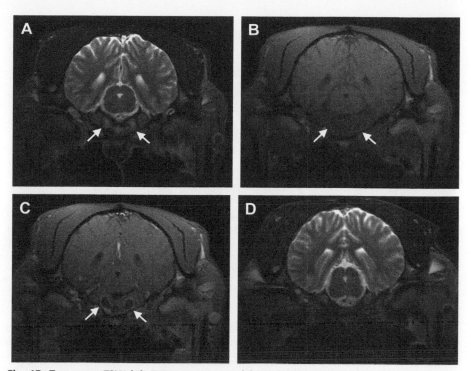

Fig. 15. Transverse T2W (*A*), T1W precontrast (*B*), and T1W postcontrast (*C*) MR images of the brain at the level of the caudal pituitary fossa in a horse with ataxia and recurrent febrile episodes. Left is to the right of the images. A mass with distinct margins and an encapsulated appearance in the pituitary fossa (*arrows*) compresses the brainstem. The mass has rim enhancement after intravenous positive contrast administration (compare *B* and *C*) consistent with an abscess. (*D*) is a transverse T2W MR image at the same location obtained 2 months later after long-term antibiotic therapy that shows resolution of the mass. Clinical signs had improved.

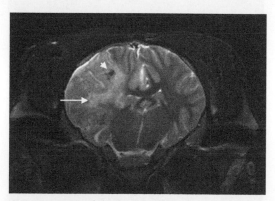

Fig. 16. Transverse T2W MR image of the brain at the level of the pituitary gland in a horse with acute development of ataxia, circling to the left, left-sided head tilt, lack of menace OS, and seizures which progressed to obtundation. Left is to the right of the image. Abnormalities in the right cerebral hemisphere include areas of hemorrhage (*arrowhead*) and inflammation (*arrow*) as well as cerebral hemisphere swelling that causes a mass effect. Postmortem examination showed multifocal infarcts and suppurative encephalitis in the right cerebral hemisphere.

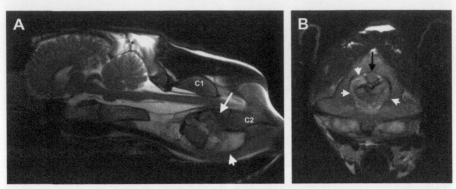

Fig. 17. Median plane (*A*) and transverse plane (*B*) T2W MR image of the cranial cervical spinal column of a foal with ataxia, a low and extended head carriage, and neck pain. Cranial is to the left of image A and left is to the right of image B, which is at the C1-C2 articulation. There is severe synovitis of the atlantoaxial joint (*arrowheads*) which compresses the spinal cord (*black arrow*) as well as abnormal signal intensity in the dens of C2 consistent with osteomyelitis (*white arrow*). These findings were confirmed at post-mortem examination.

In foals, areas of osteomyelitis, abscessation, and synovial sepsis can be identified throughout the spinal column (**Figs. 17** and **18**). This is particularly useful in foals who have vague signs of lameness or neurologic deficits whereby radiography and/or ultrasonography have failed to yield a diagnosis. Congenital abnormalities can also be identified (**Fig. 19**).[20,21]

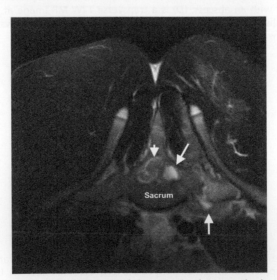

Fig. 18. Transverse plane T2W MR image of the spinal column at the level of the sacroiliac joint of a foal with left hindlimb proprioceptive deficits. Left is to the right of the image. There is heterogeneous signal intensity in the left sacrum and sacroiliac region consistent with osteomyelitis. There are more focal hyperintense areas consistent with abscessation (*arrows*) causing spinal cord compression (*arrowhead*).

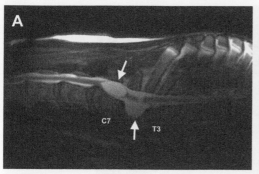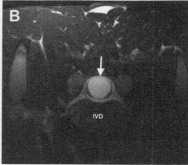

Fig. 19. T2W MR images of the spinal column at the cervicothoracic region in a foal with weakness and ataxia since birth. (*A*) is a median plane image with cranial to the left of the image. (*B*) is a transverse plane image at the level of C7-T1 with left to the right of the image. Dilated cyst-like structures (*arrows*) are present in the spinal cord, one of which extends into the vertebral body at T1-2. Postmortem examination confirmed hydromyelia. IVD: Intervertebral disc.

COMPUTED TOMOGRAPHY

Computed tomography provides excellent bony detail and the examination itself can often be completed in less than 5 minutes. Due to technological advances, systems are now available that can scan the skull of standing, sedated adult horses, reducing the need for general anesthesia. However, horses who are unable to maintain a stable standing position or who demonstrate sudden head movements may still require a skull examination to be completed under general anesthesia to obtain diagnostic-quality images and for patient safety. Many designs also permit the examination of the entire cervical spine of an adult horse. Some of these systems (typically cone

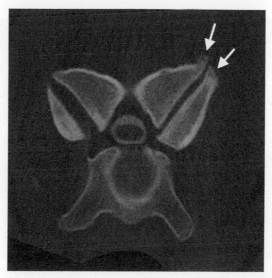

Fig. 20. Transverse CT myelographic image at the level of C6-C7. Left is to the right of the image. Osteophytes are present on the margins of the left articular processes (*arrows*).

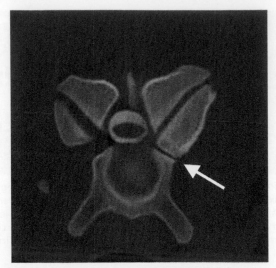

Fig. 21. Transverse CT myelographic image at the level of C6-7. Left is to the right of the image. The left articular processes are enlarged and the left intervertebral foramen is narrowed (*arrow*). The subarachnoid contrast column is normal.

beam systems) do not require general anesthesia but clinicians should be aware of the differences between cone-beam systems versus fan-beam systems.

The cross-sectional nature of CT images allows the evaluation of the cervical spinal column in all planes (with the use of reconstructions) without superimposition. This has significant advantages as the spinal column can be evaluated for the signs of osteoarthritis or osteochondral fragmentation, intervertebral foramen narrowing, intervertebral disc disease, fracture, malformation, and spinal canal narrowing (**Figs. 20–**

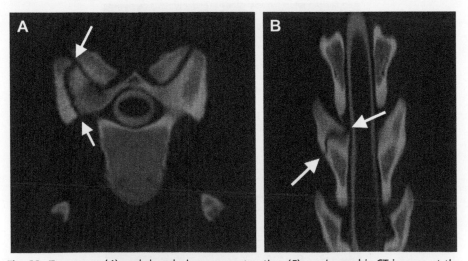

Fig. 22. Transverse (*A*) and dorsal plane reconstruction (*B*) myelographic CT images at the level of C5-6. Left is to the right of the images and cranial is to the top of image B. There is a fracture of the right cranial articular process of C6 (*arrows*).

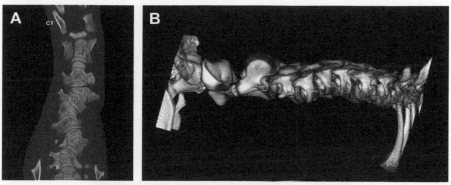

Fig. 23. Dorsal plane CT reconstruction (*A*) and 3D rendering (*B*) of a foal with severe vertebral abnormalities, including the presence of 8 cervical vertebrae. Cranial is to the top (*A*) or left (*B*) of the images.

24).[24–27] Computed tomographic myelography is particularly useful in identifying potential sites of spinal cord compression indicated by contrast column narrowing, but as CT scans of the cervical spine are generally not able to be performed with the neck in a flexed or extended position, a radiographic myelographic examination that includes these positions is recommended in conjunction with the CT myelogram.[25,27] As the use of CT for cervical spinal cord disease is relatively new, the clinical significance of some abnormalities has yet to be determined.[24,25]

The same lack of superimposition of anatomy provides is beneficial when evaluating the skull for signs of temporohyoid osteoarthropathy or skull fracture (**Figs. 25** and **26**). However, information about the brain itself is much more limited with CT as compared with MRI.

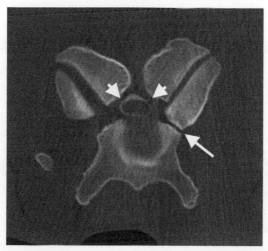

Fig. 24. Transverse CT myelographic image at the level of C6-C7. Left is to the right of the image. There is enlargement of the left articular processes, narrowing of the left intervertebral foramen (*arrow*), and circumferential narrowing of the subarachnoid contrast column (*arrowheads*). Postmortem examination confirmed compressive myelopathy at this location.

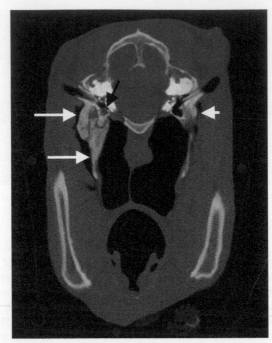

Fig. 25. Transverse CT image of the skull at the level of the temporohyoid articulation. Left is to the right side of the image. There is severe right temporohyoid osteoarthropathy with a large amount of new bone formation (*white arrows*) as well as increased opacity in the right tympanic bulla (*black arrow*). There is mild-moderate left temporohyoid osteoarthropathy (*arrowhead*).

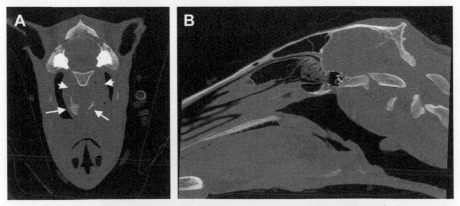

Fig. 26. Transverse (*A*) and paramedian plane reconstruction (*B*) CT images of a horse with a basioccipital and basisphenoid bone fracture. The fragments are displaced caudally and ventrally (*white arrows*) from the parent bones (*black arrow*). There is a large amount of fluid opacity consistent with hemorrhage with small gas opacities between the guttural pouches (*arrowheads*).

CLINICS CARE POINTS

- Myelography provides more definitive diagnosis of spinal canal narrowing than does plain radiography.
- Diagnosis of intra-cranial abnormalities is best accomplished with magnetic resonance imaging.
- Computed tomography (including myelography) is currently the most practical way to gain information about the cervical spine in adults.

DISCLOSURE

The author has nothing to disclose.

REFERENCES

1. Withers JM, Voute LC, Hammond G, et al. Radiographic anatomy of the articular process joints of the caudal cervical vertebrae in the horse on lateral and oblique projections. Equine Vet J 2009;41(9):895–902.
2. Veraa S, Bergmann W, van den Belt AJ, et al. Ex vivo computed tomographic evaluation of morphology variations in equine cervical vertebrae. Vet Radiol Ultrasound 2016;57(5):482–8.
3. DeRouen A, Spriet M, Aleman M. Prevalence of anatomical variation of the sixth cervical vertebra and association with vertebral canal stenosis and articular process osteoarthritis in the horse. Vet Radiol Ultrasound 2016;57(3):253 8.
4. Veraa S, Graaf K De, Wijnberg ID, et al. Caudal cervical vertebral morphological variation is not associated with clinical signs in Warmblood horses. Equine Vet J 2019;52(2):219–24.
5. Down SS, Henson FMD. Radiographic retrospective study of the caudal cervical articular process joints in the horse. Equine Vet J 2009;41(6):518–24.
6. Mayhew IG, deLahunta A, Whitlock RH, et al. Spinal cord disease in the horse. Cornell Vet 1978;68(Suppl 6):44–71.
7. Moore BR, Reed SM, Biller DS, et al. Assessment of vertebral canal diameter and bony malformations of the cervical part of the spine in horses with cervical stenotic myelopathy. Am J Vet Res 1994;55(1):5–13.
8. Hahn CN, Handel I, Green SL, et al. Assessment of the utility of using intra- and intervertebral minimum sagittal diameter ratios in the diagnosis of cervical vertebral malformation in horses. Vet Radiol Ultrasound 2008;49(1):1–6.
9. Hughes KJ, Laidlaw EH, Reed SM, et al. Repeatability and intra- and interobserver agreement of cervical vertebral sagittal diameter ratios in horses with neurological disease. J Vet Intern Med 2014;28(6):1860–70.
10. Scrivani PV, Levine JM, Holmes NL, et al. Observer agreement study of cervical-vertebral ratios in horses. Equine Vet J 2011;43(4):399–403.
11. Biervliet JV, Scrivani PV, Divers TJ, et al. Evaluation of decision criteria for detection of spinal cord compression based on cervical myelography in horses: 38 cases (1981-2001). Equine Vet J 2004;36(1):14–20.
12. Nyland TG, Blythe LL, Pool RR, et al. Metrizamide myelography in the horse: clinical, radiographic, and pathologic changes. Am J Vet Res 1980;41(2):204–11.
13. Levine JM, Scrivani PV, Divers TJ, et al. Multicenter case-control study of signalment, diagnostic features, and outcome associated with cervical vertebral malformation-malarticulation in horses. J Am Vet Med Assoc 2010;237(7):812–22.

14. Nielsen JV, Berg LC, Thoefnert MB, et al. Accuracy of ultrasound-guided intra-articular injection of cervical facet joints in horses: a cadaveric study. Equine Vet J 2003;35(7):657–61.
15. Johnson JP, Stack JD, Rowan C, et al. Ultrasound-guided approach to the cervical articular process joints in horses: a validation of the technique in cadavers. Vet Comp Orthop Traumatol 2017;30(3):165–71.
16. Mattoon JS, Drost WT, Grguric MR, et al. Technique for equine cervical articular process joint injection. Vet Radiol Ultrasound 2004;45(3):238–40.
17. Pease A, Behan A, Bohart G. Ultrasound-guided cervical centesis to obtain cerebrospinal fluid in the standing horse. Vet Radiol Ultrasound 2012;53(1):92–5.
18. Wood AD, Sinovich M, Prutton JSW, et al. Ultrasonographic guidance for perineural injections of the cervical spinal nerves in horses. Vet Surg 2021;50(4):816–22.
19. Touzot-Jourde G, Geffroy O, Tallaj A, et al. Ultrasonography-guided perineural injection of the ramus ventralis of the 7 and 8th cervical nerves in horses: A cadaveric descriptive pilot study. Front Vet Sci 2020;7:102.
20. Ferrell EA, Gavin PR, Tucker RL, et al. Magnetic resonance for evaluation of neurologic disease in 12 horses. Vet Radiol Ultrasound 2002;43(6):510–6.
21. Manso-Díaz G, Dyson SJ, Dennis R, et al. Magnetic resonance imaging characteristics of equine head disorders: 84 cases (2000-2013). Vet Radiol Ultrasound 2015;56(2):176–87.
22. Veraa S, Bergmann W, Wijnberg ID, et al. Equine cervical intervertebral disc degeneration is associated with location and MRI features. Vet Radiol Ultrasound 2019;60(6):696–706.
23. Janes JG, Garrett KS, McQuerry KJ, et al. Comparison of magnetic resonance imaging with standing cervical radiographs for evaluation of vertebral canal stenosis in equine cervical stenotic myelopathy. Equine Vet J 2014;46(6):681–6.
24. Tucker R, Hall YS, Hughes TK, et al. Osteochondral fragmentation of the cervical articular process joints; prevalence in horses undergoing CT for investigation of cervical dysfunction. Equine Vet J 2021;54:106–1113.
25. Gough SL, Anderson JDC, Dixon JJ. Computed tomographic cervical myelography in horses: Technique and findings in 51 clinical cases. J Vet Intern Med 2020;34(5):2142–51.
26. Brown KA, Davidson EJ, Johnson AL, et al. Inflammatory cytokines in horses with cervical articular process joint osteoarthritis on standing cone beam computed tomography. Equine Vet J 2020;5:9440954.
27. Lindgren CM, Wright L, Kristoffersen M, et al. Computed tomography and myelography of the equine cervical spine: 180 cases (2013–2018). Equine Vet Educ 2020;33:475–83.

Transcranial Magnetic Stimulation and Transcranial Electrical Stimulation in Horses

Henricus Louis Journée, MD, PhD[a,b,*], Sanne Lotte Journée, DVM[c,d]

KEYWORDS

- Horse • Transcranial stimulation • TMS • TES • MEP • Neurology • Ataxia

KEY POINTS

- Transcranial MEPs offer a valuable ancillary non-invasive test to assess the integrity of the motor function of the spinal cord in horses.
- Are complementary to radiological imaging techniques revealing the anatomy of the spine and spinal cord.
- Their high sensitivity for minor impact on the spinal cord likely exert the diagnostic power to also low grades of ataxia.
- Dominant late MEPs of extracranial elicited startle reflexes are characteristic for horses.
- MEPs of muscles from different segmental levels can likely be used to locate spinal cord lesions with affected motor functions

Abbreviations	
TES	transcranial electrical stimulation
TMS	transcranial magnetic stimulation
MEP	(muscle) motor evoked potential
MT	motor threshold
LMN	lower motoneuron
EDM	equine degenerative myeloencephalopathy
EPM	equine protozoal myeloencephalitus
CVSM	cervical vertebral spinal myelopathy
ECR	musculus extensor carpi radialis
TC	musculus tibialis cranialis

[a] Department of Neurosurgery, University of Groningen, Univ Med Center Groningen, Hanzeplein 1, Groningen 9713 GZ, the Netherlands; [b] Department of Orthopedics, Univ Utrecht, Univ Med Ctr Utrecht, PO-box 85500 NL-3508 GA, Utrecht, Netherlands; [c] Equine Diagnostics, Tergracht 2A, Wijns 9091 BG, the Netherlands; [d] Research Group of Comparative Physiology, Department of Translational Physiology, Infectiology and Public Health, Faculty of Veterinary Medicine, Ghent University, Merelbeke, Belgium
* Corresponding author. Department of Neurosurgery, University of Groningen, Univ Med Center Groningen, Hanzeplein 1, Groningen 9713 GZ, the Netherlands.
E-mail address: hljournee@gmail.com

Vet Clin Equine 38 (2022) 189–211
https://doi.org/10.1016/j.cveq.2022.04.002
0749-0739/22/© 2022 The Author(s). Published by Elsevier Inc. This is an open access article under the CC BY license (http://creativecommons.org/licenses/by/4.0/).

INTRODUCTION

Depending on the localization of the lesion, spinal cord ataxia is the most common type of ataxia in horses. Most prevalent diagnoses include cervical vertebral stenotic myelopathy (CVSM), equine protozoal myeloencephalitis (EPM), trauma and equine degenerative myeloencephalopathy (EDM). Other causes of ataxia and weakness are associated with infectious causes, trauma and neoplasia. A neurologic examination is indispensable to identify the type of ataxia. In addition, clinical neurophysiology offers tools to locate functional abnormalities in the central and peripheral nervous system. Clinical EMG assessment looks at the lower motoneuron function (LMN) and is used to differentiate between neuropathy in peripheral nerves, which belong to LMNs and myopathy.[1] As LMNs reside in the spinal cord, it is possible to grossly localize lesions in the myelum by muscle examination.[2] Transcranial (tc) stimulation techniques are gaining importance in all areas of medicine to assess the motor function of the spinal cord along the motor tracts to the LMNs. Applications in diagnostics, intraoperative neurophysiological monitoring (IONM), and evaluation of effects of treatment are still evolving in human medicine and offer new challenges in equine medicine. Tc stimulation techniques comprise transcranial magnetic stimulation (TMS) and transcranial electrical stimulation (TES). TMS was first applied in horses in 1996 by Mayhew and colleagues[3] and followed by TES. The methods are exchangeable for clinical diagnostic assessment but show a few differences.

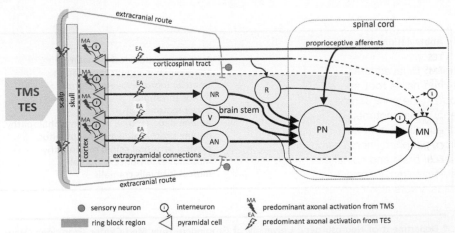

Fig. 1. TMS and TES activation of important motor tracts as expected in ungulates as horses. The scheme is speculative because no specific anatomic data on horses is available. The predominant intra and extracranial locations whereby axons are activated are indicated. When stimulation intensities increases, activated (EA) locations will shift toward the brain stem while TMS activation (MA) remains in place in the cortex. Extracranial activated sensory axons are conveyed to the neural network in the brain stem whereby startle reflexes may be elicited. The proprioceptive nucleus PN (C3-C4 levels) has a major integrating role in the depicted motor tracts and proprioceptive afferents. R, reticular neurons; NR, nucleus ruber; V, vestibular nuclei; AN, additional nuclei like the tectum; MN, motoneuron. The PN possibly also receives collaterals from corticospinal tracts. Retrograde connections of the PN to the brain stem and cerebellum are not shown.

PRINCIPLES OF TRANSCRANIAL STIMULATION, CONNECTING NEURAL CIRCUITS, AND MUSCLE MOTOR-EVOKED POTENTIALS

In horses, TMS and multipulse TES are interchangeable transcranial stimulation techniques suitable to assess the motor function of the spinal cord.[4] Elicited muscle motor-evoked potentials (MEPs) reflect the functional properties of neural elements of the route along brainstem nuclei, extrapyramidal motor tracts, propriospinal neurons, and motoneurons. Both techniques are applied to standing sedated horses, are painless and noninvasive.

Fig. 1 gives a schematic survey of which and whereby axons are activated and their routes across the brain stem and spinal cord to the motoneuron. TES and TMS share many neurophysiological properties. Small differences are attributable to dissimilarities in the interaction with the brain.

TMS generates induction currents in the brain from a magnetic coil placed on the forehead of the horse. These mainly activate axons in the cortex that in turn activate cascaded neurons of which the pyramidal cell or upper motoneuron is the end station in the cortex and gateway to the spinal cord. The pyramidal axons form the corticospinal tract and propagate a train of action potentials further down the spinal cord. These can epidurally be recorded as dominant I (indirect)-waves.[5,6] A few corticospinal axons may also become activated of which small D (direct)-waves may join.

In contrast to TMS, TES activates mainly corticospinal tract axons directly near the active anodal electrode.[6,7] This occurs below the cortex bypassing the cortical neurons. These action potentials can be recorded downstream as a large dominant D-wave. Cortical axons are activated as well and appear as subsequent repetitive relatively small I-waves. I-waves are extra attenuated or absent under sedation. The insensitivity of D-waves for anesthetic agents is an important reason why TES is used instead of TMS in IONM in humans. The predominant D-waves of TES become evident as shorter motor latency times (MLT) of muscle MEPs than in TMS whereby I-waves are predominant.[5,8–12]

Latency times of muscle MEPs are the sum of central and peripheral conduction times. Delayed latencies may also have a peripheral origin. The conduction time between nerve root and muscle must be subtracted from the muscle MEP latency to obtain the pure central motor conduction time (CMCT) between the stimulated brain and spinal motoneuron. Peripheral conduction times for correction are obtained by direct stimulation at nerve roots or from latency times of M- and F-waves of MEPs from peripheral nerve stimulation.[13–15] The CMCT specifically reflects the motor function of brain and spinal cord. An often-used term of "upper motoneuron function" is, strictly taken, incorrect as the pyramidal tract is not exclusively involved as extrapyramidal tracts also contribute to the generation of muscle MEPs.

APPLICATIONS OF TRANSCRANIAL STIMULATION IN HUMAN MEDICINE

TMS and TES provide information about the motor functions and the modulating effects of the cortex, subcortical nuclei and nuclei in the brain stem, cerebellum, and spinal cord.[14] This led to applications in areas of medicine and neuroscience, unfolding of tools for clinical diagnostic assessment like stroke, cervical myelopathy, amyotrophic lateral sclerosis (has similarities with EDM in horses), dystonia, Parkinson's disease and cerebellar ataxia,.[14,16–18] Neurophysiological measures as corticomotor threshold (MT), MEP amplitude, latency and wave morphology, cortical silent period duration or CMCT among others, can provide evidence of disease-related changes in motor cortical control output in patients. Repeated TMS (rTMS) is also considered in the treatment of many disorders in neurology and psychiatry like motor disorders such as dysphagia, anxiety and PTST, depression, neuromodulation of pain, neurologic, and psychiatric diseases.[19–21] Intraoperative neurophysiology is a specific field whereby transcranial MEPs are used in which TES is pivotal. TES has a recognized place in the fast-expanding applications for IONM and surgical and anesthetic interventions like for example, in the placement of spinal or deep brain stimulation electrodes and neuronavigation.[14,22]

In humans, TMS is used for clinical diagnosis as it is painless. Frequently used muscles for the assessment of the motor function of the spinal cord are hand muscles, extensor carpi radialis, and biceps in the upper limbs and the anterior tibial, gastrocnemius, and abductor halluces muscle in the lower limbs.[15,23,24] Intercostal and paraspinal tc-muscle MEPs can be used to determine the location of the lesion responsible for the thoracic myelopathy. Such MEPs can identify the level of origin of a myelopathic lesion in patients with a radiologically visible lesion.[25–27] Also accessible by TMS are facial, tongue, respiratory, laryngeal, pharyngeal, cricothyroid, vocal cord, pelvic, and anal sphincter muscles.[14,24,28–32]

The CMCT is correlated with the grading of myelum compression on MRI and with the degree of functional involvement of the spinal cord as observed by a neurologic examination. TMS has a sensitivity and specificity of 100% and 84.5% to detect cord compression and might even detect subclinical lesions.[18,33] TMS may clarify whether locations with anatomic cord compression as found in MRI are a functional lesion.[34–36] MEP studies can demonstrate spinal involvement even when radiological evidence for spinal cord damage is absent or equivocal.[17] Muscle MEPs allows to monitor progressive diseases. Pre, per and postoperative testing monitors neurophysiological events during surgery and reflects the status after surgery.[16,37,38] Tc muscle MEPs provide no information about the etiology of the lesion.[16]

TRANSLATIONAL ASPECTS OF HUMAN APPLICATIONS IN EQUINE MEDICINE

Many applications of transcranial MEPs in human medicine can be transposed to equine medicine. Transcranial stimulation is a valuable ancillary test to assess the integrity of the motor tracts in horses. The technique is painless and safe and shows good sensitivity to detect lesions along the descending motor pathways when used under sedation to prevent anxiety and occasional kicking.[39,40] When horses are sedated, the discomfort of TES and TMS is comparable while both techniques can grossly be considered as interchangeable.[4,41,42] In man and animals with spinal cord trauma and ischemia, TMS has proven to be a valuable diagnostic tool for the detection of lesions along the spinal cord.[43–46] TMS and TES are valuable to detect abnormal MEP characteristics at different grades of ataxia in horses.

So far, only prolonged MLTs muscle MEPs of thoracic and pelvic limbs are used and described. The large inter-stimulus variations of MEP amplitudes make these still useful but are of limited value.[39,40,42,47,48] Further diagnostic improvements and applications are expected by including more muscles.

The pure CMCT reflects specifically the motor function of the spinal cord and results from the subtraction of the peripheral nerve conduction time from muscle MEP latency. The peripheral conduction time can be determined from M and F responses or obtained by nerve root stimulation.[13,14,24]

Tc-MEPs of paraspinal muscles can be used to localize spinal cord lesions with a segmental accuracy. Other interesting muscles for the assessment of their functional integrity and innervation are facial, pharyngeal, vocal cord, and other muscles that are innervated by cranial nerves, respiratory muscles, pelvic muscles, and anal sphincters. Urination, defecation, and sexual functions depend on the anatomic and functional integrity of central and peripheral nerve pathways to the pelvic floor and the sacral region. TES may be an attractive alternative for the assessment of facial muscles to avoid coil repositioning errors and saturation effects of physiologic amplifiers caused by strong induction currents in close proximity to a TMS coil.

IONM modalities can be transposed to horses. Challenging application are IONM in spinal cord and nerve root decompression, placement of baskets, and stabilization of the spine. Sensory evoked potentials can be of complementary value. However, IONM may limit the choice of anesthetic agents.[22] Other potential applications are the assessment of the progression of symptoms and functional recovery on treatment of prognosis.

Neural Pathways from Cortex to Spinal Motoneurons

Spinal motor tracts have crossed and uncrossed connections to the spinal cord. When asymmetry exists in muscle MEPs, their lowest MTs are found at the contralateral side of the active electrode or active induced cortical current direction. The crossed corticospinal tract has a dominant role in the voluntary control of movement in man, but is less important in phylogenetically older species[49] whereby extrapyramidal pathways and associated neuronal circuits exert a major role. An outline of the main connections from literature data is given in **Fig. 1**, which depicts the dominating connections from the brain stem to motoneurons. This model is speculative because no specific anatomic data on horses is available. Although differences may exist between rodents, cats, rats, and ungulates, such as horses, it is expected that these animals share the integrating and dominating role of the proprioceptive neuron (PN) in the control of movements. Most experimental studies are performed on cats and rodents. The next outline is mainly based on studies performed on cats of which most experimental studies are published and used as a reference for horses. The reticulospinal, rubrospinal, tectospinal, and vestibulospinal tracts are important brain stem and mesencephalon leaving extrapyramidal motor tracts and are a prominent input to C2-C4 spinal PNs.[50] The PN is an important common path station. However, also direct monosynaptic connections of vestibular nuclei to motoneurons of extensor muscles of the knee are reported in cats.[51] It relays to cervical and thoracic motoneurons and back to the brain stem and cerebellum.[50,52,53] Monosynaptic connections between the nucleus ruber and motoneurons are also encountered as shown in **Fig. 1**.[54] Collateral connections of the corticospinal tract with reticular and other neurons in the brain stem provide an access port to the PN. The PN is also an important interacting station with somatosensory axons of which many are of proprioceptive origin. These exert a modulating influence on the control of movements and also on tc-MEPs.

Selective studies with epidural measurements at supramaximal TES or TMS and stimulation in the brainstem reveal that the major portion of the extrapyramidal motor conduction runs along the reticulospinal and vestibulospinal tracts in the ventral funiculus.[55–58] Tectospinal fibers are there less numerous and share the ventral funiculus until C4 level.[55] The rubrospinal pathways in cats play probably a minor role in the spinal MEPs from TMS.[57,59]

Most studies in older species show a large variety of connections via the PN and interneurons to motoneurons. The pyramidal tract is likely not a significant motor pathway (dashed connections in **Fig. 1**). It is generally accepted that the pyramidal pathways descend to the level of the first cervical segment in the horse.[60] For example, the locomotion in rats is not affected by further caudally created lesions.[61] It is presumed that the rise of the membrane potentials of LMNs after transcranial stimulation is mainly controlled by transmission through PNs, while a monosynaptic transfer via the pyramidal tract is subordinate or absent.

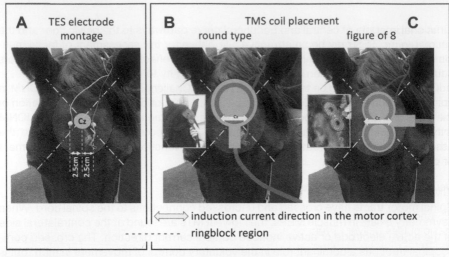

Fig. 2. Optimal montage of TES electrodes (*A*), positioning of a round TMS coil (*B*) and a butterfly or figure-of-8 TMS coil (*C*) over the head of a horse. The shown locations and given coil orientations provide the induced current direction (*B*, *C*) to focus on for lowest stimulation thresholds. The optimal currents direction in the cortex runs is centered between the vertex Cz (crossing point of dashed *lines* connecting eye and contralateral ear) and about 1 cm frontal from Cz. The corkscrew or s.c. needle electrodes are bilateral placed on a distance of about 2.5 cm from the midline (see Fig. 2A). Round coils produce circular currents while butterfly coils currents are focused between the double coils. The dashed circle indicates the location of the ringblock.

Remarkable is the large variety in conduction velocities of different motor tracts in cats. Conduction velocities in the corticospinal tract are around 60 to 70 m/s.[56,59,62] These are markedly higher in all extrapyramidal tracts with the largest velocities in the vestibulospinal and reticulospinal motor tracts in the ventral funiculus with upper ranges of respectively 164 m/s and 140 m/s.[51,56,58,63–65] This indicates that transcranial MLTs are ruled by the ventral located vestibulospinal and reticulospinal tracts.

GUIDELINES FOR TRANSCRANIAL STIMULATION
TES Electrode Montages and TMS Coil Placement

Lowest transcranial MTs are obtained by applying currents in the motor cortex in a lateral direction over the vertex Cz or a little more frontal. For TES, corkscrew or s.c. needle electrodes are bilaterally placed at a distance of about 2.5 cm from the midline (**Fig. 2**A). TMS can be performed by round (**Fig. 2**B) or figure-of-8 (butterfly) coils (**Fig. 2**C). More focal stimulation is possible with a figure-of-eight-shaped coil.[66]

Induction currents in the cortex from the changing magnetic field should run in the lateral direction as shown. Round coils produce circular currents within the rim while butterfly coils currents are focused between the double coils. When Cz is within about 1–2 cm from the frontal external edge of the round coil, the situation agrees with the optimal location nr 2 in the paper of Nollet.[67] With a typical 12 cm diameter round coil the strength is halved at 4–5 cm from the coil surface.[68] The cerebral cortex is about 1–2 cm separated from scalp surface. TMS-induced currents are severely attenuated at deeper locations of the basal ganglia or thalamus.[69] Maximum (100% intensity) magnetic field strength changes in TMS pulses are 35 to 41 kT/s for butterfly (2 × 75 mm) and round coils (~120 mm).

The shape of the TMS coil has practical consequences. The induced current direction of a round coil is defined by the coil surface, which touches the skin. The orientation of the coil handle has no relevance. In contrast, the handle of a butterfly coil points in the current direction. Its orientation is highly relevant and must keep constant to secure stimulation conditions. The current direction in the brain can be reversed by rotating the butterfly coil 180° with the handle in the opposite lateral direction. Both coil types can be used for diagnostic TMS. A nonfocal large round coil is preferred as its positioning over the target region is easier and less susceptible to minor changes in the coil position and activates a larger cortical area and depth which is important for the activation of deeper-seated primary motor areas of pelvic limb muscles.

STIMULATION PARAMETERS

TES and TMS pulses can be monophasic or biphasic. In humans, transcranial monophasic pulses deliver asymmetric MEPs and MTs when the currents in the brain run in the lateral direction. The lowest TES MTs are found at the anode,[7,9,70] which is the active stimulation electrode for muscle MEPs on the contralateral side. Biphasic transcranial pulses deliver symmetric MEPs and MTs. Asymmetry of muscle MEPs and MTs of monophasic pulses are not reported in phylogenetic older species like rodents, cats, and ungulates.

Widths of monophasic and biphasic TMS pulses are about 100 to 150 µs and 200 to 280 µs.[69] TMS in horses is mostly performed with monophasic pulses of a Magstim 200 (Eden Prairie, MN USA) stimulator at maximum intensities of 100%.[47,69,71] These are supramaximal levels whereby MEPs are symmetric anyway. Also biphasic pulses from a MagPro Compact magnetic stimulator (Medtronic Functional Diagnosis A/s) are used.[4] Published TES studies in horses are performed with 3 high biphasic pulses with 100 µs/phase pulse width and 1.3 ms interpulse interval.[41,72]

Transcranial muscle MEPs of different muscles may have different MTs.[14,24] These depend on the distance between upper motoneurons and TES electrode or TMS coil.

MUSCLE MOTOR-EVOKED POTENTIALS
Transcranial MEPs

Both TMS and TES generate trains of action potentials at the entry of descending motor tracts to motoneurons of muscles whereby MEPs are recorded. Motoneurons fire earlier at higher intensities while latencies decrease. The reduction of latencies for maximum TMS intensities is in dogs maximal −2.5 ms.[73] Stimulation by 3 high multipulse TES pulses, give an extra boost for earlier firing. Increasing TES intensities penetrate deeper in the brain. This shortens the motor route length and MLT. In humans, the latency time of D-waves is decreased to about −0.8 ms at the depth of the cerebral peduncle[10,74–77] and −1.8 ms at the foramen magnum.[78,79] At about 3 times the transcranial MT the D-wave amplitude increases by 100% to 200% as D-waves of extrapyramidal spinal motor tracts join the corticospinal D-wave.[80] The distance between vertex and brainstem of horses and cats is shorter than in man which is expected to cause smaller differences between (sub)cortical and brainstem thresholds. This is also reflected in the feline experiments of Konrad and colleagues[56] and Kawai and colleagues[59] whereby the supramaximal intensity level for the direct stimulation of the extrapyramidal tracts in cats lies close to the TES threshold to the brain stem but may exceed the depth range of TMS. This may introduce differences in muscle MEPs between TMS and TES.

Reported equine intensity-dependent of muscle MEP MLTs decreases around −1.7 ms and −2 ms for TES for increases of stimulation intensity of respective 20% and 20V above MT.[4,42]

Sedatives may suppress the synaptic transmission to motoneurons.[81–85] This can be compensated by multipulse stimulation.[4,86]

Extracranial Elicited Reflexes

A recently unfolded unique phenomenon in horses is the occurrence of late MEPs below transcranial MTs. These appear about 15 to 20 ms later than transcranial MEPs as a prominent part of muscle MEPs.[4,41,42] The late MEPs in all muscles impress as extracranially elicited startle reflexes (SR). Since these appear below transcranial MTs, these SRs originate most likely from the activation of extracranial sensory afferents as shown in **Fig. 1** and conveyed to the brain stem and spinal cord.[41] The difference between transcranial and late muscle MEPs latencies defines a transcranial time window for which the transcranial MEP is free from interference with late MEPs.

Muscle motor-evoked potential recording

Muscle MEPs are preferably measured by extramuscular electrodes as these observe the elicited electrical activity of many muscle fibers. Intramuscular needle electrodes record the activity of only a few muscle fibers can easily dislodge and impair reproducibility. However, these are still needed for deep-seated muscles.[48] Signals from subcutaneous needle and gelled surface electrodes are highly correlated. The signal quality is good when impedances are low. However, the signal quality of surface electrodes is unpredictable and may show a high background noise, which depends on the electrical properties of the skin which can be dry or wet and may contain salty debris.[48,87] Taping of both electrode types is recommended for the fixation and improvement of the signal quality but surface electrodes may show long adaptation times.[87] Subcutaneous needle electrodes are recommended as these have a predictable good signal quality. Adhesive surface electrodes are a useful alternative choice.

Segmental conduction times and velocities of paraspinal muscle motor-evoked potentials

Transcranial MEPs of paraspinal muscles can be used to determine the focus of myelopathic lesions with a segmental precision. This has been shown in humans in patients with a radiologically visible lesion.[25–27,88] Surface recordings of paraspinal muscles may be confounded by cross-talk from underlying fascicles.[89] Most appropriate are intramuscular needle or hookwire electrodes.[90] Clinical applications of paraspinal muscle MEPs in horses are not reported yet.

The mono-segmentally innervated multifidus muscle interconnects 2 subsequent vertebral bodies.[91] Other paraspinal muscles may be multisegmentally innervated which could blur the segmental accuracy.

Placement of intramuscular electrodes in the multifidus muscle in horses requires ultrasound guidance by a trained physician with good anatomic knowledge. Hitting nerve roots and blood vessels are potential risks. Paravertebral muscles aside vertebral corpora are easier to access.[92]

The segmental motor latency (SMT) over one segment is equal to the MLT difference over the segment. The SMT is a link in the CMCT chain. The segmental spinal motor conduction velocity (SMV) is defined as the segment length divided by the SMT. The SMT and SMV are suited to identify segmental links with prolonged latencies. Indirectly estimated spinal velocities are well more than 100 m/s.[4] In an unpublished scouting study using multifidus TES-MEP latencies between C3 and C6 levels in 3 horses, we found mean SMVs and SMTs between 141 to 192 m/s and 0.50 to 0.85 ms.

Significant displacement and distortion of the long needle electrodes may result from shearing forces between unequally moving muscle groups and cutaneous tissue layers. Repositioning of distorted electrodes is not always possible. It is recommended to insert all paraspinal electrodes over a segmental trajectory after finishing the MEP procedure with extramuscular MEPs and use the concluding TES intensity for latency assessment. Multichannel recording allows simultaneous measurements of paraspinal MEPs at single transcranial stimuli.

EQUIPMENT

Transcranial MEPs can be measured with a myograph intended for clinical neurophysiological assessment. Such devices mostly support conduction studies with external TMS stimulators. Build-in peripheral nerve stimulators are not powerful enough for TES. TMS devices can be replaced by an external TES device. The choice of certified TES stimulators is limited. In human medicine, TES is only used in neuromonitoring whereby the stimulator is integrated into most IONM equipment. In the remaining situations, the Digitimer D185 (Digitimer, Welwyn Garden City, UK) stimulator is mostly used as an auxiliary TES device. This voltage stimulator delivers monophasic trains with 50 µs pulse widths and can deliver the required 3 pulses per train with 1.3 ms interpulse time. Although delivered pulse voltages and shapes strongly depend on the impedance of the stimulation electrodes,[93] which affects the accuracy of MTs, the stimulator is reliable for clinical diagnostic use in horses.

A minimal inexpensive configuration consists of a single or 2-channel electromyograph connected to an auxiliary transcranial stimulator. Used myographs in TMS studies in horses are Neurostar, Sapphire, and Synergy (Medelec Ltd, Old Woking UK). These old designs can be replaced by current commercially available alternatives. In human medicine, TES is only used for neurophysiological monitoring with the TES stimulator usually integrated into the IONM equipment.

Single-channel assessment of tc MEPs in horses has practical disadvantages. TES settings need to be read from the stimulator and manually labeled to the MEP traces, which takes extra time. Four-limb assessment requires to repeat the measurements, rewiring, and labeling of muscle electrodes 4 times. This leads to unnecessary stimulations, prolongation of the sedation, and assessment time.

In contrast, to-date multichannel equipment with build-in transcranial stimulators like the NIM-Eclipse (Medtronic-Xomed, Inc USA) can be tailored for diagnostic use in horses. Multichannel MEPs offer the feature for intrastimulus comparisons of MLTs that are insensitive to varying levels of facilitation and sedation,[4,72] enable short-lasting sessions with less discomfort to the horse and don't require manual labeling of MEP traces. As being designed for IONM, the equipment may work cumbersome for diagnostic assessment and is expensive. New applications like segmental motor conduction measurements for locating spinal cord lesions in horses and specific diagnostic protocols for segmental tracing of prolonged SMTs and SMVs require software updates from the manufacturer.

To become attractive for a wide use in equine practice, there remains a need for portable, affordable, and user-friendly equipment, for use by trained equine veterinary practitioners.

SET-UP FOR 4-LIMB TRANSCRANIAL MUSCLE-MEP ASSESSMENT

A general set-up and procedure for 4-limb muscle-MEP assessment will briefly be described with illustrations of applications of TES and TMS with a multichannel and a 2-channel myographic systems in normal horses and a case with ataxia.

After a neurologic examination of the motor function and measurements of the height at withers and weight, horses are prepared for transcranial muscle MEP assessment.

The horses are initially sedated by i.v. injection of a half dose of a combination of detomidine (Detosedan, AST Farma B.V., Oudewater, The Netherlands) and butorphanol (Butomidol AST Farma B.V., Oudewater, The Netherlands). The second half is given before starting the measurement procedure (both 15-20 µg/kg in total).

To minimize extracranial reflexes, a subcutaneous ring block surrounding Cz with a diameter of about 8 cm is placed as shown in **Fig. 1**A by using 300 to 400 mg lidocaine 2% + adrenaline (Alfasan, Woerden, The Netherlands). For TES, two corkscrew electrodes (Medtronic-Xomed, Jacksonville, FL, Rhythmlink Columbia SC, Natus Medical, Middletown WI) are positioned 2.5 cm bilateral from the vertex at Cz as depicted in **Fig. 1**A. Corkscrew electrodes cannot dislodge.

Subcutaneous needle electrodes (L 13 mm 27 GA Rhythmlink Columbia SC, Natus Medical, Middletown WI, Medtronic-Xomed, Jacksonville, FL, or other manufacturers) are placed over the musculus extensor carpi radialis (ECR) (10 and 20 cm above the os carpi accessorium) and over the musculus tibialis cranialis (TC) (10 and 20 cm above the medial malleolus) with an s.c. ground needle electrode in the neck. Mono-polar recordings with an active electrode over the muscle belly and a distal located electrode are useful as well. The reference electrode should be placed. Recommended filter settings for high and low pass filters are 50 Hz and 10 kHz.

MEASUREMENT PROCEDURE

After a check of all electrode impedances, confirming correct connections, and background noise checks, repeated MEP measurements are performed by stepwise incrementing stimulation intensities starting at zero intensit with steps of 10V for voltage TES or in TMS steps of 10% from maximum intensity. Measurements are performed twice at each intensity. On the appearance of early MEPs at the first latency jump, measurements may initially show back and forth switching transitions between early and late MEPs in a transcranial segue region. This pattern disappears usually after a few intensity steps when transcranial MEPs remain always visible.

When elicited movements remain acceptable, stimulation intensities steps can be continued to 30V or 30% above the threshold when usually a supramaximal level is approached. Stimulation thresholds of pelvic limb muscles can be one or two intensity steps higher than forelimb or neck muscles because of considerable trial-to-trial variability finally, 6 consecutive muscle MEPs are recorded at the highest intensity step. The shortest latencies associated with the largest amplitude are used for the report.[14,24] For the 2-channel system in one of the presented examples the ECR and TC are first assessed on one side after followed by the assessment of the contralateral side. The second stimulation intensity series can be shortened as transcranial thresholds already are known. For the adaptation of the horse, it is recommended to start at the previously obtained transcranial motor threshold of the ECR and pursuit the series with 10V or 10% steps.

EXAMPLES

Fig. 3 gives an overview of 4-channel recorded MEP responses from the ECR (A and C) and TC (B and D) muscle groups for TES (A and B) and TMS (C and D) in landscape plots. These are illustrative examples from a normal horse without neurologic signs, depicting how MEPs unfold at increasing stimulation intensities. The first elicited

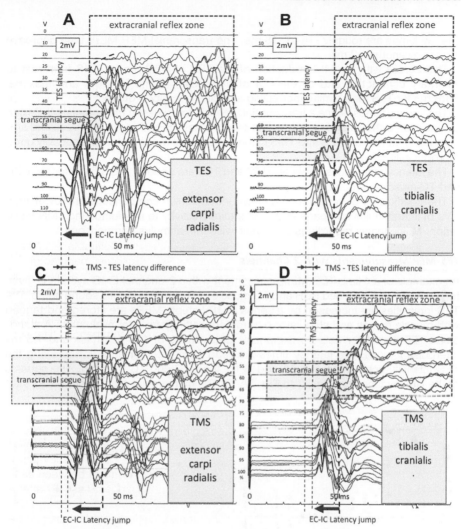

Fig. 3. Overview of MEP responses from the ECR (*A, C*) and TC (*B, D*) muscle groups for TES (*A, B*) and TMS (*C, D*) in landscape plots from a normal horse with grade 0 ataxia at stepwise increasing stimulation intensities. The first elicited MEPs are from extracranial origin and show relative long latency times which decrease by about -20 ms when reaching the transcranial thresholds for TES: ECR at about 45 V and TC at 50V and for TMS: at 55% for both muscles. The intensity width of the transcranial segue region is for the ECR 45 to 55V; for TC 50 to 60V for TES or 55% to 70% for TMS. The extra to intracranial (EC-IC) latency jumps are between about -15 to -18 ms. The early latencies of the transcranial MEP then decrease further by about ms.

MEPs are of extracranial origin and show for both TES and TMS relative long latency times at about 45 to 50 ms for the ECR and 65 to 70 ms for the TC muscle groups. These decrease by about when reaching the transcranial thresholds for TES at about 45V and 50V for the ECR and TC or for TMS at 55% for both muscle groups. The intensity range of the transcranial segue region is for TES 45 to 55V and 50 to 60V for the ECR and TC or for TMS 55% to 70% in all limbs. The extracranial to intracranial (EC-IC) latency jumps are roughly -15 to -18 ms. The transcranial MEP MLTs then decrease further by another -2 ms.

This agrees with the MLT reduction of the APB of −2.3 ms for TMS from rest to voluntary contraction and of the FDI of more than -3 ms for TMS and maximal −1.8 ms for TES for a similar increasing stimulus intensity protocol.[8,9]

The latency jumps define a transcranial time window wherein transcranial MEPs can be analyzed without interference by late extracranial MEPs. The wave shapes and amplitudes of MEPs from TES and TMS in the transcranial window show reasonably good reproducibility.

The latency differences between TMS and TES are about 3 and 3.5 ms for the ECR and TC muscles.

The coefficients of variations (CV) from intrastimulus comparisons are lower than CVs of interstimulus comparison due to the insensitivity to the fluctuating LMN facilitation. Multichannel recordings allow pair-wise intrastimulus comparisons.

TES-MEP Measurements with 2 Channels

An example of a 4 limb TES-MEP assessment with a 2-channel EMG system is given for simultaneous recorded ECR and TC muscles at the right side of a sound horse. The TES intensities are increased by a series of 10V steps. MEPs are stored and tagged with muscle names and stimulator parameters settings for later evaluation. A standalone TES stimulator delivers 3 biphasic pulse trains of 100 μs/phase and 1.5 ms interpulse interval. The latency times are read from a cursor and plotted along the TES-intensity scale in graphs 4A and B for the ECR and TC muscles. The courses of the latency times are similar to **Fig. 3**A, B. The extracranial elicited late MEPs start

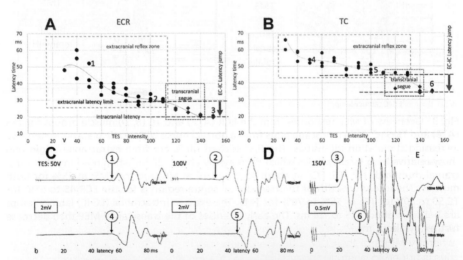

Fig. 4. Example of TES-MEP recordings of a healthy horse obtained from a standard 2-channel EMG machine modified for use in connection with a stand-alone TES voltage stimulator. The upper graphs show the course of the MEP latency times as a function of the TES intensity of the ECR (*A*) and TC (*B*) muscles on the right side. Graphs C, D, and E show the MEP traces of the ECR (upper) and the TC (lower) at TES intensities of 50, 100, and 150 V. The numbered arrows refer to the numbers in the upper plots and indicate the latency times at the onset of the responses. The measurements are performed in the Rood and Riddle horse clinic in Lexington KY and used with permission.

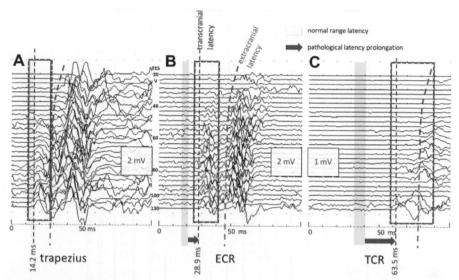

Fig. 5. Overview of TES-MEP responses from the m. trapezius (*A*), the ECR (*B*), and TC (*C*) muscle groups with from top to bottom increasing voltages. These are examples from a grade 4 ataxic horse with a spinal cord lesion. The first elicited late MEPs are of extracranial origin with relative long latency times at about 35 ms for the trapezius, 58 ms for the ECR, and strong varying latencies above 85 ms for the TC. The late latencies decrease to respectively 27 ms, 46 ms, and strong varying above 80 ms. Extra-to intracranial latencies reduction jumps are visible in all muscles between -15 and -19 ms. The gray bars represent the range of normal latencies. The red arrows indicate the prolongation of latencies from the normal. Only the trapezius latency is within the normal range.

at 30V with latencies of 50 to 60 ms for the ECR and 60 to 68 ms for the TC. These decrease to respectively 33 ms and 45 ms when reaching the transcranial threshold at 120V and 140V where extra-intra cranial latency jumps appear. Beyond the transcranial segue region, the minimum latencies and amplitudes are 19.0 ms/3.3 mV for the ECR and 35.0 ms/4.15 mV for the TC. The recorded MEPs are shown in **Fig. 4**C, D, E for TES voltages of 50, 100, and 150V.

The MLTs and amplitudes at the left side are 18.5 ms/13 mV and 32.0 ms/8.0 mV, respectively.

TES-MEPs of an Ataxic Horse

An example of MEPs in an ataxic horse with prolonged MLTs is illustrated in **Fig. 5** whereby MEPs of the ECR and TC are shown at increasing TES voltages. The trapezius is added to illustrate the possibility of locating functional motor lesions in the cervical myelum. Like in normal horses (**Fig. 3** and **4**), late MEPs of extracranial origin become first visible. Their latencies reduce to 35 ms, 58 ms and strong varying latencies more than 80 ms for respectively the trapezius, ECR, and TC at the appearance of extra-to intracranial latency reductions -15 to -19 ms. The MLT of the trapezius of 14.2 ms is within the normal range, whereas the MLTs of 28.9 ms and 63.5 ms of the ECR and TC are significantly prolonged. A functional lesion is likely located between the cervical root levels C2-C4 and C6-C7 of the trapezius and ECR.

Table 1
Survey of published reference data for tc-MEP motor latencies (MLT), heights at withers

	Withers Height Means ± SD (cm)	N	Eloc	Motor Latency Time mean ± SD (ms)		ΔMLT/Δstimint	
				ECR	TCR	ECR	TCR
TMS							
Mayhew & Washbourne,[3] 1996	NA (ponies)	10	em	19.0 ± 2.3	30.2 ± 3.4		
Nollet et al,[47] 2004	137 ± 27	84	im	19.3 ± 2.5	30.5 ± 5.3	0.078	0.17
Nollet et al,[67] 2003	152 ± 5	7	im	21 ± 1.5	32 ± 3		
Nollet et al,[40] 2003	156 ± 4.5	6	im	21.1 ± 1.0	32.6 ± 2.0		
Nollet et al,[39] 2002	NA	12	im	20.7 ± 1.8	36.1 ± 3.5		
Rijckaert et al,[48] 2018	160 ± 5	10	im	20.8 ± 1.5	39.4 ± 3.8		
			em	21.2 ± 1.4	39.2 ± 3.8		
Rijckaert et al,[71] 2019	NA	5	im&em	20 ± 1	39 ± 1		
TES							
Journée et al,[42] 2018	161 ± 10	12	em	19.4 ± 0.9	36.3 ± 2.3	0.065	0.125

Survey of published reference data for tc-MEP motor latencies (MLT), heights at withers, N: number of included horses, Eloc: electrode location: extra- (em) or intramuscular (im), ΔMLT/Δstimint: MLT increase per increment of stimulation intensity (ms/% for TMS; ms/V for TES). NA: data not available.

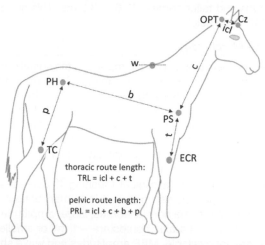

Fig. 6. Thoracic and pelvic route lengths from the vertex Cz to the ECR and TC muscles. OPT: occipital protuberance, W, height at withers; PS, point of shoulder; PH, point of hip. icl, intracranial length c, neck length; b, back length; t and p, lengths to electrodes of the thoracic and pelvic limbs. (*Modified from* Mayhew, I.G. and Washbourne, J.R. (1996) Magnetic motor evoked potentials in ponies. *J. Vet. Intern. Med.* 10, 326–9.)

INTERPRETATION OF MOTOR-EVOKED POTENTIALS
Motor Latency Times

Table 1 gives a survey of normative data of MLTs for TMS and TES of ECR and TCR muscles from the literature. Pelvic limbs show a wide latency range, which strongly depends on the length of the motor pathway between stimulation and recording. The regression coefficients ΔMLT/Δstimint expressing the MLT increase over a given increment of height at withers[47] are given in **Table 1**.

When comparing TES latencies with TMS, 3 and 3.8 ms should be subtracted from TMS-MEP latencies the MLTs for correction of the latency difference between TMS and TES for respectively the thoracic and pelvic limbs.

Motor Conduction Velocities

Motor conduction velocities (MCV) are expected to be independent of height as these are equal to the traveled route length divided by the MLT as described by Mayhew and colleagues.[3] The route lengths between TC stimulation and ECR or TC: TRL, and the TC: PRL, respectively are depicted in **Fig. 6**. These measures can be divided by the MLTs of the associated muscles for calculations of MCVs.

The velocities are compound velocities and include peripheral and central axonal motor conduction and also synaptic delays of inter- and motoneurons and neuromuscular junction. Axonal conduction velocities are therefore underestimated. MCVs of TES are higher than for TMS. This has been shown in 5 horses with heights of 160 ± 7 cm[4] whereby for TES $MCV_{ECR} = 66.2$ m/s and $MCV_{TC} = 73.7$ m/s and for TMS: $MCV_{ECR} = 58.5$ m/s and $MCV_{TC} = 63.8 \pm 8.0$ m/s.[4] The values for TMS agree with the results of Mayhew and colleagues[3] for ponies: $MCV_{ECR} = 63.4 \pm 9.3$ m/s and $MCV_{TC} = 63.8 \pm 8.0$ m/s, while MLTs of pelvic muscles are significant different: for ponies: 30.2 ± 3.4 ms and taller horses: 42.6 ± 3.5 ms. This supports the expected independence of MCVs on height.

MEP Amplitudes and Morphology

Tc-MEP amplitudes are sensitive to a minor impact on the spinal cord and are a pivotal parameter in the warning criteria in neurophysiological monitoring.[22,94] In contrast to the small variability of MLTs in horses with CVs of 3% to 9%, the CVs thoracic and pelvic muscle MEP amplitudes of 35% and 60% are markedly higher with an amplitude range of 0.5 to 20 mV. Mild cervical spinal cord lesions with ataxia in the hind limbs may be visible as clearly or sometimes only slightly prolonged MLTs.[95] For statistical analysis, MEP amplitude data should be compared in the logarithmic domain whereby they have normal distribution functions.[96]

Left-right differences may have a clinical meaning.[97] Side-to-side differences of 50% or greater can be regarded as abnormal in human patients. However, Nollet and colleagues[47] reported in some normal horses, larger amplitude asymmetries. Reported MEP amplitudes of most ataxic horses are ~1 mV or smaller.[39] Cut-off values for amplitude ratios are not available. MEP amplitudes and wave shapes of extramuscular needle or surface electrodes are equal[87] but differ markedly from intramuscular needle electrodes.[48]

Pure tc-MEP amplitudes and wave shapes can only be analyzed within the transcranial time window. Published peak-peak amplitudes and phases of MEP waves likely reflect composites of transcranial and extracranial elicited MEPs. These still may have a diagnostic meaning as both MEPs result from motor conduction along the spinal cord.

CONCLUDING REMARKS

Transcranial stimulation is a valuable ancillary test to assess the integrity of the motor tracts in horses and is complementary to imaging techniques revealing the anatomy of the spine and spinal cord. TMS and TES are 2 comparable stimulation techniques whereby TES is less sensitive to modulation by cortical activity while reproducibly errors from magnetic coil repositioning are absent.

Measurements are relatively simple to perform in skilled hands. Shortest sessions with less discomfort to the horse and improved accuracy are possible with multichannel electromyographic equipment configured for equine applications. New insights in neurophysiological characteristics which apply specifically to horses' challenges to further optimize the technique and equipment by focusing on equine use and exploring the possibility to locate spinal cord lesions by identifying regions with impaired motor conduction with segmental precision. Because of its insensitivity to geometric measures of horses, it looks worthwhile to explore the features of the MCV as an alternative parameter for the motor conduction time.

CLINICS CARE POINTS

- Electrical or magnetic transcranial stimulation is painless and safe and shows good sensitivity to detect lesions along the descending motor pathways when used under sedation.
- In horses, transcranial electric and magnetic stimulation are well known as non-invasive diagnostic tests with low discomfort, under sedated conditions.
- Both techniques are able to discern between presence or absence of possible neurological lesions and identify their focal or widespread presence.

- Only thoracic and pelvic limbs muscle MEPs from TES and TMS have been documented for diagnostic evaluation in horses; except for small differences, latencies are interchangeable.

- A not skilled user may misinterpret latencies of extracranial elicited startle responses as pathological delayed transcranial MEPs.

REFERENCES

1. Wijnberg ID. A review of the use of electromyography in equine neurological diseases. Equine Vet Educ 2010;17:123–7. Available at: https://onlinelibrary.wiley.com/doi/10.1111/j.2042-3292.2005.tb00350.x.
2. Wijnberg ID, Back W, Jong M de, et al. The role of electromyography in clinical diagnosis of neuromuscular locomotor problems in the horse. Equine Vet J 2004;36:718–22. Available at: http://www.ncbi.nlm.nih.gov/pubmed/15656503. Accessed July 8, 2021.
3. Mayhew IG, Washbourne JR. Magnetic motor evoked potentials in ponies. J Vet Intern Med 1996;10:326–9.
4. Journée SL, Journée HL, Berends HI, et al. Comparison of Muscle MEPs From Transcranial Magnetic and Electrical Stimulation and Appearance of Reflexes in Horses. Front Neurosci 2020;14:570372.
5. Amassian VE, Cracco RQ, Maccabee PJ. Focal stimulation of human cerebral cortex with the magnetic coil: a comparison with electrical stimulation. Electroencephalogr Clin Neurophysiol 1989;74:401–16. Available at: http://www.ncbi.nlm.nih.gov/pubmed/2480218.
6. Amassian VE, Quirk GJ, Stewart M. A comparison of corticospinal activation by magnetic coil and electrical stimulation of monkey motor cortex. Electroencephalogr Clin Neurophysiol 1990;77:390–401.
7. Rothwell JC, Thompson PD, Day BL, et al. Motor cortex stimulation in intact man. 1. General characteristics of EMG responses in different muscles. Brain 1987; 110:1173–90.
8. Hess CW, Mills KR, Murray NM. Magnetic stimulation of the human brain: facilitation of motor responses by voluntary contraction of ipsilateral and contralateral muscles with additional observations on an amputee. Neurosci Lett 1986;71:235–40.
9. Day BL, Thompson PD, Dick JP, et al. Different sites of action of electrical and magnetic stimulation of the human brain. Neurosci Lett 1987;75:101–6.
10. Nielsen J, Petersen N, Ballegaard M. Latency of effects evoked by electrical and magnetic brain stimulation in lower limb motoneurones in man. J Physiol 1995; 484(Pt 3):791–802.
11. Ubags LH, Kalkman CJ, Been HD, et al. A comparison of myogenic motor evoked responses to electrical and magnetic transcranial stimulation during nitrous oxide/opioid anesthesia. Anesth Analg 1999;88:568–72.
12. Lazzaro V Di, Oliviero A, Pilato F, et al. Comparison of descending volleys evoked by transcranial and epidural motor cortex stimulation in a conscious patient with bulbar pain. Clin Neurophysiol 2004;115:834–8.
13. Chen R, Cros D, Curra A, et al. The clinical diagnostic utility of transcranial magnetic stimulation: report of an IFCN committee. Clin Neurophysiol 2008;119:504–32. Available at: http://www.ncbi.nlm.nih.gov/pubmed/18063409.
14. Rossini PM, Burke D, Chen R, et al. Non-invasive electrical and magnetic stimulation of the brain, spinal cord, roots and peripheral nerves: Basic principles and procedures for routine clinical and research application. An updated report from

an I.F.C.N. Committee. Clin Neurophysiol 2015;126:1071–107. Available at: http://www.ncbi.nlm.nih.gov/pubmed/25797650.

15. Furby A, Bourriez JL, Jacquesson JM, et al. Motor evoked potentials to magnetic stimulation: technical considerations and normative data from 50 subjects. J Neurol 1992;239:152–6. Available at: http://www.ncbi.nlm.nih.gov/pubmed/1573419.

16. Nardone R, Höller Y, Brigo F, et al. The contribution of neurophysiology in the diagnosis and management of cervical spondylotic myelopathy: a review. Spinal Cord 2016;54:756–66. Available at: http://www.nature.com/articles/sc201682.

17. Nardone R, Höller Y, Thomschewski A, et al. Central motor conduction studies in patients with spinal cord disorders: a review. Spinal Cord 2014;52:420–7. Available at: http://www.ncbi.nlm.nih.gov/pubmed/24752292.

18. Lo YL, Chan LL, Lim W, et al. Systematic correlation of transcranial magnetic stimulation and magnetic resonance imaging in cervical spondylotic myelopathy. Spine (Phila Pa 1976) 2004;29:1137–45. Available at: http://www.ncbi.nlm.nih.gov/pubmed/15131444.

19. Cirillo P, Gold AK, Nardi AE, et al. Transcranial magnetic stimulation in anxiety and trauma-related disorders: A systematic review and meta-analysis. Brain Behav 2019;9:e01284. Available at: http://www.ncbi.nlm.nih.gov/pubmed/31066227.

20. Simons A, Hamdy S. The Use of Brain Stimulation in Dysphagia Management. Dysphagia 2017;32:209–15. Available at: http://www.ncbi.nlm.nih.gov/pubmed/28353151.

21. O'Connell NE, Wand BM, Marston L, et al. Non-invasive brain stimulation techniques for chronic pain. Cochrane Database Syst Rev 2018;CD008208. Available at: http://www.ncbi.nlm.nih.gov/pubmed/29652088.

22. MacDonald DB, Skinner S, Shils J, et al. Intraoperative motor evoked potential monitoring - a position statement by the American Society of Neurophysiological Monitoring. Clin Neurophysiol 2013;124:2291–316.

23. Funaba M, Kanchiku T, Imajo Y, et al. Transcranial magnetic stimulation in the diagnosis of cervical compressive myelopathy: comparison with spinal cord evoked potentials. Spine (Phila Pa 1976) 2015;40:E161–7. Available at: http://www.ncbi.nlm.nih.gov/pubmed/25384053.

24. Groppa S, Oliviero A, Eisen A, et al. A practical guide to diagnostic transcranial magnetic stimulation: report of an IFCN committee. Clin Neurophysiol 2012;123:858–82. Available at: http://www.ncbi.nlm.nih.gov/pubmed/22349304.

25. Hashimoto T, Uozumi T, Tsuji S. Paraspinal motor evoked potentials by magnetic stimulation of the motor cortex. Neurology 2000;55:885–8. Available at: http://www.ncbi.nlm.nih.gov/pubmed/10994018.

26. Ertekin C, Uludag B, On A, et al. Motor-evoked potentials from various levels of paravertebral muscles in normal subjects and in patients with focal lesions of the spinal cord. Spine (Phila Pa 1976) 1998;23:1016–22.

27. Misawa T, Ebara S, Kamimura M, et al. Evaluation of thoracic myelopathy by transcranial magnetic stimulation. J Spinal Disord 2001;14:439–44. Available at: http://www.ncbi.nlm.nih.gov/pubmed/11586145.

28. Rödel RMW, Laskawi R, Markus H. Tongue representation in the lateral cortical motor region of the human brain as assessed by transcranial magnetic stimulation. Ann Otol Rhinol Laryngol 2003;112:71–6. Available at: http://www.ncbi.nlm.nih.gov/pubmed/12537062.

29. Ertekin C, Turman B, Tarlaci S, et al. Cricopharyngeal sphincter muscle responses to transcranial magnetic stimulation in normal subjects and in patients

with dysphagia. Clin Neurophysiol 2001;112:86–94. Available at: http://www.ncbi.nlm.nih.gov/pubmed/11137665. Accessed August 10, 2021.

30. Rödel RMW, Olthoff A, Tergau F, et al. Human cortical motor representation of the larynx as assessed by transcranial magnetic stimulation (TMS). Laryngoscope 2004;114:918–22. Available at: http://www.ncbi.nlm.nih.gov/pubmed/15126757.

31. Thumfart WF, Pototschnig C, Zorowka P, et al. Electrophysiologic investigation of lower cranial nerve diseases by means of magnetically stimulated neuromyography of the larynx. Ann Otol Rhinol Laryngol 1992;101:629–34. Available at: http://www.ncbi.nlm.nih.gov/pubmed/1497266.

32. Khedr EM, Aref E-EM. Electrophysiological study of vocal-fold mobility disorders using a magnetic stimulator. Eur J Neurol 2002;9:259–67. Available at: http://www.ncbi.nlm.nih.gov/pubmed/11985634.

33. Travlos A, Pant B, Eisen A. Transcranial Magnetic Stimulation for Detection of Pre-clinical Cervical Spondylotic Myelopathy. Arch Phys Med Rehabil 1992;73:442-6.

34. Deftereos SN, Kechagias EA, Panagopoulos G, et al. Localisation of cervical spinal cord compression by TMS and MRI. Funct Neurol 2009;24:99–105. Available at: https://www.semanticscholar.org/paper/Localisation-of-cervical-spinal-cord-compression-by-Deftereos-Kechagias/53096e40407480d6212d092df988ce8f5bcf0e1a.

35. Chan KM, Nasathurai S, Chavin JM, et al. The usefulness of central motor conduction studies in the localization of cord involvement in cervical spondylytic myelopathy. Muscle Nerve 1998;21:1220–3. Available at: http://www.ncbi.nlm.nih.gov/pubmed/9703453.

36. Lazzaro V Di, Restuccia D, Colosimo C, et al. The contribution of magnetic stimulation of the motor cortex to the diagnosis of cervical spondylotic myelopathy. Correlation of central motor conduction to distal and proximal upper limb muscles with clinical and MRI findings. Electroencephalogr Clin Neurophysiol 1992;85:311–20. Available at: http://www.ncbi.nlm.nih.gov/pubmed/1385091.

37. Visser J, Verra WC, Kuijlen JM, et al. Recovery of TES-MEPs during surgical decompression of the spine: a case series of eight patients. J Clin Neurophysiol 2014;31:568–74. Available at: http://www.ncbi.nlm.nih.gov/pubmed/25462144.

38. Nakanishi K, Tanaka N, Kamei N, et al. Electrophysiological evidence of functional improvement in the corticospinal tract after laminoplasty in patients with cervical compressive myelopathy: clinical article. J Neurosurg Spine 2014;21:210–6. Available at: http://www.ncbi.nlm.nih.gov/pubmed/24855997.

39. Nollet H, Deprez P, Ham L Van, et al. The use of magnetic motor evoked potentials in horses with cervical spinal cord disease. Equine Vet J 2002;34:156–63.

40. Nollet H, Ham L Van, Gasthuys F, et al. Influence of detomidine and buprenorphine on motor-evoked potentials in horses. Vet Rec 2003;152:534–7.

41. Journée SL, Journée HL, Bruijn CM de, et al. Design and Optimization of a Novel Method for Assessment of the Motor Function of the Spinal Cord by Multipulse Transcranial Electrical Stimulation in Horses. J Equine Vet Sci 2015;35:793–800.

42. Journée SL, Journée HL, Bruijn CM de, et al. Multipulse transcranial electrical stimulation (TES): normative data for motor evoked potentials in healthy horses. BMC Vet Res 2018;14:121.

43. Levy WJ. Spinal evoked potentials from the motor tracts. J Neurosurg 1983;58:38–44. Available at: http://www.ncbi.nlm.nih.gov/pubmed/6847907.

44. Levy WJ, York DH. Evoked Potentials from the Motor Tracts in Humans. Neurosurgery 1983;12:422–9. Available at: https://academic.oup.com/neurosurgery/article-lookup/doi/10.1227/00006123-198304000-00009.

45. Fehlings MG, Tator CH, Linden RD, et al. Motor evoked potentials recorded from normal and spinal cord-injured rats. Neurosurgery 1987;20:125–30. Available at: http://www.ncbi.nlm.nih.gov/pubmed/3808252.

46. Rossini PM, Caramia MD, Zarola F. Mechanisms of nervous propagation along central motor pathways: noninvasive evaluation in healthy subjects and in patients with neurological disease. Neurosurgery 1987;20:183–91. Available at: http://www.ncbi.nlm.nih.gov/pubmed/3808260.

47. Nollet H, Deprez P, Ham L van, et al. Transcranial magnetic stimulation: normal values of magnetic motor evoked potentials in 84 normal horses and influence of height, weight, age and sex. Equine Vet J 2004;36:51–7.

48. Rijckaert J, Pardon B, Ham L Van, et al. Magnetic Motor Evoked Potential Recording in Horses Using Intramuscular Needle Electrodes and Surface Electrodes. J Equine Vet Sci 2018;68:101–7.

49. Kuypers HGJM, Martin GF. Anatomy of descending pathways to the spinal cord. In: Armand J, editor. The Origin, Course and Terminations of Corticospinal Fibers in Various Mammals. Amsterdam: Elsevier; 1982. p. 329–60.

50. Alstermark B, Isa T, Pettersson L-G, et al. The C3-C4 propriospinal system in the cat and monkey: a spinal pre-motoneuronal centre for voluntary motor control. Acta Physiol 2007;189:123–40.

51. Grillner S, Hongo T, Lund S. The vestibulospinal tract. Effects on alpha-motoneurones in the lumbosacral spinal cord in the cat. Exp Brain Res 1970; 10:94–120. Available at: http://link.springer.com/10.1007/BF00340521.

52. Alstermark B, Ogawa J, Isa T. Lack of Monosynaptic Corticomotoneuronal EPSPs in Rats: Disynaptic EPSPs Mediated Via Reticulospinal Neurons and Polysynaptic EPSPs Via Segmental Interneurons. J Neurophysiol 2004;91:1832–9.

53. Nielsen JB, Perez MA, Oudega M, et al. Evaluation of transcranial magnetic stimulation for investigating transmission in descending motor tracts in the rat. Eur J Neurosci 2007;25:805–14.

54. Fujito Y, Aoki M. Monosynaptic rubrospinal projections to distal forelimb motoneurons in the cat. Exp Brain Res 1995;105:181–90. Available at: http://www.ncbi.nlm.nih.gov/pubmed/7498371.

55. Petras JM. Cortical, tectal and tegmental fiber connections in the spinal cord of the cat. Brain Res 1967;6:275–324. Available at: http://www.ncbi.nlm.nih.gov/pubmed/6060511.

56. Konrad PE, Tacker WA. Suprathreshold brain stimulation activates non-corticospinal motor evoked potentials in cats. Brain Res 1990;522:14–29. Available at: http://www.ncbi.nlm.nih.gov/pubmed/2224506.

57. Levy WJ, McCaffrey M, York DH, et al. Motor evoked potentials from transcranial stimulation of the motor cortex in cats. Neurosurgery 1984;15:214–27. Available at: http://www.ncbi.nlm.nih.gov/pubmed/6090971.

58. Kitagawa H, Takano H, Takakuwa K, et al. Origins and conducting pathways of motor evoked potentials elicited by transcranial (vertex-hard palate) stimulation in cats. Neurosurgery 1991;28:358–63. Available at: http://www.ncbi.nlm.nih.gov/pubmed/2011217. Accessed August 9, 2021.

59. Kawai N, Nagao S. Origins and conducting pathways of motor evoked potentials elicited by transcranial magnetic stimulation in cats. Neurosurgery 1992;31: 520–6 [discussion: 526-7]. Available at: http://www.ncbi.nlm.nih.gov/pubmed/1407432.

60. Barone R. Observations sur le faisceau pyramidal des équides. Bull Soc Sci Vet Lyon 1959;61:135–40.

61. Muir GD, Whishaw IQ. Complete locomotor recovery following corticospinal tract lesions: Measurement of ground reaction forces during overground locomotion in rats. Behav Brain Res 1999;103:45–53.

62. Lloyd DPC. The spinal mechanism of the pyramidal system in cats. J Neurophysiol 1941;4:525–46.

63. Eccles JC, Scheid P, Táboríková H. Responses of red nucleus neurons to antidromic and synaptic activation. J Neurophysiol 1975;38:947–64. Available at: http://www.ncbi.nlm.nih.gov/pubmed/1159474.

64. Ito M, Hongo T, Yoshida M, et al. Antidromic and trans-synaptic activation of deiters' neurones induced from the spinal cord. Jpn J Physiol 1964;14:638–58. Available at: http://www.ncbi.nlm.nih.gov/pubmed/14252836.

65. Matsuyama K, Drew T. Vestibulospinal and reticulospinal neuronal activity during locomotion in the intact cat. I. Walking on a level surface. J Neurophysiol 2000;84: 2237–56. Available at: http://www.ncbi.nlm.nih.gov/pubmed/11067969.

66. Cohen LG, Bandinelli S, Topka HR, et al. Topographic maps of human motor cortex in normal and pathological conditions: mirror movements, amputations and spinal cord injuries. Electroencephalogr Clin Neurophysiol Suppl 1991;43: 36–50. Available at: http://www.ncbi.nlm.nih.gov/pubmed/1773774.

67. Nollet H, Ham L Van, Dewulf J, et al. Standardization of transcranial magnetic stimulation in the horse. Vet J 2003;166:244–50.

68. Hess CW, Mills KR, Murray NM. Responses in small hand muscles from magnetic stimulation of the human brain. J Physiol 1987;388:397–419.

69. Nollet H, Ham L Van, Deprez P, et al. Transcranial magnetic stimulation: review of the technique, basic principles and applications. Vet J 2003;166:28–42.

70. Szelényi A, Kothbauer KF, Deletis V. Transcranial electric stimulation for intraoperative motor evoked potential monitoring: Stimulation parameters and electrode montages. Clin Neurophysiol 2007;118:1586–95.

71. Rijckaert J, Pardon B, Saey V, et al. Determination of magnetic motor evoked potential latency time cutoff values for detection of spinal cord dysfunction in horses. J Vet Intern Med 2019;33:2312–8. Available at: https://onlinelibrary.wiley.com/doi/full/10.1111/jvim.15576. Accessed May 4, 2021.

72. Journée SL, Delesalle CJG, Bruijn CM de, et al. Multipulse transcranial electrical stimulation (TES) to diagnose spinal cord injury in horses. Equine Vet J 2018;50: 30. Available at: https://onlinelibrary.wiley.com/doi/10.1111/evj.55_13008. Accessed July 6, 2021.

73. Sylvestre AM, Cockshutt JR, Parent JM, et al. Magnetic Motor Evoked Potentials for Assessing Spinal Cord Integrity in Dogs with Intervertebral Disc Disease. Vet Surg 1993;22:5–10.

74. Burke D, Hicks RG, Stephen JP. Corticospinal volleys evoked by anodal and cathodal stimulation of the human motor cortex. J Physiol 1990;425:283–99.

75. Edgley SA, Eyre JA, Lemon RN, et al. Excitation of the corticospinal tract by electromagnetic and electrical stimulation of the scalp in the macaque monkey. J Physiol 1990;425:301–20.

76. Li DL, Journee HL, van Hulzen A, et al. Computer simulation of corticospinal activity during Transcranial Electrical Stimulation in neurosurgery. Stud Health Technol Inform 2007;125:292–7.

77. Rothwell J, Burke D, Hicks R, et al. Transcranial electrical stimulation of the motor cortex in man: further evidence for the site of activation. J Physiol 1994;481: 243–50.

78. King JL. The pyramid tract and other descending paths in the spinal cord of the sheep. Quart J Expt Phys 1911;4:133–49.

79. Hess CW, Ludin HP. [Transcranial cortex stimulation with magnetic field pulses: methodologic and physiologic principles]. EEG EMG Z Elektroenzephalogr Elektromyogr Verwandte Geb 1988;19:209–15.

80. Journee H, Dijk M, Berends H, et al. 26. High intensity transcranial electrical stimulation: Brainstem fugal motor tracts may augment epidural D-waves of the cortico-spinal system. Clin Neurophysiol 2014;125:e21. Available at: https://www.sciencedirect.com/science/article/abs/pii/S1388245713012650.

81. Nicoll RA, Madison DV. General anesthetics hyperpolarize neurons in the vertebrate central nervous system. Science 1982;217:1055–7.

82. Zentner J, Albrecht T, Heuser D. Influence of halothane, enflurane, and isoflurane on motor evoked potentials. Neurosurgery 1992;31:298–305.

83. Zentner J, Thees C, Pechstein U, et al. Influence of nitrous oxide on motor-evoked potentials. Spine (Phila Pa 1976) 1997;22:1002–6.

84. Sloan TB, Heyer EJ. Anesthesia for intraoperative neurophysiologic monitoring of the spinal cord. J Clin Neurophysiol 2002;19:430–43.

85. Zhou HH, Jin TT, Qin B, et al. Suppression of spinal cord motoneuron excitability correlates with surgical immobility during isoflurane anesthesia. Anesthesiology 1998;88:955–61.

86. Journée HL, Polak HE, Kleuver M De. Conditioning stimulation techniques for enhancement of transcranially elicited evoked motor responses. Neurophysiol Clin 2007;37:423–30.

87. Journée SL, Journée HL, Reed SM, et al. Extramuscular Recording of Spontaneous EMG Activity and Transcranial Electrical Elicited Motor Potentials in Horses: Characteristics of Different Subcutaneous and Surface Electrode Types and Practical Guidelines. Front Neurosci 2020;14:652. Available at: http://www.ncbi.nlm.nih.gov/pubmed/32765207. Accessed May 4, 2021.

88. Urban PP, Vogt T. Conduction times of cortical projections to paravertebral muscles in controls and in patients with multiple sclerosis. Muscle Nerve 1994;17:1348–9. Available at: http://www.ncbi.nlm.nih.gov/pubmed/7935559.

89. Tsao H, Danneels L, Hodges PW. Individual fascicles of the paraspinal muscles are activated by discrete cortical networks in humans. Clin Neurophysiol 2011;122:1580–7. Available at: https://www.sciencedirect.com/science/article/abs/pii/S1388245711000988.

90. Donisch EW, Basmajian JV. Electromyography of deep back muscles in man. Am J Anat 1972;133:25–36. Available at: http://www.ncbi.nlm.nih.gov/pubmed/5008883.

91. Macintosh JE, Bogduk N. The biomechanics of the lumbar multifidus. Clin Biomech (Bristol, Avon) 1986;1:205–13. Available at: http://www.ncbi.nlm.nih.gov/pubmed/23915551.

92. Rijckaert J, Pardon B, Ham L Van, et al. Magnetic motor evoked potentials of cervical muscles in horses. BMC Vet Res 2018;14:290. Available at: https://bmcvetres.biomedcentral.com/articles/10.1186/s12917-018-1620-z.

93. Journée HL, Shils J, Bueno De Camargo A, et al. Failure of Digitimer's D-185 transcranial stimulator to deliver declared stimulus parameters. Clin Neurophysiol 2003;114:2497–8. Available at: http://www.ncbi.nlm.nih.gov/pubmed/14652109.

94. MacDonald DB. Overview on Criteria for MEP Monitoring. J Clin Neurophysiol 2017;34:4–11. Available at: http://www.ncbi.nlm.nih.gov/pubmed/28045852.

95. Nollet H, Ham L Van, Verschooten F, et al. Use of magnetic motor-evoked potentials in horses with bilateral hind limb ataxia. Am J Vet Res 2003;64:1382–6.

96. Journée HL, Berends HI, Kruyt MC. The Percentage of Amplitude Decrease Warning Criteria for Transcranial MEP Monitoring. J Clin Neurophysiol 2017;34: 22–31.
97. Weber M, Eisen AA. Magnetic stimulation of the central and peripheral nervous systems. Muscle Nerve 2002;25:160–75. Available at: http://www.ncbi.nlm.nih. gov/pubmed/11870682.

Equine Neuroaxonal Dystrophy and Degenerative Myeloencephalopathy

Carrie J. Finno, DVM, PhD[a],*, Amy L. Johnson, DVM[b]

KEYWORDS

- A-tocopherol • Ataxia • Genetic • Horse • Inherited • Vitamin E
- Neurodegenerative • Spheroids

KEY POINTS

- Equine neuroaxonal dystrophy/degenerative myeloencephalopathy (eNAD/EDM) is described in horses of many different breeds, with genetic causes suspected in many, which seems to be associated with an early onset vitamin E (α-tocopherol) deficiency and oxidative stress.
- The genetic cause for eNAD/EDM is currently unknown, and a definitive diagnosis requires histologic evaluation of the spinal cord and brainstem at necropsy.
- The typical clinical presentation of eNAD/EDM is a young (<2 year-old) horse with symmetric proprioceptive ataxia, but some horses, particularly Warmbloods, are affected later in life and show behavior changes in addition to progressive ataxia.
- A protein biomarker test, phosphorylated neurofilament heavy, was recently developed that has a high specificity but low sensitivity in the serum for the diagnosis of eNAD/EDM in young non Warmblood breeds with eNAD/EDM.

HISTORY AND NOMENCLATURE

Equine degenerative myeloencephalopathy (EDM) is a progressive, symmetric disease of neuronal degeneration first described by Drs Ian Mayhew, Alexandra deLahunta, and Robert Whitlock in a group of horses of mixed breeding in 1977.[1] In these cases, horses were first observed to be ataxic before the age of 12 months. Neurologic deficits consisted of abnormal limb positioning, pelvic limb ataxia, thoracic limb hypermetria, and decreased strength and spasticity of the limbs and were characterized as upper motor neuron and general proprioceptive tract lesions. There was

[a] Department of Veterinary Population Health and Reproduction, School of Veterinary Medicine, University of California Davis, Room 4206 Vet Med 3A One Shields Avenue, Davis, CA 95616, USA; [b] Department of Clinical Studies, University of Pennsylvania School of Veterinary Medicine- New Bolton Center, 382 West Street Road, Kennett Square, PA 19348, USA
* Corresponding author.
E-mail address: cjfinno@ucdavis.edu

Vet Clin Equine 38 (2022) 213–224
https://doi.org/10.1016/j.cveq.2022.04.003
0749-0739/22/© 2022 Elsevier Inc. All rights reserved.

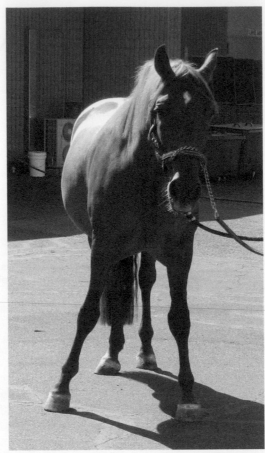

Fig. 1. An abnormal stance at rest is often evident in eNAD/EDM (8-year-old Andalusian gelding with postmortem-confirmed eNAD/EDM).

no evidence of cranial nerve, cerebral, or cerebellar involvement, and affected horses were clinically indistinguishable from those with other focal, multifocal, or diffuse myelopathies affecting the cervical spinal cord. Antemortem diagnostics in each of the horses included a routine hemogram, chemistry panel, urinalysis, cerebrospinal fluid (CSF) analysis, lateral radiographs, and a cervical venogram and myelogram under general anesthesia. Hematologic and biochemical values were within normal limits and, although some cases demonstrated abnormalities in cervical radiographs and/ or myelogram, there was no evidence of compression of the spinal cord at postmortem examination. Histologically, all animals had a diffuse degenerative myeloencephalopathy, with degeneration of the neuronal processes of the white matter of all spinal cord funiculi, especially in the dorsal spinocerebellar tract. Dystrophic axons were found at most spinal cord levels and were most severe in the nucleus of the dorsal spinocerebellar tract, especially in the thoracic segments (T10 to T15). Axonal dystrophy was also noted in the caudal medulla within the nucleus gracilis, medial cuneate nucleus and lateral (accessory) cuneate nucleus (LACN) and was most severe in the latter. In this initial case report, two of the horses were half siblings by the same sire.

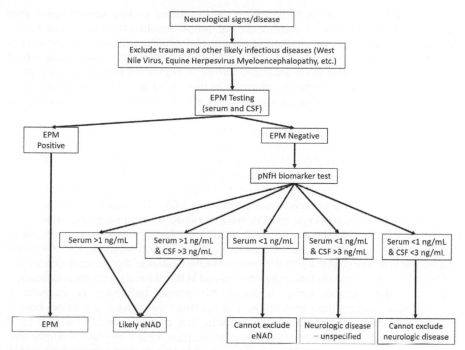

Fig. 2. Recommended flowchart for pNfH testing.

In 1978, Mayhew and colleagues[2] undertook a large-scale prospective case study of ataxic and normal horses using routine historical, clinical, radiographic, clinicopathologic, and pathologic findings in each ataxic horse. Additional diagnostics in these cases included contrast radiography, electromyography, targeted serum and CSF chemistry, long-bone-specific gravity estimations, specialized neuropathologic procedures, and neurochemistry, and these findings were compared with those of normal horses. Of the 96 horses with spinal cord disease examined in an 18-month period, 23 (24%) were classified as EDM cases, which was the second most common diagnosis in this study. Despite extensive testing, there were no antemortem abnormalities consistent with the EDM phenotype.

Five years later, Beech and colleagues[3] described a similar, but less diffuse, disease in a family of Morgan horses. Data were collected from 37 Morgan horses with varying degrees of spinal ataxia. Most of the severely affected cases were noted to be abnormal by 6 months of age. An abnormal stance was noted in the severe cases, and the degree of pelvic limb ataxia was worse than that of the thoracic limbs. Pelvic limb spasticity was reported, and horses were unable to stop smoothly from any gait. Some mildly affected cases were observed over 2 to 5 years and their gait deficits worsened over time, although progression was slow and no horses ever became recumbent. Hemograms were again normal in evaluated cases. Necropsy results again revealed no gross lesions in the 37 abnormal horses. Histologic evaluation revealed neuronal cell body and axonal degeneration in the LACN in all cases and horses were diagnosed with equine neuroaxonal dystrophy (eNAD). Rarely, sparsely scattered degenerating axons were noted in the spinocerebellar tract and, in one horse, in the fasciculus cuneatus and medial cuneate nuclei. Interestingly, these pathologic findings were representative of damage to the proprioceptive tracts of the neck and thoracic limbs but all of these cases demonstrated a more severe pelvic limb ataxia, raising the question of whether clinical deficits resulted from functional abnormalities or subtle, easily overlooked structural abnormalities. Lipofuscin deposits in affected nuclei were noted in some of the Morgan horses with eNAD; however, it was clumped and unable to be assessed further. A significant correlation was made between the amount of lipofuscin pigment in the LACN and the age at necropsy. This was the first case series to suggest that eNAD was an inherited condition in the horse.

In subsequent reports, it was apparent that eNAD was clinically indistinguishable from EDM, and the current consensus is that the conditions have such striking clinical and pathologic similarities that eNAD could be considered a localized form of EDM or EDM a more diffuse form of eNAD. Although histologic lesions in both eNAD and EDM consisted of dystrophic neurons and axons, vacuolization, and spheroid formation,[3] the distribution of the lesions was more diffuse in EDM. The disease was classified as eNAD if the histopathologic lesions were confined to the brainstem, specifically within the LACN, medial cuneate, and gracilis nuclei,[3–5] whereas a diagnosis of EDM was assigned when axonal necrosis and demyelination extended into the dorsal and ventral spinocerebellar tracts and ventromedial funiculi of the cervicothoracic spinal cord.[1,6–11] The cuneate fasciculus is involved in discriminative touch and proprioception of the thoracic limbs, whereas the gracile fasciculus is involved in discriminative touch of the pelvic limbs. The nucleus thoracicus of the spinal cord is the origin of the dorsal spinocerebellar tracts. The dorsal spinocerebellar tract is also involved in proprioception of the pelvic limbs. Thus, based on disease similarities, in all likelihood, eNAD and EDM are the same disease and thus classified as eNAD/EDM.

CLINICAL PRESENTATION

There is no sex predilection to eNAD/EDM, and the disease has been reported in a variety of horse breeds, including Andalusians,[12] Appaloosa horses,[9] Arabians,[2,6,12] a Fell pony,[12] Haflingers,[5] Lusitanos,[13] Mongolian horses,[11] Morgans,[14,15] Norwegian Fjord Horses,[16] Paso Fino horses,[8] Paint horses,[12,16] a Pony of the Americas,[17] Quarter horses (QHs),[4,7,18] a Shire,[19] Standardbreds,[8] Tennessee Walking Horses,[16] Thoroughbreds,[2] Warmbloods,[12,20] a Welsh Pony,[16] and various mixed breeds.[1,10,12] Although the histologic lesions seem similar across breeds, distinct clinical differences can be observed between Warmbloods versus other breeds.

Clinical Signs

In most breeds, eNAD/EDM is characterized by symmetric ataxia, abnormal base-wide stance at rest and proprioceptive deficits in all limbs, signs that can develop from a few weeks to 3 years of age, although most horses develop clinical signs by 6 to 12 months of age (**Fig.1**). The ataxia is often more severe in the pelvic limbs than the thoracic limbs. As the neuroanatomic tracts affected in eNAD/EDM primarily involve sensory tracts,[15] the clinical presentation is consistent with a sensory ataxia. Horses with severe eNAD/EDM may be tetraparetic because the neuroanatomic tracts involved in these cases also include motor tracts in the ventromedial funiculi. In some reports, hyporeflexia of the cervical, cervicofacial, laryngeal adductor (slap), and cutaneous trunci reflexes is described, in addition to obtunded mentation and a decreased or inconsistent bilateral menace response with no apparent loss of vision.[18,21] Affected horses maintain normal symmetric musculature, and recumbency is rare unless the horse suffers from concurrent equine motor neuron disease (EMND).[12,20,22]

Horses affected at a young age with eNAD/EDM commonly exhibit stable lifelong neurologic deficits.

Unpublished data from one of the author's (Sherry A. Johnson, 2022) institution (NBC) suggest that horses histologically diagnosed with eNAD/EDM frequently have a clinical presentation that differs from descriptions of EDM in earlier literature. Clinical signs are frequently recognized in older sport horses, between the ages of 5 and 15 years, after a period of successful competition or training. The other notable feature is that affected horses often are presented for abnormal behavior rather than ataxia. Many horses are reported to display "bad behavior" under saddle, including excessive or unpredictable spookiness, bucking, bolting, rearing, or stopping at fences. Some horses show changes in overall demeanor, from lethargic or dull to anxious. Abnormal interactions with other horses, animals, or people are sometimes recognized, ranging from aggression to loss of interest in social interaction. Riders and caregivers sometimes make observations consistent with abnormal sensory function, from loss of normal sensation to hyperreactivity. Affected horses also display gait and stance abnormalities consistent with mild to moderate proprioceptive ataxia, most commonly graded 1 to 2/5 on the modified Mayhew scale.

With an inconsistent menace reflex and potential visual abnormalities causing spookiness noted in both QH and Warmbloods, full ophthalmic examinations have been performed in a cohort of postmortem-confirmed eNAD/EDM cases across both breeds. Although there was no evidence of lipofuscin deposits and electroretinograms were unremarkable in QHs affected with eNAD/EDM,[21] a pigment retinopathy was observed in young Warmbloods with eNAD/EDM.[20] This contrast may be due to underlying genetic differences in the etiology of eNAD/EDM in QHs versus Warmbloods or the overall disease severity as the Warmbloods were much more deficient in α-tocopherol and had more severe clinical ataxia than the QHs. Regardless, a careful fundic evaluation is warranted in suspect eNAD/EDM cases.

In the past few years, it has been recognized that clinical and postmortem features of concurrent eNAD/EDM and EMND can be identified in young horses.[20,22,23] Clinically, these cases often present primarily as a sensory ataxia (ie, eNAD/EDM) or a lower motor neuron phenotype (ie, EMND), yet they will have lesions consistent with both diseases at postmortem evaluation. Careful histologic assessment at necropsy is recommended to determine if lesions consistent with both disease phenotypes are present.

PREVALENCE

A prospective study at the Cornell University College of Veterinary Medicine found that EDM (n = 23/96) was the second leading cause of equine spinal cord disease among all necropsied spinal cord disease cases between 1974 and 1976.[2] In this population of horses, equine protozoal myeloencephalitis (EPM) (n = 32) was the leading cause of neurologic disease. Eleven years later, a retrospective study of 19 ataxic horses was published by the University of Montreal College of Veterinary Medicine. In this study, cervical vertebral compressive myelopathy (CVCM) was the leading cause of ataxia (n = 11), and EDM was the second most common (n = 4).[24] Recently, a retrospective analysis was performed on postmortem diagnosis of spinal ataxia in 316 horses in California.[23] In this study, CVCM was the most common diagnosis (n = 77), followed by no diagnosis (n = 56) and eNAD/EDM (n = 38). Horses with spinal ataxia with CVCM were more likely to be Thoroughbreds (odds ratio [OR], 2.54), whereas horses with eNAD/EDM were more likely to be QHs (OR, 2.95) and less likely to be Thoroughbreds (OR, 0.11). Based on these three studies with postmortem-confirmed diagnoses of spinal ataxia, it can be concluded eNAD/EDM should remain a top differential for spinal ataxia in horses.

Supporting this assertion, in one of the author's (ALJ's) caseloads, eNAD/EDM was pathologically diagnosed as the cause of neurologic disease in a quarter of patients over a 5-year period (24%, 28/119 horses submitted for necropsy from 2014-2018). Over the past 5 years (2017–2021), the number of horses in the author's referral caseload histologically diagnosed with eNAD/EDM has been increasing steadily, with 6 horses diagnosed in 2017, 12 in 2018, 28 in 2019, and 40 in 2020. Whether this increase represents a true increase in incidence, improving awareness of the disease, or more accurate pathologic diagnosis is uncertain.

INHERITANCE AND GENETICS

Beech and colleagues[14] followed the initial pathologic investigation with a prospective breeding trial in the Morgan horse, demonstrating that eNAD in the Morgan seems to have a significant familial component. Nine out of 15 offspring from affected horses were affected as compared with 0/22 offspring from control Morgan horses. There seemed to be no sex predilection. A recessive mode of inheritance was excluded as breeding two affected horses produced normal offspring and breeding affected horses did not increase the frequency of affected horses. A dominant mode of inheritance with variable expression or a polygenic mode of inheritance was suggested; however, there were no outcrosses to verify this theory.

In addition to this breeding trial, clusters of cases in related horses[1,5,8,14] provided strong evidence for a genetic basis to eNAD/EDM. A study of risk factors associated with the development of EDM found that foals from dams that had had an EDM-affected foal were at a significantly higher risk (25x more likely) of developing EDM than were foals from other dams.[25] Chromosomal analyses in Appaloosa horses with EDM demonstrated normal karyotypes.[9]

In a family of clinically phenotyped QHs with eNAD/EDM, sharing the same underlying risk factor of α-tocopherol deficiency, heritability was estimated at 70%.[26] Complex segregation analysis excluded both an X-linked pattern of inheritance and a fully penetrant (ie, 100% of cases with the genetic mutation display the disease phenotype) autosomal dominant mode of inheritance. Thus, it appears in QHs that eNAD/EDM may be inherited as an incompletely penetrant autosomal dominant trait with vitamin E, specifically α-tocopherol, concentrations during the first year of life modifying the overall phenotype of affected horses.

Comparatively, the clinical and histologic findings in horses with eNAD/EDM resemble ataxia with vitamin E deficiency (AVED) in humans. Human AVED is caused by various mutations in the α-tocopherol transfer protein gene (TTPA),[27,28] which encodes for the protein responsible for vitamin E transport in the liver and incorporation of α-tocopherol into very low density lipoproteins for transport throughout the body. The candidate gene TTPA was excluded in eNAD/EDM in a family of QHs.[26] Subsequent genome-wide association studies have attempted to identify the genetic variant associated with eNAD/EDM in the QH.[29,30] A recent association study identified a genomic region on chromosome 7 and a positional candidate gene was excluded.[30] Additional genes in this region are currently being investigated.

Through the use of RNA sequencing of spinal cord tissue from eNAD/EDM affected horses, including QHs, a Warmblood, and a Shire, downregulation of glutamate receptor and synaptic vesicle tracking pathways was identified.[19] Cholesterol biosynthesis pathways were also downregulated, with the evidence of upregulation of a specific nuclear transcription factor, the liver X receptor. This suggested a potential dysregulation of cholesterol homeostasis within the central nervous system of eNAD/EDM horses, which is likely due to excessive oxidized cholesterol products (ie,.oxysterols). Subsequently, specific oxysterols, including 7-ketocholesterol, 7-hydroxycholesterol, and 7-keto-27-hydroxycholesterol, were found to be increased within the spinal cord of eNAD/EDM affected horses (QHs, Shire, and a Lusitano).[31] Unfortunately, these biomarkers were not altered in serum or CSF with eNAD/EDM, precluding their use as diagnostic tests.

ROLE OF VITAMIN E AND OXIDATIVE STRESS

At the time of the early reports of eNAD/EDM, a similarity between the histologic lesions noted in these cases and those observed in rats with experimental vitamin E deficiency was made. However, the association between vitamin E, specifically α-tocopherol, and EDM was first truly assessed in a group of Mongolian wild horses in 1983.[11] Six Mongolian wild horses were diagnosed with EDM on histologic evaluation, and these horses were found to be deficient in serum α-tocopherol (mean 0.04 ± 0.01 mg/dL; reference range > 0.5 mg/dL). Of note, seven unaffected horses were also deficient in serum α-tocopherol in this study (mean 0.11 ± 0.02 mg/dL).

Although vitamin E deficiency has been reported in some cases of eNAD/EDM,[7–9] low vitamin E levels are not present consistently in all cases. Serum vitamin E concentrations were not significantly different between EDM-affected horses and control horses in many studies.[10,14,25] It seems, however, that vitamin E supplementation of susceptible horses (ie, on the same farm as previously diagnosed horses), lowers the severity and overall incidence of eNAD/EDM. It has been demonstrated that, during the first year of life, vitamin E supplementation of genetically susceptible foals (from a dam/sire that produced affected foals), lowers the overall incidence (40% to 10%) and severity of eNAD/EDM.[9,25] A study by Blythe and colleagues[32] determined by an oral vitamin E absorption test that foals with EDM do not demonstrate significant differences in oral vitamin E absorption as compared with controls.

A recent study followed 14 QH α-tocopherol deficient foals throughout the first year of life.[33] Four of these foals were genetically susceptible to develop eNAD/EDM based on their pedigree. Although all 14 foals were deficient in α-tocopherol by 6 months of age, the foals that were genetically susceptible to develop eNAD/EDM were α-tocopherol deficient in both serum and CSF at earlier time points (ie, 10 days of age and 30 days of age, respectively). These four foals were later confirmed to have eNAD/EDM at necropsy performed at 1.5 years of age. This study clearly demonstrated that both a genetic susceptibility and a temporal α-tocopherol deficiency are required for the phenotype to develop in QHs.

These findings, combined with the knowledge of comparative diseases in humans caused by genetic mutations in genes that encode proteins involved in vitamin E transfer, led to the hypothesis that horses with eNAD/EDM may metabolize vitamin E faster due to an underlying genetic defect. To investigate this further, an assay was developed to quantify isoforms of vitamin E (α-tocopherol, γ-tocopherol, α-tocotrienol, and γ-tocotrienol), along with the respective metabolites (α-CMBHC, α-CEHC, γ-CEHC), in equine serum, plasma, CSF, and urine.[34,35] This assay was then used to perform a proof-of-concept study, followed by a validation study, that demonstrated that QHs with eNAD/EDM had an increased rate of α-tocopherol metabolism.[36] This highlights the need for high-dose supplementation to prevent the clinical phenotype in genetically susceptible horses.

In addition to a deficiency in available vitamin E, an essential antioxidant, it is also plausible that excessive oxidative stress due to environmental (or other) factors could contribute to disease development. A case–control study identified several risk factors associated with the development of EDM, including the use of insecticide (insect repellent) applied to foals, exposure of foals to wood preservatives/sealers (creosote, oil-based stain), and foals spending time on dirt lots while outside.[25] Similar environmental factors or even individual horse factors (medical diseases or treatments) that lead to increased oxidative stress in a susceptible horse could overwhelm protective antioxidant defense mechanisms and influence disease development. This type of oxidative imbalance or cumulative oxidative stress over time could help explain the later onset of clinical disease in some horses. Further evidence for oxidative stress or antioxidant deficiency comes from work demonstrating oxidative injury within the cervical spinal cords of two horses with EDM by using histochemical staining for 3-nitrotyrosine and 4-hydroxynonenal.[37]

DIAGNOSIS

At present, definitive diagnosis of eNAD/EDM is only possible on postmortem histologic evaluation of spinal cord and brainstem tissue. The disease may be underdiagnosed in equine practice because an antemortem diagnostic test is not readily available, and many neurologic cases that are evaluated at postmortem do not undergo comprehensive histologic evaluation of the spinal cord and brainstem to identify lesions consistent with eNAD/EDM. With increased recognition of the lesions consistent with eNAD/EDM, diagnosis of unknown origin of spinal equine ataxia has decreased.[23] In addition, the use of calretinin as an immunohistochemical marker of axonal swellings, or spheroids, associated with eNAD/EDM has assisted with the postmortem diagnosis.[15]

Antemortem diagnosis is largely based on clinical signs and exclusion of other potential disease processes. Most horses with symmetric tetra-ataxia consistent with a cervical, multifocal, or diffuse myelopathy fall into one of three disease categories: spinal cord compression due to cervical vertebral stenotic myelopathy (CVSM), spinal cord inflammation due to infectious disease such as EPM, or neurodegenerative disease (eNAD/EDM). Compressive myelopathies can usually be diagnosed through imaging, including cervical radiography, myelography, and computed tomography. Infectious disease status can usually be ascertained through cytology and immunologic (antibody) testing of CSF and serum. Certain clinical signs heighten the degree of suspicion for these diseases; for example, a horse with neck pain is more likely to have CVSM, and a horse with asymmetrical ataxia or concurrent focal muscle atrophy is more likely to have EPM. As aforementioned, unpredictable or aberrant behavior is more commonly observed in horses with eNAD/EDM than those with CVSM or EPM.

Unfortunately, imaging is not always definitive, with false positive results possible, and antibody testing can be hard to interpret in horses tested after periods of treatment. In addition, horses are not limited to one disease process at a time, and some might have eNAD/EDM plus CVSM or EPM. Therefore, any additional tests that could support a diagnosis of eNAD/EDM would be helpful. On antemortem evaluation of potential cases, no abnormalities are observed on CSF cytology, although spinal fluid α-tocopherol concentrations are often low if the horse has low serum α-tocopherol concentrations. Some horses with eNAD/EDM have CSF total protein levels higher than the reference range, but this is not a consistent clinical feature. Muscle and peripheral nerve biopsies are unremarkable. Recently, a protein biomarker test was evaluated for the antemortem diagnosis of eNAD/EDM. Phosphorylated neurofilament heavy chain (pNfH) protein was assessed in serum and CSF from horses with postmortem-confirmed eNAD/EDM, postmortem-confirmed CVCM, and clinically neurologically healthy control horses.[38] Serum pNfH concentrations greater than 1 ng/mL were significantly associated with eNAD/EDM, with only 12% sensitivity but 99% specificity. In the CSF, increased pNfH concentrations (>3 ng/mL) were observed with either eNAD/EDM or CVCM. Importantly, a value of less than 1 ng/mL (serum) and/or less than 3 ng/mL (CSF) did not exclude a diagnosis of eNAD/EDM. In fact, all Warmbloods with eNAD/EDM had normal serum pNfH concentrations. Assessment of additional protein biomarkers in serum and CSF is currently underway to improve on our ability to provide an accurate antemortem diagnosis of eNAD/EDM. An important point to consider when using the pNfH test is that these results can only be interpreted once infectious and traumatic causes for neurological disease have been excluded (Fig. 2). Additionally, this test should not be used during pre-purchase examinations.

TREATMENT

In families of horses in which eNAD/EDM has been diagnosed, supplementation of pregnant broodmares and foals with α-tocopherol at 10 IU/kg PO once daily during the last trimester (mares) and first 2 years of life (foals) is advisable. If fresh pasture is not available to provide α-tocopherol, the cost of direct supplementation for one genetically susceptible foal over the course of 2 years is approximately $3500.[39] This supplementation should be in the form of RRR-α-tocopherol, which has the greatest bioavailability[40] and can increase α-tocopherol concentrations in the CSF.[33,41,42] It is important to realize, however, that the foal may still be mildly affected with neurologic deficits secondary to eNAD/EDM despite adequate α-tocopherol supplementation. Introduction of new genetic lines into the herd is necessary to completely prevent new eNAD/EDM cases.

Horses suspected of having eNAD/EDM are often treated empirically with α-tocopherol; however, this rarely results in any improvement of neurologic status. At present, there are no effective therapies for eNAD/EDM and, although neurologic deficits seem to stabilize by 2 to 3 years of age in horses affected at a young age, these horses remain neurologically abnormal and unfit for performance activity. Horses with a later onset of clinical signs, particularly those with behavior changes, often show slow worsening of both ataxia and behavior over months to years. In one of the author's (ALJ's) experience, horses with ataxia and behavior changes associated with eNAD/EDM rarely can stay in work or even be retired safely for any length of time, as their erratic and unpredictable behavior frequently poses a substantial safety hazard, even under routine management conditions.

CLINICS CARE POINTS

- NAD/EDM is a common cause of ataxia in horses.
- Vitamin E deficiency and a genetic predisposition play a role in eNAD/EDM.
- Currently, a definitive diagnosis of eNAD/EDM can only be achieved at necropsy.

DISCLOSURE

The authors have nothing to disclose. Support for C.J.F. was provided by the National Institutes of Health (NIH) L40 TR001136.

REFERENCES

1. Mayhew IG, deLahunta A, Whitlock RH, et al. Equine degenerative myeloencephalopathy. J Am Vet Med Assoc 1977;170:195–201.
2. Mayhew IG, deLahunta A, Whitlock RH, et al. Spinal cord disease in the horse. Cornell Veterinarian 1978;68(Suppl 6):1–207.
3. Beech J. Neuroaxonal dystrophy of the accessory cuneate nucleus in horses. Vet Pathol 1984;21:384–93.
4. Adams AP, Collatos C, Fuentealba C, et al. Neuroaxonal dystrophy in a two-year-old quarter horse filly. Can Vet J La Revue Veterinaire canadienne 1996;37:43–4.
5. Baumgartner W, Frese K, Elmadfa I. Neuroaxonal dystrophy associated with vitamin E deficiency in two Haflinger horses. J Comp Pathol 1990;103:114–9.
6. Siso S, Ferrer I, Pumarola M. Abnormal synaptic protein expression in two Arabian horses with equine degenerative myeloencephalopathy. Vet J 2003; 166:238–43.
7. Gandini G, Fatzer R, Mariscoli M, et al. Equine degenerative myeloencephalopathy in five Quarter Horses: clinical and neuropathological findings. Equine Vet J 2004;36:83–5.
8. Mayhew IG, Brown CM, Stowe HD, et al. Equine degenerative myeloencephalopathy: a vitamin E deficiency that may be familial. J Vet Intern Med 1987;1:45–50.
9. Blythe LL, Hultgren BD, Craig AM, et al. Clinical, viral, and genetic evaluation of equine degenerative myeloencephalopathy in a family of Appaloosas. J Am Vet Med Assoc 1991;198:1005–13.
10. Dill SG, Kallfelz FA, deLahunta A, et al. Serum vitamin E and blood glutathione peroxidase values of horses with degenerative myeloencephalopathy. Am J Vet Res 1989;50:166–8.
11. Liu SK, Dolensek EP, Adams CR, et al. Myelopathy and vitamin E deficiency in six Mongolian wild horses. J Am Vet Med Assoc 1983;183:1266–8.
12. Hales EN, Aleman M, Marquardt SA, et al. Retrospective study of postmortem diagnoses of equine spinal ataxia in California (2005-2017). J Am Vet Med Assoc 2020;258(12):1386–93. In press.
13. Finno CJ, Higgins RJ, Aleman M, et al. Equine degenerative myeloencephalopathy in Lusitano horses. J Vet Intern Med 2011;25:1439–46.
14. Beech J, Haskins M. Genetic studies of neuraxonal dystrophy in the Morgan. Am J Vet Res 1987;48:109–13.
15. Finno CJ, Valberg SJ, Shivers J, et al. Evidence of the Primary Afferent Tracts Undergoing Neurodegeneration in Horses With Equine Degenerative Myeloencephalopathy Based on Calretinin Immunohistochemical Localization. Vet Pathol 2016;53:77–86.
16. Blythe LL, Craig AM. Equine degenerative myelencephalopathy: part I. Clinical signs and pathogenesis. Comp Cont Educ Pract Vet 1992;14:1215–21.
17. Brosnahan MM, Holbrook TC, Ritchey JW. Neuroaxonal dystrophy associated with cerebellar dysfunction in a 5-month-old Pony of the Americas colt. J Vet Intern Med 2009;23:1303–6.
18. Aleman M, Finno CJ, Higgins RJ, et al. Evaluation of epidemiological, clinical, and pathological features of neuroaxonal dystrophy in Quarter Horses. J Am Vet Med Assoc 2011;239:823–33.
19. Finno CJ, Bordbari MH, Valberg SJ, et al. Transcriptome profiling of equine vitamin E deficient neuroaxonal dystrophy identifies upregulation of liver X receptor target genes. Free Radic Biol Med 2016;101:261–71.

20. Finno CJ, Kaese HJ, Miller AD, et al. Pigment retinopathy in warmblood horses with equine degenerative myeloencephalopathy and equine motor neuron disease. Vet Ophthalmol 2017;20:304–9.

21. Finno CJ, Aleman M, Ofri R, et al. Electrophysiological studies in American Quarter horses with neuroaxonal dystrophy. Vet Ophthalmol 2012;15(Suppl 2):3–7.

22. Finno CJ, Miller AD, Siso S, et al. Concurrent Equine Degenerative Myeloencephalopathy and Equine Motor Neuron Disease in Three Young Horses. J Vet Intern Med 2016;30:1344–50.

23. Hales EN, Aleman M, Marquardt SA, et al. Postmortem diagnoses of spinal ataxia in 316 horses in California. J Am Vet Med Assoc 2021;258:1386–93.

24. Nappert G, Vrins A, Breton L, et al. A retrospective study of nineteen ataxic horses. Can Vet J La Revue Veterinaire Canadienne 1989;30:802–6.

25. Dill SG, Correa MT, Erb HN, et al. Factors associated with the development of equine degenerative myeloencephalopathy. Am J Vet Res 1990;51:1300–5.

26. Finno CJ, Famula T, Aleman M, et al. Pedigree analysis and exclusion of alpha-tocopherol transfer protein (TTPA) as a candidate gene for neuroaxonal dystrophy in the American Quarter Horse. J Vet Intern Med 2013;27:177–85.

27. Gotoda T, Arita M, Arai H, et al. Adult-onset spinocerebellar dysfunction caused by a mutation in the gene for the alpha-tocopherol-transfer protein. N Engl J Med 1995;333:1313–8.

28. Yokota T, Shiojiri T, Gotoda T, et al. Retinitis pigmentosa and ataxia caused by a mutation in the gene for the alpha-tocopherol-transfer protein. N Engl J Med 1996;335:1770–1.

29. Finno CJ, Aleman M, Higgins RJ, et al. Risk of false positive genetic associations in complex traits with underlying population structure: a case study. Vet J 2014; 202:543–9.

30. Hales EN, Esparza C, Peng SH, et al. Genome-Wide Association Study and Subsequent Exclusion of ATCAY as a Candidate Gene Involved in Equine Neuroaxonal Dystrophy Using Two Animal Models. Genes (Basel) 2020;11:82.

31. Finno CJ, Estell KE, Winfield L, et al. Lipid peroxidation biomarkers for evaluating oxidative stress in equine neuroaxonal dystrophy. J Vet Intern Med 2018;32: 1740–7.

32. Blythe LL, Craig AM, Lassen ED, et al. Serially determined plasma alpha-tocopherol concentrations and results of the oral vitamin E absorption test in clinically normal horses and in horses with degenerative myeloencephalopathy. Am J Vet Res 1991;52:908–11.

33. Finno CJ, Estell KE, Katzman S, et al. Blood and Cerebrospinal Fluid alpha-Tocopherol and Selenium Concentrations in Neonatal Foals with Neuroaxonal Dystrophy. J Vet Intern Med 2015;29:1667–75.

34. Habib H, Finno CJ, Gennity I, et al. Simultaneous quantification of vitamin E and vitamin E metabolites in equine plasma and serum using LC-MS/MS. J Vet Diagn Invest 2021;33:506–15.

35. Favro G, Habib H, Gennity I, et al. Determination of vitamin E and its metabolites in equine urine using liquid chromatography-mass spectrometry. Drug Test Anal 2021;13:1158–68.

36. Hales EN, Habib H, Favro G, et al. Increased alpha-tocopherol metabolism in horses with equine neuroaxonal dystrophy. J Vet Intern Med 2021;35(5):2473–85.

37. Wong DM, Ghosh A, Fales-Williams AJ, et al. Evidence of oxidative injury of the spinal cord in 2 horses with equine degenerative myeloencephalopathy. Vet Pathol 2012;49:1049–53.

38. Edwards LA, Donnelly CG, Reed SM, et al. Serum and cerebrospinal fluid phosphorylated neurofilament heavy protein concentrations in equine neurodegenerative diseases. Equine Vet J 2021;54(2):290–8.
39. Burns EN, Finno CJ. Equine degenerative myeloencephalopathy: prevalence, impact, and management. Vet Med (Auckl) 2018;9:63–7.
40. Finno CJ, Valberg SJ. A comparative review of vitamin E and associated equine disorders. J Vet Intern Med 2012;26:1251–66.
41. Brown JC, Valberg SJ, Hogg M, et al. Effects of feeding two RRR-alpha-tocopherol formulations on serum, cerebrospinal fluid and muscle alpha-tocopherol concentrations in horses with subclinical vitamin E deficiency. Equine Vet J 2017;49:753–8.
42. Pusterla N, Puschner B, Steidl S, et al. alpha-Tocopherol concentrations in equine serum and cerebrospinal fluid after vitamin E supplementation. Vet Rec 2010; 166:366–8.

Cervical Vertebral Stenotic Myelopathy

Brett Woodie, DVM, MS[a],*, Amy L. Johnson, DVM[b], Barrie Grant, DVM, MS, MRCVS[c]

KEYWORDS

- Cervical vertebral stenotic myelopathy • Minimum sagittal diameter • Myelography
- Cervical vertebral body • Thoracic vertebral body

INTRODUCTION

Cervical vertebral stenotic myelopathy (CVSM) is a common cause of ataxia in horses secondary to spinal cord compression. Early articles describing this problem indicate genetic predisposition as a known risk factor.[1] Further studies have shown the problem is a developmental abnormality, which might have genetic predisposition and environmental influences. CVSM is characterized by ataxia and weakness, caused by narrowing of the cervical vertebral canal and compression of the spinal cord often in combination with malalignment and malformation of the cervical vertebrae. Stenosis of the vertebral canal, anywhere from the first cervical vertebral body (C1) to the first thoracic vertebral body (T1), is the most important abnormality in CVSM.

Neurologic gait deficits in horses have been recognized since at least 1860,[2] and the term "Wobblers syndrome" was introduced in 1938 to describe several clinically observed abnormalities.[3] CVSM is the main cause of "Wobblers syndrome," and older synonyms for CVSM include equine sensory ataxia, equine incoordination, and spinal ataxia.[4] As malformation, malarticulation, or malalignment of one or more cervical vertebrae generally lead to CVSM, the disease has also been referred to as cervical vertebral malformation (CVM) or cervical vertebral instability. Cervical vertebral compressive myelopathy (CVCM) or CVSM seems to be the most commonly used and appropriate terms when referring to this condition.

Types of Cervical Vertebral Stenotic Myelopathy

Rooney distinguished three types of CVSM.[5] In type I, the vertebral column is fixed in flexed position at the site of malarticulation/malformation, which generally occurs at C2–C3, but has been observed at other sites. Type I CVSM is less common and often presents at birth. In type II CVSM, symmetric overgrowth of the articular processes

[a] Surgery, Rood and Riddle Equine Hospital, 2150 Georgetown Road, Lexington, KY 40511, USA; [b] Department of Clinical Studies, University of Pennsylvania School of Veterinary Medicine- New Bolton Center, 382 West Street Road, Kennett Square, PA 19348, USA; [c] 31624 Wrightwood Road, Bonsall, California, 92003-4708, USA
* Corresponding author.
E-mail address: bwoodie@roodandriddle.com

Vet Clin Equine 38 (2022) 225–248
https://doi.org/10.1016/j.cveq.2022.05.002
0749-0739/22/© 2022 Elsevier Inc. All rights reserved.

vetequine.theclinics.com

causes spinal cord compression during flexion of the neck. Type II lesions occur most often in foals and weanlings and are generally found in the mid-cervical region. Type III CVSM is characterized by asymmetrical overgrowth of one articular process that leads to compression of the spinal cord either directly by bony proliferation or indirectly by associated soft tissue hypertrophy. Type III is most often seen in mature horses but can begin as early as 1 to 3 years of age. This lesion most often affects C5– C6 and C6–C 7.[6]

CVSM has been divided into two broad categories or classes of horses: one is affecting young horses (Type I, which correlates with Rooney's Type II) and one is affecting older horses (Type II, which correlates with Rooney's Type III).[7,8] In both types of CVSM, morphologic changes of the cervical vertebrae cause stenosis of the vertebral canal and spinal cord compression. Type I CVSM, the condition of young horses, is observed most often in Thoroughbreds and is a multifactorial disease including such factors as gender, inheritance, diet, trauma, and rate of growth.[9,10] These factors cause developmental abnormalities of the cervical vertebral column including malformation of the vertebral canal, enlargement of the physes, extension of the dorsal aspect of the vertebral arch, angulation sometimes with fixation between adjacent vertebrae, and malformation of the articular processes as a result of osteochondrosis.[11] Type II CVSM, the condition of older horses, affects all breeds and involves osteoarthritic changes of the articular processes. These changes often include malformation with degenerative joint disease of the articular processes, wedging of the vertebral canal, periarticular proliferation with or without a synovial or epidural cyst and overt fractures of the articular processes.[11,12] It is important to note that many older horses will have bony abnormalities of the cervical vertebral column, however, only a small percentage of horses develop clinical signs as a result of spinal cord compression.[13]

Epidemiology

CVSM is the leading cause of noninfectious spinal ataxia in the horse[9,14–17] and is estimated to affect 1.3% to 2% of Thoroughbred horses[5] but has also been identified in many other breeds including Arabians, Morgans, and Appaloosas.[9,16,18,19] Breeds described as predisposed to CVCM include Thoroughbred, Quarter Horse, Warmblood, and Tennessee Walking Horse.[11,12,16] A large case-control study showed that Thoroughbreds, Tennessee Walking Horses, and Warmbloods were overrepresented compared with Quarter Horses, whereas Arabians and Standardbred were underrepresented.[20]

Male horses are more likely to be affected than female horses with a ratio of 3:1.[6,8,9,12,14–16,20,21] Age is significantly associated with a diagnosis of CVSM; horses less than 7 years of age are more likely to be diagnosed with CVCM than horses 10 years or older.[20] Horses with type 1 CVSM are generally younger at time of diagnosis than horses with type 2 CVSM.[8] Although the horse is often 1 to 2 years of age at presentation, the onset of the condition was likely much earlier. The onset of clinical signs depends on the degree of compression or repeated trauma to the spinal cord.

Clinical Examination

History

Young horses often have a history of a recent period of rapid growth or weight gain, and foals might have high milk-producing dams or be larger than similarly aged unaffected foals. Although a common historical finding is an acute onset of ataxia or gait abnormalities following trauma, that is, a fall or halter-breaking accident, in many cases the horse will have been mildly ataxic before the observed trauma. In fact, the mild neurologic deficits might have caused the traumatic incident that resulted in exacerbation of the neurologic signs. In other cases, the onset is more insidious and weeks or months pass before neurologic deficits are recognized. Often clinical signs are noted when yearlings are being worked in preparation for commercial sale. Older horses (with type II CVSM) more commonly have a more chronic history of performance problems, inability to progress in training, possible lameness, reluctance to bend, neck stiffness, tripping, or even behavior issues.

Physical examination

Physical examination might reveal abrasions around the heels or medial aspect of the thoracic limbs due to interference, and short, squared hooves due to excessive toe-dragging. Although the physical examination is often unremarkable, many young horses affected with CVSM have signs of developmental orthopedic diseases such as physitis or physeal enlargement of the long bones, joint effusion secondary to osteochondrosis, and flexural limb deformities. Stewart and colleagues showed the increased incidence of osteochondrosis in horses with CVSM.[22,23] Evidence of damage to nerve roots or spinal nerves such as cervical pain, atrophy of cervical musculature, and cutaneous hypalgesia adjacent to affected cervical vertebrae is rare in young horses. These signs are more common in older horses with arthropathies of the caudal cervical vertebrae; these horses might demonstrate focal muscle wasting, focal sweating, or palpable bony abnormalities of the vertebral articular processes. Reluctance to raise or lower the head or bend the neck laterally is more commonly observed in older horses.

Neurologic examination

Complete neurologic examination is described elsewhere but in general horses with CVSM should have a normal attitude/mental status, normal cranial nerve function, and normal spinal reflexes.

Gait examination will reveal upper motor neuron paresis and general proprioceptive ataxia compatible with compression and damage of the cervical spinal cord white matter. Ataxia and spasticity followed by weakness are usually observed in the pelvic limbs first and then progress to the thoracic limbs.[16,24] Signs tend to remain more severe in the pelvic than thoracic limbs and are often relatively symmetric, although many horses with CVSM show some asymmetry. Asymmetric signs are more common in horses with significant degenerative joint disease of the articular processes and lateral compression of the spinal cord.[17] In a standing horse, general proprioceptive deficits might be present such as an abnormally wide-based stance, abnormal limb placement, and delayed limb positioning. Ataxia and paresis are more easily observed at a walk than at faster gaits, and horses often demonstrate truncal sway, irregular and unpredictable stride length and foot placement with a tendency to have a longer stride, an overreaching or "floating" thoracic limb gait, circumduction of the outside limb, pivoting on the inside limb, toe-dragging, delayed protraction, and stumbling. The horse may exhibit an exaggerated, stiff-legged, or spastic movement. These signs will be exacerbated when the horse is circled, led up and down a hill or over obstacles, and when the horse's head is elevated during the neurologic examination. In young horses, clinical signs of ataxia often progress and then stabilize. This cycle of progression followed by stabilization can occur several times before final confirmation of the diagnosis.

Neuropathophysiology

The characteristic signs of CVSM are the result of lesions in the white matter of the cervical spinal cord, specifically damage to the ascending general proprioception pathways (causing ataxia) and the descending upper motor neuron pathways (causing paresis).[4] Progression of disease is due to prolonged compression or repeated trauma to the spinal cord, with initial damage to superficial white matter followed by gradual spread to deeper areas. The lateral funiculi are especially susceptible to degeneration by pressure or compression.

A cervical spinal cord compressive lesion produces more severe pelvic limb than thoracic limb ataxia in part because of the more superficial anatomic location of the proprioceptive tracts from the pelvic limbs, the dorsal and ventral spinocerebellar tracts, compared with those of the thoracic limbs, and the cuneocerebellar and cranial (rostral) spinocerebellar tracts.[4,25] Disparity in signs between the pelvic and thoracic limbs might also be explained by the greater distance of the pelvic limbs from the center of gravity of the horse and the greater percentage of upper motor neuron synapses in the gray matter of the cervical intumescence.[4] Obvious signs of disturbance of the ascending general somatic afferent pathway, characterized by decreased nociception, occur rarely.

Differential Diagnoses for Spinal Ataxia

Important differential diagnoses for spinal ataxia in a young horse include CVSM, equine protozoal myeloencephalitis (EPM), trauma, equine degenerative myeloencephalopathy (EDM), and equine herpesvirus 1 myeloencephalopathy. Less common causes of spinal ataxia and weakness include rabies, viral encephalitides (Eastern, Western, Venezuelan, and West Nile), brain abscesses, neoplasia, and hepatoencephalopathy. Congenital anomalies and malformations of the vertebral column which could cause compression of the cervical spinal cord are reported infrequently, including occipitoatlantoaxial malformation, butterfly vertebrae, hemivertebrae, block vertebrae, atlantoaxial subluxation, and atlantoaxial instability.[19] Spinal cord compression can also result from traumatic injury,[26] vertebral fracture,[27–29] vertebral neoplasia,[30] discospondylitis,[31,32] diskospondylosis,[33] intervertebral disk protrusion,[31,34] arachnoid diverticulum,[35] unusual parasite migration,[36] and spinal hematomas.[37]

Diagnostic Techniques

The diagnosis of CVSM is generally based on a detailed history, the signalment, recognition of spinal ataxia on neurologic examination, imaging findings consistent with vertebral canal stenosis, and elimination of other possible causes of spinal ataxia. The "gold standard" for confirmation of the diagnosis remains a postmortem examination.[6,9]

Plain radiography

Lateral radiographs of the cervical vertebrae, obtained in the standing horse, can be subjected to subjective, semiquantitative, and objective analyses. Most horses with CVSM have bony malformations of the cervical vertebrae, although exceptions exist. The five characteristic bony malformations of the cervical vertebrae in horses with CVSM are "flare" of the caudal vertebral epiphysis of the vertebral body, abnormal ossification of the articular processes, malalignment between adjacent vertebrae, extension of the dorsal laminae, and degenerative joint disease of the articular processes.[9,14–16,19]

Degenerative joint disease characterized by osteochondrosis and/or osteoarthrosis of the articular processes is a common lesion identified on cervical vertebral radiographs in horses affected with both type I and type II CVSM and is a defining feature of type II CVSM.[9,12] Despite this, not all horses that have osteochondrosis or osteoarthrosis lesions involving the articular process joints have spinal cord compression.

Several caveats exist to subjective interpretation of equine cervical radiographs. Most importantly, subjective assessment of cervical radiographs does not adequately discriminate between horses with and without CVSM.[15] Compressive lesions can develop at vertebral sites that are not affected by bony malformation, and sites with malformation do not always cause compression.[16,22] Evaluation of degenerative joint disease is particularly challenging, both in terms of radiographic technique and interpretation. Articular process disease is most common in the caudal cervical region, where overlying muscle is thickest and dorsoventral views difficult to obtain. There is limited visualization of the articular process joints in laterolateral radiographs, and oblique views are difficult to interpret unless ideal technique is used.[38] Even when degenerative joint disease is radiographically obvious, the significance of such change is often unclear. Age of the horse appears to contribute to the presence of degenerative joint disease, but disease has not been shown to correlate with clinical signs of neurologic disease.[39]

Many investigators have attempted to improve radiographic interpretation by obtaining more objective values. Minimum sagittal diameter (MSD) values were published for horses under anesthesia;[16] however, magnification made these values impossible to interpret and unreliable in cervical vertebral radiographs obtained in standing horses. Subsequently, a noninvasive, semiquantitative, radiographic CVSM scoring system was developed for foals in which multiple radiographic characteristics were considered, one of which was stenosis of the vertebral canal. The presence of stenosis was assessed by the corrected MSD (ratio of MSD: vertebral body length) in which the MSD was measured either intravertebral or intervertebral.[11] Using this scoring system, foals with signs of CVSM were successfully distinguished from normal foals.[11]

An intravertebral ratio method of canal diameter assessment was developed for use in adult horses based on a similar method that improved accuracy of diagnosis of cervical spinal stenosis in people.[12] This method is still frequently used and requires direct lateral radiographs. The sagittal ratio is the ratio of the MSD:sagittal height of the maximum dimension of the cranial aspect of the vertebral body (**Figs. 1** and **2**). Assessment of this ratio is therefore independent of radiographic magnification. A ratio of less than 50% at C4–C6 or a ratio of less than 52% at C7 is associated with a high likelihood (likelihood ratio: 26.1–41.5) of having cervical stenotic myelopathy. The sensitivity and specificity of this ratio method is >89% at each vertebral site using suggested cutoffs of <52% for C4–C6 and <56% for C7.[12] Although this method is

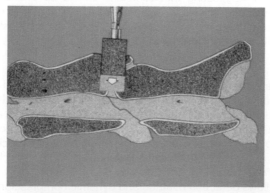

Fig. 1. Diagram of the original Cloward technique.

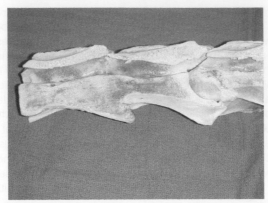

Fig. 2. Sagittal section of the cervical spine of a fusion done 20 years previously.

relatively accurate in detecting CVSM, it does not accurately identify the site(s) of compression for any individual horse.[7]

More recently, inclusion of intervertebral MSD measurements for assessing canal height has been proposed as a way to increase the accuracy of using standing survey radiographs to diagnose CVSM in horses and assist in identifying sites of compression.[33,40,41] When intravertebral and intervertebral MSD ratios were applied to a small group of horses, including 8 horses with necropsy-confirmed CVSM and 18 horses without CVSM, all horses with CVSM had at least one MSD ratio ≤ 0.485, and the smallest intervertebral ratio always indicated a site of compression.[41] One reason that intervertebral MSD ratios were more accurate at determining site of compression could be that most (11/14) sites of compression were intervertebral rather than intravertebral. However, when this method was used to compare ratios of compressed sites with non-compressed sites in both CVSM and non-CVSM cases, there was a significant overlap between values.[7]

Overall, MSD ratios are relatively accurate at predicting a diagnosis of CVSM, with intervertebral MSD ratios slightly superior to intravertebral MSD ratios, but neither should be used to predict the site of compression in a CVSM case due to unacceptable sensitivity and specificity.[7,12,24] Furthermore, an observer agreement study using two examiners revealed that cervical vertebral ratios varied by 5% to 10% within and between examiners, suggesting that clinicians should be cautious when applying these ratios in practice to avoid misdiagnosis.[42] Therefore, myelography and contrast-enhanced computed tomography (CECT) are the diagnostic tools of choice for antemortem diagnosis of CVSM and identifying the specific sites of compression.

Myelography

Myelography is required to confirm a diagnosis of focal spinal cord compression and to identify the location and number of lesions, particularly if surgical treatment is to be considered or pursued.[6,12,14,43,44] The technique for performing a myelogram has been described using a nonionic, water-soluble contrast agent (iopamidol, iohexol) administered through the atlanto-occipital space into the subarachnoid space after withdrawal of an equal volume of cerebrospinal fluid (CSF).[43,45–48] Radiographs are taken in neutral, flexed, and extended positions of the neck.

Myelography allows detection of static and dynamic compression. Static compression is defined by narrowing of the vertebral canal with subsequent compression of the spinal cord regardless of neck position, whereas dynamic compression is only evident in certain neck positions. By definition static stenosis is noticeable in neutral views, but extension of the neck may exacerbate this compression suggesting a degree of coexisting dynamic compression. The most common sites for static stenosis are at C5–C6 and C6–C7[6,9,49] (**Fig. 3**). Dynamic compression is most commonly seen in flexed views at more cranial sites, including C3–C4 and C4–C5 (**Fig. 4**). However, narrowing of the vertebral canal can occur at any site within the cervical vertebral column, and stenosis at more than one site is not uncommon.[9,12,14,16]

Several criteria for evaluating equine myelograms have been proposed but continue to be the source of debate. These criteria include a reduction of thickness of the contrast columns to less than 2 mm[47] and attenuation of both the dorsal and ventral contrast columns by greater than 50% at diametrically opposed sites.[15] Currently, complete attenuation of the ventral contrast column with 50% attenuation of the dorsal contrast column compared with the maximal height of the dorsal contrast column within the cranial vertebral body is most commonly used as myelographic evidence of compression.[50] The accuracy of this criterion has been questioned, and use of the minimal sagittal dural diameter (MSDD), which is the sagittal diameter of the dural space measured intervertebrally, has been advocated to more precisely define the sites of spinal cord compression.[24,40,51] MSDD greater than 20% smaller than the largest dural diameter measured within the cranial vertebra has been suggested as a potentially more accurate criterion.[52] However, when these various myelographic criteria for compression are critically evaluated, it becomes clear that none yields high sensitivity and specificity at all cervical articulations.[7,52,53]

It is important to recognize that standard myelographic views, performed in lateral recumbency, are best at identifying dorsoventral compression and not ideal for identifying lateral or dorsolateral compression.

As can be seen, although myelography is currently considered one of the most accurate antemortem tests, it has several limitations. As described, no consensus for diagnosis of compression exists. Most myelographic studies only include laterolateral images of the vertebral column despite the fact that horses often have dorsolateral spinal cord compression, which would be best viewed with ventrodorsal or oblique radiographic images.[52,54,55]

Computed tomography
CECT is considered to be more useful than myelography to diagnose and characterize vertebral stenosis in humans and has been evaluated in the horse.[17] In a postmortem

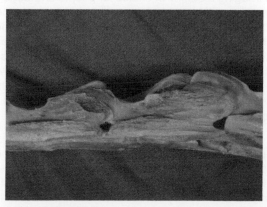

Fig. 3. Dorsal aspect of horse in **Fig. 2**.

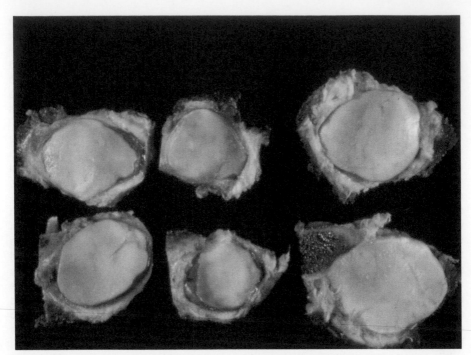

Fig. 4. Articular facets 8 months after fusion with Bagby basket. **Fig. 3** and 4 show the atrophy of the articular facets at the fusion level.

study involving six horses with CVSM, CECT images could be obtained from C1–T1. CVSM lesions were accurately detected, and significant additional information was obtained regarding location and severity of the lesions.[17] The main indications for CECT are presurgical evaluation of the cervical vertebral column and spinal cord at sites that are suspected to have dynamic compressive lesions and evaluation of lateral compressive lesions in horses strongly suspected to have CVSM without myelographic evidence. Depending on the patient aperture and table size, evaluation of C1–C7 is possible with CECT.

Magnetic resonance

MR imaging is the imaging modality of choice for people and dogs with compressive myelopathy and has been evaluated for horses.[56] A postmortem study was performed on 39 ataxic and 20 neurologically normal horses using a 1.5 T magnet after removal of the head and neck from the body at T1 or T2. Although subjective evaluation of MR images allowed differentiation of horses with cervical vertebral disease from horses with other causes of ataxia and normal horses, MR imaging did not allow accurate identification of the site of compression, as an MR diagnosis of spinal cord compression had only poor to slight agreement with histology. This finding is somewhat surprising when compared with results in people and dogs.

Endoscopy

A technique for epiduroscopy and myeloscopy has been developed using an open approach to the epidural and subarachnoid spaces.[57] Cervical vertebral canal endoscopy potentially allows identification of compressive lesions as well as spinal cord lesions that could only be identified by direct visualization. Successful completion of the procedure has been described in six healthy horses and one neurologic horse.[58,59]

Complications included an increase in mean arterial pressure during epiduroscopy, minor hemorrhage at the insertion site and introduction of air into the subarachnoid space during myeloscopy, transient ataxia in one horse after recovery, and transient subclinical meningitis.[58] Although the sensitivity and specificity of this technique are unknown, myeloscopy correctly identified the site of compression, which was misdiagnosed by myelography, in the single clinical case evaluated.[59]

A technique for arthroscopic evaluation of cervical articular process joints has been described.[60] Good visualization of the cartilage surfaces was achieved and complications were minimal, although only three clinical cases were reported.

To summarize the current state of diagnostic testing, no single modality is sufficient for accurate diagnosis.[61] The most accurate diagnosis for any individual horse is achieved through careful consideration of all available information, including history, signalment, neurologic examination findings, imaging studies, and other ancillary tests to eliminate other possible differential diagnoses. Of all the widely available imaging modalities, MSD ratios best predict a diagnosis of CVSM, but do not reliably identify sites of compression. Myelography is necessary for surgical planning but does not have well established criteria for compression; experience of the observer likely contributes to diagnostic accuracy. As for many neurologic diseases, histopathology remains the gold standard diagnostic test.

Treatment

Medical treatment

The choice of medical treatment of CVSM depends in part on type of lesion, severity and chronicity of clinical signs, and age of the horse. In the immediate period following an acute onset of ataxia and paresis, medical therapy is aimed at reducing cell swelling and edema formation, thereby reducing compression on the spinal cord. Anti-inflammatory drugs, such as corticosteroids, nonsteroidal anti-inflammatory drugs, and dimethyl sulfoxide, are the most commonly used treatments.

For horses less than 1 year of age, changes in management may influence the development of CVSM. These changes include restricted exercise and diet, along with alterations in the concentrations of trace nutrients such as copper and zinc in the diet. The "paced growth" program, for which efficacy has been suggested in young horses with early clinical or radiographic signs of CVSM,[62] includes stall rest and a diet that restricts protein and carbohydrate intake. Proponents of this diet suggest that bone growth should be retarded, bone metabolism should be enhanced, and the vertebral canal diameter should enlarge and relieve spinal cord compression. However, controlled studies demonstrating efficacy are lacking and it is unclear whether the strict diet provides any additional benefit to time alone. It is important that the selected diet meet minimum requirements of essential nutrients, and during the period of growth retardation, the patient should be under careful nutritional supervision.[63] In young horses, supplementation with vitamin E/selenium is recommended as EDM is an important differential diagnosis which might improve following vitamin E administration.[64] General recommendations for a paced diet include restricting protein and carbohydrates to 65% to 75% National Research Council (NRC) recommendations, maintaining balanced vitamin and mineral intake (minimum 100% NRC requirements), supplementing vitamins A and E at three times NRC recommendations, and supplementing selenium to 0.3 ppm.

In adult horses with compressive lesions of the spinal cord, the options for medical therapy are restricted to stabilizing a horse with acute neurologic deterioration and injecting the articular joints with corticosteroids, chemical mucopolysaccharides such as hyaluronate sodium, or both in an attempt to reduce soft tissue swelling and stabilize or prevent bony proliferation.[65,66] Injecting articular joints is most beneficial in horses that demonstrate zero or only minimal neurologic deficits (grade 0–2) and that have moderate to significant degenerative joint changes evident on radiographs of the cervical vertebral column. Horses that fit into this last category are generally older horses (>5 years) that are in training and have developed osteoarthritic changes, usually in the caudal cervical vertebral joints.

Surgical treatment

General considerations. The aim of surgical treatment is to stop repetitive trauma to the spinal cord, which is caused by narrowing of the vertebral canal, and thereby to allow the inflammation in and around the spinal cord to resolve. Restoration or maintenance of adequate blood supply to the spinal cord is vital to reduction of edema and removal of inflammatory mediators from the affected site. Surgical management of horses that have been diagnosed with spinal cord compression involves the use of a ventral stabilization procedure. The surgical technique was initially described in 1979[67] and in the hands of some surgeons is now considered a routine procedure. However, several factors must be considered carefully and discussed with the patient's owners and caregivers before recommending surgical treatment for any individual horse. These include whether or not the horse is a good surgical candidate, expectations for improvement and return to use, cost of surgical treatment and rehabilitation, insurance issues, and safety and liability concerns.

The best surgical candidates are young horses with only one or two myelographic lesions, a short duration of mild-to-moderate clinical signs, and no evidence of concurrent disease such as EPM. However, surgical success has been reported in less than ideal candidates, including horses undergoing trilevel interbody fusion.[68,69] Horses that might have EPM based on antibody titers in CSF should undergo antiprotozoal therapy before considering cervical surgery.

It is important for the owner and trainer to have realistic expectations and to be aware that the final determination of the results might not be known until the end of the recovery period, which usually takes 6 months–1 year. Following interbody fusion surgery, an improvement of 1 to 2 out of 5 grades is expected. There is a low probability that a horse will improve more than 3 out of 5 grades, so severely affected horses (grade 4 or 5) are highly unlikely to return to normal neurologic function. Although normal neurologic function is not always required for breeding stock, the potential heritability of vertebral canal stenosis must be considered.

Discussion of cost with the owner must include estimates of initial diagnostic testing, transportation costs for the horse to ship to a surgical facility or an experienced surgeon to travel to a local facility, surgical expenses, postoperative care and rehabilitation, and general maintenance costs of the horse for the duration of the recovery period. A structured rehabilitation program is essential to success, and the owner must commit to spending time with the horse daily or paying for this service.

Horses with CVSM and insurance policies present an additional set of issues for the owner and the veterinarian. In the authors' opinion, there are several important insurance aspects for consideration. The most common questions encountered are whether the horse is a candidate for medical or surgical treatment and when the horse becomes a candidate for humane destruction. The response to the first question is impacted by several factors including the severity of clinical signs, the number of sites affected, the owners' commitment to the horse, and the economic value of the horse combined with the cost for performing surgery. Whether a horse is a candidate for humane destruction is governed by guidelines established by the American Association of Equine Practitioners (AAEP) Insurance committee on behalf of the AAEP. Important criteria for euthanasia include inhumane suffering, chronic and incurable pain neces-sitating pain-relieving medication, a chronic and incurable condition, and an animal that is a danger to itself, other animals, or its handlers. Some insurance underwriters have established a "wobbler clause" which in general says that for a horse with CVSM to be a candidate for humane destruction it must have severe clinical signs (at least grade 3/5) as well as myelographic confirmation of a surgical lesion. This statement is a generality and in no way do the authors intend to interpret the policy guidelines of any insurance underwriter or company. Depending on the policies issued, mortality claims may or may not be granted. It is uncommon but not unprecedented for insur-ance agencies to take over ownership of the affected horse and salvage it for athletic or breeding purposes. Severely affected animals and affected animals for which treat-ment is not an option or not effective are generally humanely destroyed.

Safety is of utmost importance both before and after surgical treatment of CVSM. In the authors' opinion, it is essential for everyone involved with the patient, including all potential handlers and caregivers, to be aware of what signs a horse with neurologic disease might show. In most cases, a horse with neurologic gait deficits less than a grade 4 can be managed in a fashion similar to other horses. A horse with grade 4 neurologic gait deficits may fall with normal movements and therefore needs to be handled in a very careful fashion. Opposition to surgical treatment of CVSM has gener-ally been focused on postoperative safety concerns during performance. Concerns regarding safety of the horse following surgery are based on the assumption that neu-rons do not regenerate completely following vertebral body stabilization, and thus even if the compression is alleviated, irreversible neuronal damage could make a horse unsuitable for performance activities. There is clear evidence in people, dogs, and horses with cervical compressive myelopathies that surgical intervention results in improvement in neurologic signs in most of the patients.[10,70–72] A determination of safety for the horse's intended use should be evaluated on a case-by-case basis by performance of thorough neurologic examinations.

Surgical technique. There have been several technical changes as an adaptation of the Cloward technique (anterior interbody fusion) was first described as a treatment of CVM.[67] The Cloward technique used the principle of dynamic compression that re-sults from having a circular bone dowel hammered into a slightly smaller diameter hole drilled between adjacent vertebra that need to be stabilized (see **Fig. 1**). The next sig-nificant modification was the use of a stainless steel circular implant (Bagby basket) that had numerous holes to allow for the cancellous bone from the drilling procedure to be used as an autologous graft resulting in an osseous fusion.[73,74] (see **Figs. 2** and **3**). This technique was used for over two decades with great success, although there was occasional implant migration and an increased incidence of postoperative verte-bral fractures from forcing the oversized implant into pathologic bone.

The use of the threaded Bagby and Kuslich (BAK) implant for the stabilization of lum-bar vertebrae in people led to the development of the Seattle Slew (kerf-cut cylinder [KCC]) implant in 2000 (see **Fig. 4**). This implant, a partially or fully threaded cylinder, is screwed into a previously drilled and threaded site. The implant site is prepared us-ing a combination of core saws and kerf wideners so that an isthmus of bone is left to accelerate fusion.

This procedure should be performed in an appropriate surgical facility where the pa-tient can be placed on a table in dorsal recumbency with the neck in a cervical brace. An appropriate surgical facility, capability for general anesthesia and monitoring, and intraoperative imaging are required for performing this procedure. The use of the KCC implant requires several specifically designed instruments. In addition, a general instrument pack for standard opening and closing, large curved osteotome, orthopedic hammer, Inge laminectomy retractors, nitrogen hoses and tank and regulators, and large roungers are all necessary.

Before performing the surgical procedure, an endoscopic examination is performed to evaluate recurrent laryngeal nerve function. Other routine preoperative evaluations such as screening clinicopathologic tests are also recommended.

Preoperative antibiotics and tetanus prophylaxis are administered as standard for the surgical facility. Nonsteroidal anti-inflammatory drugs are also administered preoperatively. Corticosteroids are usually only administered to the very ataxic patients (>3.5/5 grade). Clipping and preliminary cleaning of the ventral cervical area before anesthesia will assist in reducing anesthesia time. After induction and intubation, the patient is placed in dorsal recumbency on a well-padded surgical table. The neck is placed in a cervical brace. It is absolutely critical that the horse be positioned so that the neck is perfectly straight and does not move (**Fig. 5**). After standard clipping and skin preparation, the surgical site (ie, cervical vertebrae that are to be fused) is identified by placing 14 gauge needles subcutaneously in the skin over the vertebrae and obtaining radiographs to "mark" the surgical site(s) (**Fig. 6**). The vertebral bodies are approximately a hands' width apart. Care should be taken to have the needles on the cassette side of the cervical area to reduce any parallax problem. The second cervical vertebra needs to be included so the characteristic formation of C2 can be used as a reference. Standard draping technique is used as for any sterile procedure.

A 20-cm skin incision is made on ventral midline centered over the intervertebral area that is to be fused. The ventral cervical subcutaneous muscle is also incised down to the sternothyrohyoideus muscles. The thickness of these muscles is quite variable depending on the patient's age and degree of neurologic deficits. The adventitia over the trachea is separated, and blunt dissection using fingers alongside of the trachea is used to gain access to the dorsal surface of the trachea. Care must be taken not to damage the carotid artery, recurrent laryngeal nerve, and/or vagosympathetic trunk. These structures must be avoided during dissection and protected from trauma during retraction. The trachea is retracted to the side to expose the longus colli muscles. The longus colli muscles overly the vertebral bodies and has a septum on midline. The ventral spine vertebral body can be palpated on midline. An incision is made over the ventral spine parallel with the muscle fibers down to the spine. The muscle insertion on the spine is elevated with a Cobb elevator. The spine is isolated using two pairs of Inge retractors (**Fig. 7**). The spine is removed using a large curved

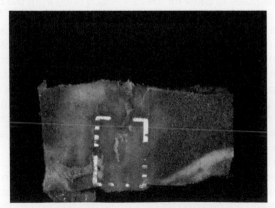

Fig. 5. Sagittal section 12 months after fusion with Bagby basket shows the ingrowth of the bone graft.

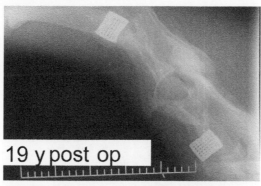

19 y post op

Fig. 6. Double-level fusion at C2–C3 and C4–C5 performed 19 years earlier.

osteotome and orthopedic hammer down to the level of the intervertebral disc. A sufficient amount of ventral spine must be removed in order to create a flat platform for the drill guide to be positioned. The intervertebral space must be identified in order to properly position the drill guide. Two K-wires are placed and intraoperative lateral radiographs are taken. The K-wire that is aligned with the intervertebral space is selected and a centering sleeve is positioned over the K-wire followed by the drill guide being positioned over the centering sleeve (**Fig. 8**). The drill guide is driven into place, and a lateral radiograph is taken to confirm that the drill guide is centered over the intervertebral space. The implant site is prepared by using core saws, kerf cleaners, and a 25 mm diameter drill to lower the isthmus of bone in the center of the implant site. The final depth of the implant site should be approximately 15 mm from the spinal canal. Intraoperative radiographs should be taken to ensure the site is of appropriate depth (**Fig. 9**). The implant site is tapped and either a partially threaded or fully treaded KCC is twisted into place using an implant driver (**Figs. 10 and 11**).

Cancellous bone graft that is harvested during preparation of the implant site from the drill and kerf wideners is placed into the opening of the KCC. A radiograph is taken. The longus colli muscle is closed using #1 synthetic absorbable suture in a simple

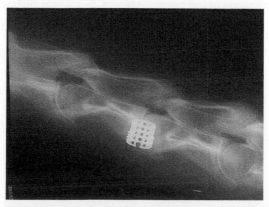

Fig. 7. A 12-month postoperative radiograph of a fusion using a Seattle Slew implant. Note collapse of intervertebral joint space and ossification of the bone graft ventral to the implant.

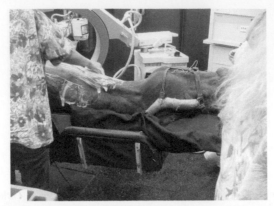

Fig. 8. Patient in dorsal: a dorsal recumbent position with mid-cervical area supported by the wooden cervical brace. A C-Arm is in place for obtaining intraoperative images.

continuous pattern. The surgery site is then examined for any foreign debris and thoroughly lavaged and suctioned. The ventral cervical muscles are reapposed in layers using #1 synthetic absorbable suture material a simple continuous pattern. The subcutaneous tissue layer is closed in using a continuous pattern of synthetic absorbable suture material. The skin is closed using skin staples. An assisted recovery using a head rope and tail rope is recommended (**Figs. 12–14**).

Locking compression plate fixation has been proposed as an alternative to KCC fixation. This method has been reported in a 3-month-old foal; revision surgery was required 11 days postoperatively due to screws backing out, but the foal's neurologic signs eventually improved by 2.5 grades.[75] In vitro studies were conducted to compare the strength of the locking compression plate fixation to traditional KCC fixation.[76,77] The mechanical properties of the LCP constructs were considered superior to the KCC in this model, although it did not assess the effect of repetitive loading nor could it predict in vivo behavior, as bony ingrowth occurs through the holes of the KCC and increases stability.

Cervical stabilization using polyaxial pedicle screw and rod construct in horses has been described.[78] In this study, the authors evaluated the safety and efficacy of this technique for stabilization of the cervical spine. C3– C4 was distracted with a porous

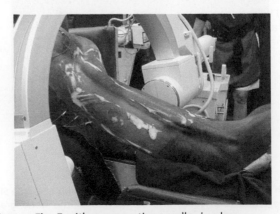

Fig. 9. Same patient as **Fig. 5** with preoperative needles in place.

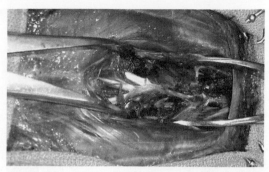

Fig. 10. Retractors. Postmortem dissection showing in the ventral spine at C3–C4 with the longus colli muscles elevated.

metal interbody fusion device and stabilized with a polyaxial screw and rod construct in four normal adult horses. The horses were evaluated monthly and euthanized 8 months postoperatively. Following euthanasia, the surgical site was evaluated for osseointegration and implant safety using microcomputed tomography, histology, and histomorphometry in each horse. There was not migration or failure of any implants. There was no instability of the surgical site in any of the horses. New bone formation was present within the interbody fusion device in each horse but there was variable osseointegration present.

The outcome using this technique for cervical interbody fusion in 10 horses diagnosed with CVCM was recently published.[79] Three horses had a single-level fusion, and seven horses had a double-level fusion. Overall, this technique resulted in at least 1 grade of improvement in 6/8 cases with ≥1 year of follow-up. Two horses were euthanized secondary to postoperative complications. This technique provides another means to achieve intervertebral fusion in the horse.

Reported nonfatal complications associated with surgical intervention include transient worsening of ataxia, seroma formation, implant failure or migration, vertebral fracture, laryngeal hemiplegia, and colitis.[10,75] Fatal complications included vertebral body fracture, spinal cord edema, and implant failure.[10]

Postoperative Care

Recommendations for aftercare vary according to surgeon preference as well as case specifics. In general, at least 1 month of strict stall rest is recommended. A second month of stall rest with hand-walking follows; the horse is initially walked for 5 to 10 minutes twice daily and gradually increased to 30 minutes two to three times daily. If the horse is comfortable and healing is progressing well, small paddock turnout is

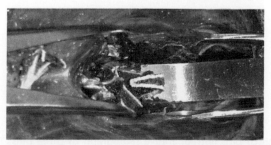

Fig. 11. Osteotome-removing spine. Preparing a flat drilling surface with an osteotome.

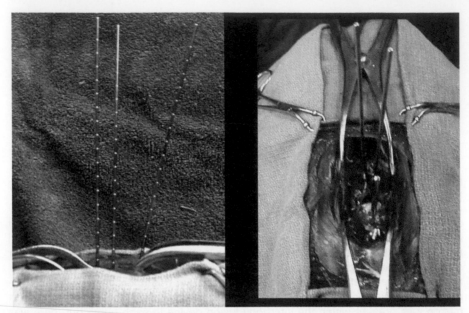

Fig. 12. Pin placement. Lateral and dorsal images of showing pin placement to determine ideal site for the placement of the drill guide over the centering pin.

introduced during the third month. Neurologic reevaluation by a veterinarian is recommended before beginning turnout. Cervical radiographs are often repeated monthly for the first 3 months postoperatively to assess healing during recuperation.

Usually, a month or more of unlimited turnout is provided before return to forced exercise (long-lining, lunging, or riding) at 4 to 6 months postoperatively. During this turnout period, ground work in hand should be performed as a form of physical therapy to improve proprioception and balance. This ground work should be performed without restriction of the horse's head and neck movements, so that the horse is free to assume a comfortable head and neck position. Exercises include walking

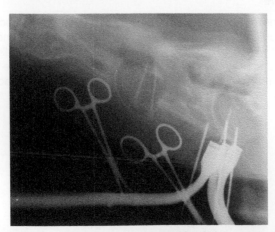

Fig. 13. Radiograph of pins. Intraoperative radiograph of three pins. The #1 K-Pin is too anterior, and the #2 K-Pin is too casual. The pins were changed in position.

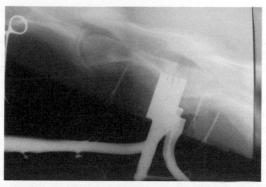

Fig. 14. Kerf Cutter Depth. Intraoperative radiograph of the same patient as **Fig. 9** showing the proper depth and ideal positioning after the pin placements were changed.

patterns (circles, serpentines, figure eights) on flat surfaces and inclines, as well as walking over cavaletti poles or other 4 to 6″ obstacles. In addition, standing exercises such as "carrot stretches" to improve the horse's cervical range of motion can be added during this time period; again, the horse should be encouraged but not forced to move its head and neck in any given direction.

Exercise under saddle most commonly begins about 6 months postoperatively but less severely ataxic horses with good recoveries sometimes can be ridden 4 months postoperatively, and more severely ataxic horses might not regain enough function to be ridden until 9 to 12 months. Full neurologic examination by a veterinarian is strongly recommended before beginning work under saddle. A slow return to previous level of exercise is recommended. Owners should anticipate a full year of recovery time before the horse being in "normal" work, although obviously some horses require less or more time than this.

Prognosis

Regardless of treatment selected, the response and the prognosis depend largely on the age of the horse, the severity of neurologic deficits, the duration of neurologic signs, and the expected level of performance. Generally, a horse with CVSM will be able to survive but performance might be impaired. Without treatment, the prognosis in all types of CVSM is usually poor to guarded, as there is continued damage to the cervical spinal cord with an increasing chance of severe cord destruction following trauma.

The initial response to medical therapy with anti-inflammatory drugs in cases of acute spinal cord damage is generally good, however, if bony malformations or soft tissue proliferations exist, neurologic deficits will remain. Young horses treated medically with a low-protein, low-energy "paced" diet, and stall confinement showed good results; in a study population of 18 young horses (<1 year of age) with a presumptive diagnosis of CVSM, 83% improved and had at least one racing start.[11] These cases were not confirmed by myelography or histology and it is unclear whether diet, exercise restriction, or time led to the perceived improvement, if there was any change at all. When medical treatment was evaluated in a population of Thoroughbreds containing slightly older horses (mainly 1–2 years of age), only 21/70 (30%) had at least one racing start.[78] For older horses with significant arthropathies, articular joint injections with corticosteroids often result in reduced soft tissue swelling.[65,66] However, these injections generally need to be repeated at variable intervals. Again, the prognosis depends on the severity of neurologic deficits and the severity of the degenerative joint changes.

The clinical response to ventral stabilization depends on the ability to detect all compressed sites and the accuracy of the diagnosis. Optimal outcomes are achieved if surgical intervention is pursued shortly after the first clinical signs develop. Overall, if return to use is considered, a success rate of 45% to 60% is estimated based on review of the literature.[68] An early study[10] evaluating 73 horses with CVSM that had surgical intervention (cervical vertebral interbody fusion [n = 63] or dorsal laminectomy [n = 10]) indicated that neurologic function improved in 77% of horses, and 46% achieved athletic function. Only 4/10 horses undergoing dorsal laminectomy improved. A shorter duration of clinical signs before intervention was positively associated with neurologic improvement and return to function, whereas age and number of compressive lesions did not affect outcome. Based on the experiences of the authors, owners and veterinarians can expect clinical improvement in approximately 80% of horses undergoing surgery.[79,80] (Reed SM, Robertson J, Grant B. Unpublished observations, 2015) Although clinical improvement can be somewhat variable, approximately 63% of the horses return to athletic function and another 15% are suitable for breeding. About 10% have poor response to treatment but can be turned out and live a relatively normal life at pasture, whereas the final 12% fail to improve sufficiently.[79]

Pathogenesis

The pathogenesis of CVSM is not fully understood but seems to be multifactorial, potentially involving genetic predisposition, trauma, exercise, and nutrition. Early on a genetic predisposition to CVSM in horses was suspected based on the frequency of CVSM in certain families of Thoroughbreds[3,81]; however, lack of many close relationships in a group of 47 horses with CVSM gave rise to thoughts on other etiologic factors.[1] Although some investigators have failed to demonstrate genetic determination of CVSM,[82,83] others believe that genetic factors that determine the length of the neck, cervical vertebral biomechanics, and body size play a significant role in the development of CVSM.[5,84,85] In the most recent investigation of the heritability of CVSM, Reed reported a suspicion that affected horses inherited a predisposition for increased sensitivity to environmental factors influencing cartilage growth.[86]

Cartilage growth and osteochondrosis dissecans are likely linked to the development of CVSM because osteochondrotic type lesions are frequently seen in vertebrae involved in myelocompressive lesions.[85] Osteochondrosis of the articular processes might result in instability and malalignment of adjacent vertebrae, secondary osteoarthritis of the articular processes, and hypertrophy of soft tissue structures. All of these changes might contribute to spinal cord compression.[9,21,22,87–91] Multiple investigators have shown that horses with CVSM have an increased incidence and severity of degenerative joint changes in the axial skeleton[1,16,22,87] and Wagner *and colleagues* demonstrated that although offspring from horses with CVSM did not develop myelocompressive lesions themselves, this group did have a high incidence (45%) of osteochondrotic lesions in both the axial and appendicular skeleton.[85]

In contrast to young horses in which the role of degenerative joint disease in the pathogenesis of CVSM seems controversial, in older horses (>4 years) CVSM is generally associated with significant arthropathies of the caudal cervical articular processes. In these horses, the compression of the spinal cord can be attributed to the bony and soft tissue proliferation at the affected articular processes. This finding is supported by the improvement; many of these horses show when medical and surgical treatment leads to reduction of the bony proliferation as evidenced radiographically. The genesis of the degenerative joint disease in older horses with CVSM is speculative but external trauma is thought to be important,[33] and exercise might have a role.

Dietary factors might also contribute to the development of osteochondrosis and CVSM.[62,92,93] An accelerated rate of gain but not of growth has been related to osteochondrosis and CVSM in horses, however, controlled investigations have failed to confirm this relationship.[94] Nutritional factors that have been associated with the incidence of developmental orthopedic disease are an imbalance in the calcium/phosphorus ratio, copper deficiency, excessive zinc, excessive protein, and excessive carbohydrate. The three most important nutritional factors seem to be excessive digestible energy, excessive phosphorus, and copper deficiency.[95,96]

A dietary calcium/phosphorus imbalance has been implicated in CVSM,[87] and particularly excessive phosphorus (388% of the requirement) seems to be correlated with an increased incidence and severity of osteochondrotic lesions in foals.[97]

SUMMARY

CVSM is the most common noninfectious cause of spinal ataxia in the horse. Stenosis of the cervical vertebral canal and subsequent myelocompression is the cause of this neurologic disease. Although the etiology of CVSM is not fully understood, diagnostic and therapeutic options for affected horses have continued to improve. The specificity and sensitivity of predicting CVSM from survey radiographs using the sagittal ratio method are high; however, myelography and cross sectional imaging (computed tomography) remains necessary for localization of compressive lesions. Further research is required in antemortem diagnostic testing to define criteria to evaluate myelograms and the use of advanced imaging techniques such as MR and CT. Ventral interbody fusion has proven to be an effective surgical procedure; however, complete recovery does not occur in all horses, and risks associated with postoperative performance must be carefully considered by the owners.

CLINICS CARE POINTS

- An accurate diagnosis is critical in achieving a positive outcome when treating cases with suspected CVM.
- CT myelography is very helpful as part of the diagnostic workup in cases with suspected CVM.
- Post operative rehabilitation is a very important part of the healing process. Owners and trainers must be patient and realize that the improvement in clinical signs takes time (up to 1 year) post surgery.
- Vertebral fusion is a viable technique used to stop spinal cord compression and allow improvment in clinical signs in horses with CVM.

REFERENCES

1. Dimock WW, Errington BJ. Incoordination of equidae: Wobblers. J Am Vet Med Assoc 1939;95:261–7.
2. Mayhew E. The illustrated horse doctor. London: W.H. Allen and Co; 1860.
3. Errington BJ. Causes of "Wobblers". Vet Bull Supp Army Med Bull 1938;32:153–5.
4. De Lahunta A. In: Veterinary neuroanatomy and clinical neurology. Philadelphia: W. B. Saunders Co; 1977;25–45.

5. Rooney JR. Disorders of the nervous system. In: Rooney JR, editor. Biomechanics in lameness. Baltimore: Williams and Wilkins; 1969. p. 219–33.

6. Wagner PC, Grant BD, Reed SM. Cervical vertebral malformation. Vet Clin North Am Equine Pract 1987;3:385–96.

7. Van Biervliet J. An evidence-based approach to clinical questions in the practice of equine neurology. Vet Clin North Am Equine Pract 2007;23:317–28.

8. Oswald J, Love S, Parkin TD, et al. Prevalence of cervical vertebral stenotic myelopathy in a population of thoroughbred horses. Vet Rec 2010;166:82–3.

9. Powers BE, Stashak TS, Nixon AJ, et al. Pathology of the vertebral column of horses with cervical static stenosis. Vet Pathol 1986;23:392–9.

10. Rush Moore B, Reed SM, Robertson JT. Surgical treatment of cervical stenotic myelopathy in horses: 73 cases (1983-1992). J Am Vet Med Assoc 1993;203:108–12.

11. Mayhew IG, Donawick WJ, Green SL, et al. Diagnosis and prediction of cervical vertebral malformation in thoroughbred foals based on semi-quantitative radiographic indicators. Equine Vet J 1993;25:435–40.

12. Rush Moore B, Reed SM, Biller DS, et al. Assessment of vertebral canal diameter and bony malformations of the cervical part of the spine in horses with cervical stenotic myelopathy. Am J Vet Res 1994;55:5–13.

13. Van Biervliet, Mayhew J, de LaHunta A. Cervical vertebral compressive myelopathy. Clin Tech Equine Prac 2006;5:54–9.

14. Nixon AJ, Stashak TS, Ingram J. Diagnosis of cervical vertebral malformation in the horse. Proc Amer Assoc Equine Pract 1982;28:253–66.

15. Papageorges M, Gavin PR, Sande RD, et al. Radiographic and myelographic examination of the cervical vertebral column in 306 ataxic horses. Vet Rad 1987;28:53–9.

16. Mayhew IG, De Lahunta A, Whitlock RH, et al. Spinal cord disease in the horse. Cornell Vet 1978;68(Suppl 6).

17. Rush Moore B, Holbrook TC, Stefanacci JD, et al. Contrast-enhanced computed tomography and myelography in six horses with cervical stenotic myelopathy. Equine Vet J 1992;24:197–202.

18. Wilson WD, Hughes SJ, Ghoshal NG, et al. Occipitoatlantoaxial malformation in two non-Arabian horses. J Am Vet Med Assoc 1985;187:36.

19. Reed SM, Rush BR. Developmental vertebral anomalies. In: Auer JA, Stick JA, editors. Equine surgery. Philadephia: W.B.Saunders; 1999. p. 423–8.

20. Levine JM, Ngheim PP, Levine GJ, et al. Associations of sex, breed, and age with cervical vertebral compressive myelopathy in horses: 811 cases (1974-2007). J Am Vet Med Assoc 2008;233:1453–8.

21. Gerber H, Ueltschi G, Diehl M, et al. Untersuchungen an der Halswirbelsäule des Pferdes - eine klinisch-radiologische Studie. Schweiz Arch Tierheilkd 1989;131:311–21.

22. Stewart RH, Reed SM, Weisbrode SE. Frequency and severity of osteochondrosis in horses with cervical stenotic myelopathy. Am J Vet Res 1991;52:873–9.

23. Newton-Clarke MJ, Divers TJ, De Lahunta A, et al. Evaluation of the thoracolaryngeal reflex ('slap test') as an aid to the diagnosis of cervical spinal cord and brainstem disease in horses. Equine Vet J 1994;26:358–61.

24. Tomizawa N, Nishimura R, Sasaki N, et al. Efficacy of the new radiographic measurement method for cervical vertebral instability in wobbling foals. J Vet Med Sci 1994;56:1119–22.

25. Andrews FM, Adair HS III. Anatomy and physiology of the nervous system. In: Auer JA, Stick JA, editors. Equine surgery. Philadelphia: W.B. Saunders; 1999. p. 405–12.

26. Mayhew IG. Equine neurology and nutrition. Proc. A.E.V.A. Bain-Fallon Memorial Lectures 1996;18:1–73.

27. Chiapetta JR, Baker JR, Feeney DA. Vertebral fracture, extensor hypertonia of thoracic limbs, and paralysis of the pelvic limbs (Schiff-Sherrington syndrome) in an Arabian foal. J Am Vet Med Assoc 1985;186:387.

28. Rashmir-Raven A, DeBowes RM, Hudson L, et al. Vertebral fracture and paraplegia in a foal. Prog Vet Neurol 1991;2:197–202.

29. Pinchbeck G, Murphy D. Cervical vertebral fracture in three foals. Equine Vet Educ 2001;1:24–8.

30. Schott HC II, Major MD, Grant BD, et al. Melanoma as a cause of spinal cord compression in two horses. J Am Vet Med Assoc 1990;196:1820–2.

31. Furr MO, Anver M, Wise M. Intervertebral disk prolapse and diskospondylitis in a horse. J Am Vet Med Assoc 1991;198:2095–6.

32. Colbourne CM, Raidal SL, Yovich JV, et al. Cervical Discospondylitis in two horses. Aust Vet J 1997;75:477–9.

33. Mayhew IGJ. The diseased spinal cord. Proc Amer Assoc Equine Pract; 1999. p. 66–84.

34. Yovich JV, Powers BE, Stashak TS. Morphologic features of the cervical intervertebral disks and adjacent vertebral bodies of horses. Am J Vet Res 1985;46: 2372–7.

35. Allison N, Moeller RB Jr. Spinal ataxia in a horse caused by an arachnoid diverticulum (cyst). J Vet Diagn Invest 2000;12.279–81.

36. Hestvik G, Ekman S, Lindberg R. Onchocercosis of an intervertebral joint capsule causing cervical vertebral stenotic myelopathy in a horse. J Vet Diagn Invest 2006;18:307–10.

37. Gold JR, Divers TJ, Miller AJ, et al. Cervical vertebral spinal hematomas in 4 horses. J Vet Intern Med 2008;22:481–5.

38. Withers JM, Voûte LC, Hammond G, et al. Radiographic anatomy of the articular process joints of the caudal cervical vertebrae in the horse on lateral and oblique projections. Equine Vet J 2009;41:895–902.

39. Down SS, Henson FM. Radiographic retrospective study of the caudal cervical articular process joints in the horse. Equine Vet J 2009;41:518–24.

40. Mayhew IG, Green SL. Radiographic diagnosis of equine cervical vertebral malformation. Proc Annu Meet Amer Coll Vet Intern Med 2002;20:382–3.

41. Hahn CN, Handel I, Green SL, et al. Assessment of the utility of using intra- and intervertebral minimum sagittal diameter ratios in the diagnosis of cervical vertebral malformation in horses. Vet Radiol Ultrasound 2008;49:1–6.

42. Scrivani PV, Levine JM, Holmes NL, et al. Observer agreement study of cervical-vertebral ratios in horses. Equine Vet J 2011;43:399–403.

43. Neuwirth L. Equine myelography. Compend Contin Educ Pract Vet 1992;14:72–8.

44. Rose PL, Abutarbush SM, Duckett W. Standing myelography in the horse using a nonionic contrast agent. Vet Radiol Ultrasound 2007;48:535–8.

45. Andrews FM, Matthews HK, Reed SM. The ancillary techniques and tests for diagnosing equine neurologic disease. Vet Med 1990;1325–30.

46. Furr MO, Tyler RD. Cerebrospinal fluid creatine kinase activity in horses with central nervous system disease: 69 cases (1984-1989). J Am Vet Med Assoc 1990; 197:245–8.

47. Furr M, Chickering WR, Robertson J. High resolution protein electrophoresis of equine cerebrospinal fluid. Am J Vet Res 1997;58:939–41.

48. Pusterla N, Wilson WD, Conrad PA, et al. Comparative analysis of cytokine gene expression in cerebrospinal fluid of horses without neurologic signs or with selected neurologic disorders. Am J Vet Res 2006;67:1433–7.

49. Reed SM, Newberry J, Norton K, et al. Pathogenesis of cervical vertebral malformation. Proc Amer Assoc Equine Pract 1985;31:37–42.

50. Nyland TG, Blythe LL, Pool RR, et al. Metrizamide myelography in the horse: clinical, radiographic, and pathologic changes. Am J Vet Res 1980;41:204–11.

51. Van Biervliet J, Scrivani PV, Divers TJ, et al. Evaluation of a diagnostic criterion for spinal cord compression during cervical myelography. Proc Annu Meet Coll Vet Intern Med 2002;20:769.

52. van Biervliet J, Scrivani PV, Divers TJ, et al. Evaluation of decision criteria for detection of spinal cord compression based on cervical myelography in horses: 38 cases (1981-2001). Equine Vet J 2004;36:14–20.

53. Mayhew IG. Tetraparesis, paraparesis and ataxia of the limbs, and episodic weakness. In: Mayhew IG, editor. Large animal neurology: a handbook for veterinary clinicians. 1st edition. Philadelphia: Lea and Febiger; 1989. p. 246–58.

54. Schmidburg I, Pagger H, Zsoldos RR, et al. Movement associated reduction of spatial capacity of the equine cervical vertebral canal. Vet J 2012;192:525–8.

55. Mayhew IG, Green SL. Accuracy of diagnosing CVM from radiographs. Proc Br Equine Vet Assoc Annu Congress, Equine Vet J Ltd., Newmarket 2000;39:74–5.

56. Mitchell CW, Nykamp SG, Foster R, et al. The use of magnetic resonance imaging in evaluating horses with spinal ataxia. Vet Radiol Ultrasound 2012;53:613–20.

57. Prange T, Derksen FJ, Stick JA, et al. Endoscopic anatomy of the cervical vertebral canal in the horse: a cadaver study. Equine Vet J 2011;43:317–23.

58. Prange T, Derksen FJ, Stick JA, et al. Cervical vertebral canal endoscopy in the horse: intra- and post operative observations. Equine Vet J 2011;43:404–11.

59. Prange T, Carr EA, Stick JA, et al. Cervical vertebral canal endoscopy in a horse with cervical vertebral stenotic myelopathy. Equine Vet J 2012;44:116–9.

60. Pepe M, Angelone M, Gialletti R, et al. Arthroscopic anatomy of the equine cervical articular process joints. Equine Vet J 2013. https://doi.org/10.1111/evj.12112.

61. Hudson NPH, Mayhew IG. Radiographic and myelographic assessment of the equine cervical vertebral column and spinal cord. Equine Vet Educ 2005;17:34–8.

62. Donawick WJ, Mayhew IG, Galligan DT, et al. Early diagnosis of cervical vertebral malformation in young Thoroughbred horses and successful treatment with restricted, paced diet and confinement. Proc Amer Assoc Equine Pract 1989;35:525–8.

63. Kronfeld DS, Meacham TN, Donoghue S. Dietary aspects of developmental orthopedic disease in young horses. Vet Clin North Am Equine Pract 1990;6:451–65.

64. Mayhew IG, Brown CM, Stowe HD, et al. Equine Degenerative Myeloencephalopathy: A vitamin E deficiency that may be familial. J Vet Int Med 1987;1:45–50.

65. Grisel GB, Grant BD, Rantanen NW. Arthrocentesis of the equine cervical facets. Proc Amer Assoc Equine Pract 1996;42:197–8.

66. Grant BD. Surgical treatment of developmental disorders of the spinal column. In: Auer JA, Stick JA, editors. Equine surgery. 1st edition. Philadelphia: W.B. Saunders; 1999. p. 429–35.

67. Wagner PC, Bagby GW, Grant BD, et al. Surgical stabilization of the equine cervical spine. Vet Surg 1979;8:7–12.
68. Walmsley JP. Surgical treatment of cervical spinal cord compression in horses: A European experience. Equine Vet Educ 2005;17:39–43.
69. Huggons N. Tri-level surgical treatment of cervical spinal cord compression in a Thoroughbred yearling. Can Vet J 2007;48:635–8.
70. Kumar VG, Rea GL, Mervis LJ, et al. Cervical spondylotic myelopathy: functional and radiographic long-term outcome after laminectomy and posterior fusion. Neurosurgery 1999;44:771–7 ; discussion 777-778.
71. Hacker RJ. Threaded cages for degenerative cervical disease. Clin Ortho Relat Res 2002;394:39–46.
72. Rusbridge C, Wheeler SJ, Torrington AM, et al. Comparison of two surgical techniques for the management of cervical spondylomyelopathy in Dobermans. J Small Anim Pract 1998;39:425–31.
73. DeBowes RM, Grant BD, Bagby GW, et al. Cervical vertebral interbody fusion in the horse: a comparative study of bovine xenografts and autografts supported by stainless steel baskets. Am J Vet Res 1984;45:191–9.
74. Nixon AJ, Stashak TS. Dorsal laminectomy in the horse. I. Review of the literature and description of a new procedure. Vet Surg 1983;12:172–6.
75. Reardon R, Kummer M, Lischer C. Ventral locking compression plate for treatment of cervical stenotic myelopathy in a 3-month-old warmblood foal. Vet Surg 2009;38:537–42.
76. Reardon R, Bailey R, Walmsley J, et al. A pilot in vitro biomechanical comparison of locking compression plate fixation and kerf-cut cylinder fixation for ventral fusion of fourth and fifth equine cervical vertebrae. Vet Comp Orthop Traumatol 2009;22:371–9.
77. Reardon RJ, Bailey R, Walmsley JP, et al. An in vitro biomechanical comparison of a locking compression plate fixation and kerf cut cylinder fixation for ventral arthrodesis of the fourth and the fifth equine cervical vertebrae. Vet Surg 2010; 39:980–90.
78. Aldrich E, Nout-Lomas Y, Seim HB, et al. Cervical stabilization with polyaxial pedicle screw and rod construct in horses: A proof of concept study. Vet Surg 2018;47:932–41.
79. Pezzanite LM, Easley JT, Bayless R, et al. Outcomes after cervical vertebral interbody fusion using an interbody fusion device and polyaxial pedicle screw and rod construct in 10 horse (2015-2019). Equine Vet J 2022;54:347–58.
80. Hoffman CJ, Clark CK. Prognosis for racing with conservative management of cervical vertebral malformation in Thoroughbreds: 103 cases (2002-2010). J Vet Intern Med 2013;27:317–23.
81. Dimock WW. Wobblers" -an hereditary disease in horses. J Hered 1950;41: 319–23.
82. Falco MJ, Whitwell K, Palmer AC. An investigation into the genetics of "Wobbler disease" in thoroughbred horses in Britain. Equine Vet J 1976;8:165–9.
83. Wagner PC, Grant BD, Watrous BJ, et al. A study of the heritability of cervical vertebral malformation in horses. Proc Amer Assoc Equine Pract 1985;31:43–50.
84. Rooney JR. Etiology of the wobbler syndrome. Mod Vet Pract 1972;53:42.
85. Stashak TS, Nixon AJ, Powers BE. Pathology associated with cervical vertebral malformation (CVM) in the horse, Proceedings of the Veterinary Orthopedic Society, 1984;12:41.
86. Reed SM. Cervical vertebral stenotic myelopathy: pathogenesis. Proc Inter Equine Neurol Conf 1997;45–9.

87. Binkhorst GJ. Het ataxie syndroom bij jonge paarden. Inaugural Dissertation, Utrecht University.
88. Gruys E, Beynen AC, Binkhorst GJ, et al. Neurodegeneratieve aandoeningen van het centrale zenuwstelsel bij het paard. Tijdschr Diergeneesknd 1994;119:561–7.
89. Yovich JV, Gould DH, LeCouteur RA. Chronic cervical compressive myelopathy in horses: patterns of astrocytosis in the spinal cord. Aust Vet J 1991;68:334–7.
90. Tomizawa N, Nishimura R, Sasaki N, et al. Relationships between radiography of cervical vertebrae and histopathology of the cervical cord in wobbling 19 foals. J Vet Med Sci 1994;56:227–33.
91. Summers BA, Cummings JF, de Lahunta A. Veterinary Neuropathology 1977;101–102.
92. Glade MJ, Belling TH Jr. Growth plate cartilage metabolism, morphology and biochemical composition in over- and underfed horses. Growth 1984;48:473–82.
93. Glade MJ, Luba NK. Serum triiodothyronine and thyroxine concentrations in weanling horses fed carbohydrate by direct gastric infusion. Am J Vet Res 1987;48:578–82.
94. Hurtig MB, Pool RR. Pathogenesis of equine osteochondrosis. In: McIllwraith CW, Trotter GW, editors. Joint disease in the horse. Philadephia: W.B. Saunders; 1996. p. 335–8.
95. Savage CJ. Etiopathogenesis of osteochondrosis. In: White NA II, Moore JN, editors. Current techniques in equine surgery and lameness. Philadephia: W.B. Saunders; 1998. p. 318–22.
96. Knight D, Weisbrode SE, Schmall LM, et al. The effects of copper supplementation on the prevalence of cartilage lesions in foals. Equine Vet J 1990;22:426–32.
97. Savage CJ, McCarthy R, Jeffcott L. Effects of dietary energy and protein on induction of dyschondroplasia in foals. Equine Vet J 1993;16:74–9.

Equine Protozoal Myeloencephalitis

Robert J. MacKay, BVSc (Dist), PhD[a], Daniel K. Howe, PhD[b],*

KEYWORDS

- *Sarcocystis* • *Neospora*, opossum • Protozoa • EPM • Central nervous system

KEY POINTS

- Equine protozoal myeloencephalitis is an infectious neurologic disease of horses in North, Central, and South America. The disease is caused by the coccidian parasite *S neurona* and less frequently by the related pathogen *N. hughesi*.
- Horses are infected with *S neurona* by ingesting food or water that has been contaminated with feces from an infected opossum. The modes of transmission remain uncertain for *N. hughesi*, although it appears that foals can be infected by transplacental passage of the parasite.
- In many geographic areas of the Americas, *S neurona* infection is common, as evidenced by the proportion of horses exhibiting antibodies against the parasites. However, clinical disease is relatively uncommon (<1% of seropositive horses).
- Anticoccidial drugs will halt infection, but early diagnosis and treatment are critical to minimize immune-mediated damage to the central nervous system.

INTRODUCTION

An unusual neurologic condition of horses termed "segmental myelitis" was first observed by Rooney in Kentucky in 1964.[1] Rooney renamed the syndrome "focal encephalitis-myelitis" because of brain involvement and Prickett, Rooney and others reported on 44 cases at the annual meeting of the American Association of Equine Practitioners in 1968[2] and on 52 cases in 1970.[1] In 1974, protozoa were first seen in association with characteristic lesions,[3] and the disease was given its current name, equine protozoal myeloencephalitis (EPM) by Mayhew and colleagues, who reported on 45 cases at the AAEP meeting in 1976.[4] Over the years, a better understanding of EPM etiology and epidemiology has been obtained. However, EPM pathogenesis remains uncertain.

[a] Department of Large Animal Clinical Sciences, College of Veterinary Medicine, University of Florida, 2015 Southwest 16th Avenue, PO Box 100136, Gainesville, FL 32610-0125, USA;
[b] Department of Veterinary Science, M.H. Gluck Equine Research Center, University of Kentucky, 108 Gluck Equine Research Center, Lexington, KY 40546-0099, USA
* Corresponding author.
E-mail addresses: dkhowe2@uky.edu; Daniel.howe@uky.edu

Vet Clin Equine 38 (2022) 249–268
https://doi.org/10.1016/j.cveq.2022.05.003
0749-0739/22/© 2022 Elsevier Inc. All rights reserved.

ETIOLOGIC AGENTS

S. neurona[5] and N. hughesi[6–10] are the 2 known causative agents of EPM, although the great majority of cases are due to infection with S. neurona. Both are protozoan parasites in the phylum Apicomplexa, which is a broad and important group of obligate intracellular pathogens that cause significant disease in humans and animals.

All species of Sarcocystis have a two-host life cycle that alternates between definitive and intermediate hosts. The opossum (Didelphis virginiana) is the definitive host for S. neurona in North America.[11] As well, South American opossums can act as definitive hosts for S. neurona.[12] The parasite undergoes sexual reproduction in the intestinal epithelium of the infected opossum, resulting in the production of sporozoite-containing sporocysts that are passed in the feces and are infectious for the intermediate hosts. Striped skunks,[13] raccoons,[14] armadillos,[15] and cats[16] have been identified as relevant intermediate hosts for S. neurona. A variety of marine mammals have been found susceptible to infection by S. neurona,[17] although it seems unlikely that these animals contribute appreciably to the natural life-cycle of the parasite. In the natural intermediate hosts, S. neurona forms sarcocysts in the muscle tissue, which is the source of infection for the opossum definitive hosts. Opossums are commonly infected with S. neurona,[18] so there can be significant contamination of the environment in locations whereby opossums are frequently observed.

Horses get infected with S. neurona when they ingest food or water contaminated with feces from an infected opossum. Horses are considered to be incidental/dead-end hosts that do not contribute to the parasite's life cycle as S. neurona sarcocysts are not found routinely in these animals. However, S. neurona sarcocysts were described in one case of a 4-month-old foal with clinical signs of EPM.[19] While it remains unlikely that horses play a major role in the life cycle of S. neurona, this finding suggests that the parasite has the capacity to establish long-term latent infection in these animals. It is very important to note that S. neurona cannot be transmitted horizontally between horses, nor can it be transmitted to horses from the intermediate hosts. There is some evidence of vertical transmission of S. neurona from mare to foal,[20,21] but this is seemingly uncommon.

The complete life cycle of N. hughesi is unknown, so the mode(s) of transmission of this parasite to horses remains uncertain. Canids are known to be a definitive host for the related species Neospora caninum,[22] but it has not been established that N. hughesi uses dogs as a definitive host. Vertical transmission of N. caninum is very efficient in cattle, and studies indicate that transplacental passage of both N. hughesi and N. caninum can also occur in horses,[20,21,23–26] occasionally causing the abortion of the foal.[25,26] Thus far, N. caninum has not been found to be associated with neurologic disease in horses but was the apparent cause of myeloencephalitis in a captive-bred zebra.[27]

EPIDEMIOLOGY

The first national epidemiologic survey of EPM used postmortem data gathered retrospectively from 10 diagnostic centers throughout the US and Canada.[28] Most horses (61.8%) were 4 years of age or less and 19.8% were 8 years of age or older. Although Thoroughbreds, Standardbreds, and Quarter Horses were most commonly affected, no breed, gender, or seasonal bias was established. In a smaller retrospective study, 82 horses with histologic lesions compatible with EPM were reviewed.[29] Disease risk was highest among male Standardbred horses compared with the gender and breed distributions of the attendant hospital population. The mean age of affected horses was 3.6 ± 2.8 years, similar to the findings of Fayer and colleagues.[28]

Early seroprevalence studies of *S. neurona* in horses from the US varied widely, ranging from as low as 15% to a high of 89%, depending on geographic location.[30–34] A more recent comprehensive study of more than 5000 serum samples from healthy horses and ponies across the US revealed antibodies against *S. neurona* in 78% of horses, confirming the general belief that exposure to the parasite is common.[35] Seroprevalences ranging from approximately 35% to 69% have been reported in horses from Central and South America,[36–39] thus suggesting that horses in these regions are also commonly exposed to the parasite.

Although there are notable discrepancies among seroprevalence study results, all studies suggest that horses are less commonly exposed to *Neospora* spp. than they are to *S. neurona.* More than 10% of horses have been reported to exhibit antibodies against *Neospora* spp.,[6,40–44] with a recent large study reporting seroprevalence of 34%.[35] In contrast, other studies detected antibodies in much smaller proportions of horses (less than 3%).[36–39,45,46] A recent systematic review and meta-analysis of 57 studies reporting *Neospora* spp. serology in 26,160 horses and donkeys yielded a weighted global seroprevalence of 13.46% (95% CI: 10.26%–17.42%) with significant effects of assay type, age, sex, and geographic location.[47] *N. hughesi* has never been isolated outside the Americas while *N. caninum* is found worldwide. Most seroprevalence studies analyzed used IFAT or direct agglutination test formats that do not reliably distinguish between the 2 *Neospora* species,[48,49] so true *N. hughesi* seroprevalence remains unclear. It will be important for future seroprevalence surveys to use serologic tests (eg, NhSAG1 ELISA) that can help to distinguish antibodies against the 2 *Neospora* species.[46]

A survey conducted by the National Animal Health Monitoring System (NAHMS) estimated that the average annual incidence of EPM in horses 6 months of age or older was 14 ± 6 cases per 10,000 horses.[50] It is apparent that equine neosporosis caused by *N. hughesi* can manifest as a neurologic disease,[6–10] but EPM cases that can be attributed to this parasite species are rare.

Many clinical reports of EPM suggest that the disease occurs sporadically and seldom involves more than one horse on an operation.[4,51] Clusters of cases can occur, however.[52,53] A retrospective study conducted at The Ohio State University found that young adult horses (1–5 years) and older horses (>13 years) had a higher risk of developing EPM than did other horses.[54] The number of cases was lowest in the winter, with the risk 3 times higher in spring and summer and 6 times higher in the fall. Other factors associated with increased risk on given premises were the presence of opossums (2.5-fold), previous diagnosis of EPM (2.5-fold), and presence of woods (2-fold). In contrast, the likelihood of EPM was reduced by one-third by preventing wildlife access to feed and by one-half by the presence of a creek or river as a water source for wildlife.

Stress or advanced age may predispose to the development of EPM via immune compromise.[55] A strong dose–response relationship was found between various "stressful" events (eg, heavy exercise, transport, injury, surgery, or parturition) and the risk of EPM.[54] After such an event, the risk of manifesting the disease increased with time. Racehorses and show horses had a higher risk of developing EPM compared with breeding and pleasure horses. Not surprisingly, horses with EPM that were treated were ten times more likely to improve than were untreated horses.[55]

From the NAHMS equine study,[50] EPM was found more likely to occur on premises where opossums were identified. Interestingly, the presence of mice or rats also was associated with increased risk for horses to develop EPM. High human population density also increased the risk of developing EPM, which may be related to the encroachment of humans on opossum habitats.

PATHOGENESIS

While all horses are thought to be susceptible, it is apparent that infection with *S. neurona* or *N. hughesi* does not equate with EPM, with only a very small proportion of seropositive horses developing clinical disease. Unfortunately, it is not clear what can cause a simple, asymptomatic infection to progress to severe neurologic disease, which has confounded EPM diagnosis in the past and continues to hamper efforts to prevent and control the disease. As mentioned, factors such as parasite inoculum and stress-induced immune suppression have been implicated in the occurrence of EPM.[55–57] However, efforts to increase stress by use of a second transport and treatment with immunosuppressive steroids did not exacerbate disease,[58,59] so the interplay between immune suppression and infection is more complex than currently understood. Modest genetic and antigenic diversity exists among strains of *S. neurona* that have been isolated,[60–62] and there is some suggestion that particular parasite genotypes may be more virulent than others.[63] This finding was based on a large collection of *S. neurona* isolates from marine mammals, however, and the association between parasite genotype and disease was not apparent in the more limited sample set of isolates from horses suffering from EPM. Consequently, further work is needed to assess whether some strains of *S. neurona* have a greater capacity to cause neurologic disease in horses. The possibility of comorbidity due to dual protozoal infection has been examined as a factor in EPM. One study comparing antibodies in neurologic horses with antibodies in normal, nonneurologic horses suggested a role for *Toxoplasma gondii* in EPM.[64] In contrast, the results from a second study showed no association between EPM and the presence of antibodies against this parasite.[65] It should be noted that equids commonly exhibit antibodies against *T gondii*,[66] but only a single case of clinical toxoplasmosis in a horse has been documented.[67]

Experimental Infections

Resistance to many intracellular pathogens is dependent on the generation of a normal Th1 cellular immune response, including the expression of cytokines such as interferonγ (IFNγ) and interleukin 12. Consistent with the importance of cell-mediated immunity, protozoal encephalitis with *S. neurona* has been induced in athymic "nude" mice, IFNγ knockout mice, and CD8 knockout mice by subcutaneous or intraperitoneal injection of cultured merozoites or by gavage with sporocysts.[68–70] Strains of immunocompetent mice (eg, C57BL/6 and BALB/c) are seemingly resistant to *S. neurona* infection, even after corticosteroid treatment. Severe combined immunodeficient (SCID) BALB/c and ICR mice, which completely lack adaptive immune systems but have a population of natural killer cells capable of producing IFNγ, are partially resistant to neurologic disease caused by *S. neurona*, despite persistent, low-level infection.[69,71] C57BL/6 SCID mice, which apparently are unable to mount a competent innate IFNγ response in this setting, are fully susceptible to *S. neurona* encephalitis.[72] As expected, adoptive transfer of IFNγ-competent T-lymphocytes into these mice conferred protection against *S. neurona*. It has been suggested that a defective IFNγ response also may underlie susceptibility to EPM in horses,[72,73] although convincing supportive data for this notion are yet to be adduced.

Initial work aimed at reproducing EPM in horses used as challenge inoculum a mixture of uncharacterized sporocysts collected from 10 feral opossums.[74] When molecular markers were identified that were able to differentiate the various *Sarcocystis* spp. sporocysts found in opossums,[75] it became possible to use challenge inocula containing known quantities of *S. neurona* sporocysts.[56,58] In all of these studies, horses produced antibodies to *S. neurona* in serum and cerebrospinal fluid (CSF), and mild to moderately severe neurologic signs were observed in some but not all challenged horses. In many cases, signs were progressive initially and then stabilized or even improved. Evidence of mild to moderate subacute to chronic multifocal changes was generally found in the CNS, but protozoa were not observed in blood or CNS tissue nor were they detected by immunohistological staining, PCR, culture, or mouse inoculation. Interestingly, immunosuppression by dexamethasone administration reduced the time to the appearance of antibodies in the CSF, and clinical signs and histologic lesions were equivalent to or even milder than those observed in the challenged control horses.[58]

With the establishment of the *S. neurona* life cycle in the laboratory, it became possible to infect horses with a homogeneous inoculum of parasite sporocysts.[57] This study found that a large inoculum (10^5–10^6 sporocysts) was needed to consistently obtain evidence of CNS infection (antibodies in CSF). Similar to the prior challenge studies, mild to moderate clinical signs were observed, but organisms were not seen histologically.

In vitro infection of buffy coat cells and intravenous inoculation of the infected cells back into horses has been used as a challenge model for EPM.[76] Similar to the prior studies using a natural route of infection, challenged horses developed moderate clinical signs and antibodies were detected in serum and CSF. Although parasites were not observed histologically within CNS lesions, culture isolation of organisms from tissues was described.

The collective results from the various experimental horse infection studies indicate that horses are relatively resistant to *S. neurona* infection and development of neurologic disease, and the role of the immune response in the progression from simple infection to acute EPM is complicated. Whereas severe immunosuppression may promote CNS invasion by *S. neurona,* components of the immune response are seemingly required for the development of EPM (**Box 1**).

CLINICAL SIGNS

EPM is often a progressively debilitating disease affecting the CNS of horses. Clinical signs vary from acute to chronic with insidious onset of focal or multifocal signs of neurologic disease involving the brain and/or spinal cord.[51] Affected horses may initially exhibit unusual signs such as dysphagia, evidence of abnormal upper airway function, unusual or atypical lameness, or even seizures.[77] Severely affected horses may have difficulty standing, walking, or swallowing and the disease may progress very rapidly. In other cases, the clinical signs seem to stabilize, only to relapse days or weeks later.

Box 1
Etiology and Epidemiology of EPM

- EPM is caused primarily by the protozoan parasite *S neurona*, although some cases have been associated with the related pathogen *Neospora hughesi*

- *S neurona* is transmitted to horses via food or water contamination with feces from infected opossums. The different modes of transmission of *N. hughesi* remain uncertain, but transplacental passage from mare to foal can occur.

- Infection of horses is fairly common, but EPM is relatively rare. The factors influencing disease susceptibility remain unknown.

The variability of clinical signs is due to the parasite's ability to infect both white and gray matter in a seemingly random fashion at multiple sites along the entire CNS. Signs of gray matter involvement include focal muscle atrophy (**Fig. 1**) and severe muscle weakness, while damage to white matter frequently results in ataxia and weakness in limbs caudal to the site of damage. The early signs of the disease, such as stumbling and frequent interference between limbs, can be confused easily with lameness. Horses affected with EPM commonly experience a gradual progression in the severity and range of clinical signs, including ataxia. In some cases, however, a gradual onset may give way to a sudden exacerbation in the severity of clinical illness, resulting in recumbency.

The vital signs in affected horses are usually normal and animals seem bright and alert. Some horses with EPM may seem thin and mildly obtunded. Neurologic examination often reveals asymmetric ataxia, asymmetric stride length particularly in the pelvic limbs, and weakness involving one to all limbs. Areas of hyporeflexia, hypalgesia, or complete sensory loss may be found. The most commonly observed signs of brain disease include the primary brainstem signs of obtundation, head tilt, facial nerve paralysis, and difficulty in swallowing. Any of an almost infinite number of other neurologic signs is possible.[78] Gait abnormalities most often result from lesions in the spinal cord and may be variable in severity, depending on the location and extent of tissue damage.

PATHOLOGY

On necropsy examination of cases of EPM, lesions may be grossly visible on cut surfaces of the CNS; these may vary from clearly demarcated discoloration (usually of gray matter) to massive necrotic even hemorrhagic lesions which destroy large portions of the brain or multiple segments of the spinal cords.[79] Histologically, parasites are seen in less than 50% of cases. When present, they can be difficult to detect using standard staining procedures (eg, hematoxylin and eosin), but may be more apparent after immunohistochemical (IHC) staining (**Fig. 2**). Histologic lesions are remarkably consistent regardless of the presence of associated organisms. Typically, there is cuffing of blood vessels by mononuclear cells, necrosis of parenchyma with phagocytosis and gitter cell formation, astrocyte proliferation, and gemistocytes formation. Eosinophils are seen commonly, as are multinucleated cells, which may be giant in size. Lesions may extend to produce nonsuppurative meningitis. Lesions

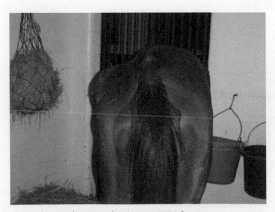

Fig. 1. Asymmetric gluteal muscle atrophy in an EPM horse.

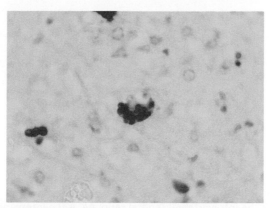

Fig. 2. Immunohistochemical labeling with anti-*S. neurona* rabbit serum showing multiple stained parasites in equine CNS tissue.

may vary from peracute to chronic with prominent lymphoid vascular cuffing with minimal tissue destruction in the former situation and marked tissue loss, prominent astrocyte proliferation, and minimal inflammatory response in chronic cases. The amount of fiber degeneration in ascending and descending pathways below and above the lesions is dependent on the duration of CNS infection.

DIAGNOSIS

EPM should always be considered in any horse exhibiting signs of CNS disease. Horses displaying such signs should be subjected to a thorough neurologic examination and appropriate laboratory tests undertaken both to support a diagnosis of EPM and to exclude other likely diagnoses. Laboratory testing should be considered ancillary and not a substitute for an in-depth clinical examination. In many cases of EPM, there is asymmetry of gait and focal muscle atrophy; when present, EPM should be high on the list of possible causes. This combination of signs has proved to be a very useful distinguishing feature of the disease and is helpful in clinically differentiating EPM from similar neurologic conditions affecting the horse.

Differential Diagnoses

Virtually any neurologic disease of horses can produce clinical signs that mimic those associated with cases of EPM. Cervical vertebral stenotic myelopathy (CVSM) is a frequently encountered disease that results from developmental compression of the cervical spinal cord. CVSM signs usually are symmetric and, typically, the pelvic limbs are more severely affected than the thoracic limbs. Focal muscle atrophy is not a clinical feature of CVSM. In horses with clinical signs that localize neuroanatomically to the cervical spinal cord, radiographs of the cervical vertebrae should be taken to determine the intervertebral and intravertebral sagittal ratios (**Fig. 3**). Trauma also can cause spinal cord damage at any level, potentially causing abnormal neurologic signs in from one to all limbs.

A history of respiratory disease or an outbreak of abortion is a common prelude to the occurrence of EHV-1-myelopathy (EHM). Affected horses may be febrile shortly before or at the sudden onset of neurologic signs. Neurologic signs most commonly are symmetric with primary pelvic limb weakness and ataxia, bladder distention,

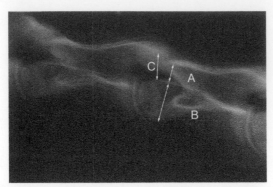

Fig. 3. Radiograph of the cervical vertebrae to assess intervertebral and intravertebral sagittal ratios. A/B is the intravertebral sagittal ratio. A/C is the intervertebral sagittal ratio.

usually without incontinence, and, more rarely, perineal and tail hypalgesia, tail and penile paralysis, and fecal retention. Signs of brain involvement are seen rarely.

Equine motor neuron disease (EMND) also produces signs that initially may be confused with those observed in horses affected with EPM. Severe limb weakness with muscle fasciculations and tremors are typical, early signs of EMND. With chronicity, there is widespread, profound, muscle atrophy.

Other causes of spinal cord disease that may result in similar clinical signs include extradural masses (neoplasms, abscesses, synovial cysts, hematomas, and granulomas), spinal cord or meningeal tumors, trauma, migrating metazoan parasites, rabies, West Nile viral encephalomyelitis, equine neuroaxonal dystrophy/equine degenerative myeloencephalopathy (eNAD/EDM), lead poisoning, creeping indigo toxicity, vascular malformations, and discospondylopathies. Any of the many equine diseases of the brain or cranial nerves must be considered as potential rule-outs in cases of EPM showing signs attributable to the dysfunction of the brain or cranial nerves. This list includes viral encephalitis, neoplasia, head trauma, Lyme neuroborreliosis, brain abscess, migrating parasites, temporohyoid osteoarthropathy, polyneuritis equi, cholesterinic granuloma, thromboembolic encephalopathy, acquired epilepsy, metabolic derangement, and hepatic encephalopathy.

Postmortem Diagnosis

Confirmation of EPM on postmortem examination is based on the demonstration of protozoa in CNS lesions, although the histologic diagnosis frequently is made presumptively even when parasites are not detected if the characteristic inflammatory changes are found. In 2 reported series, organisms were seen in H&E sections of CNS tissue in 10% to 36% of suspected cases.[29,80] Sensitivity was increased from 20% to 51% by immune-staining with antibody against S. neurona.[80] The likelihood of finding organisms is reduced by prior treatment with antiprotozoal drugs and may be increased by treatment with corticosteroids.

Immunodiagnostic Testing

As described, EPM occurs only in a small proportion of horses infected with either S. neurona or N. hughesi.[50] As a consequence, the simple detection of antibodies against these parasites has minimal diagnostic value. Even the presence of antibodies in the CSF is not a definitive indicator of EPM since there is a normal passive transfer of antibody across an intact blood–brain barrier (BBB).[81] Therefore, immunodiagnostic testing was eschewed for many years by some veterinary practitioners due to the lack of confidence in the test results.

Immunodiagnosis of EPM has improved greatly in recent years due to the development of semiquantitative assays and the utilization of diagnostic methodologies that detect intrathecal production of specific protozoal antibodies, indicative of active protozoal infection in the CNS. The Goldmann–Witmer coefficient (C-value) and the antigen-specific antibody index (AI) are tests of proportionality that assess whether there is a greater amount of pathogen-specific antibody in the CSF than would be present due to normal passive transfer across the BBB. Application of these tests to a sample set of 29 clinical cases demonstrated the value of this methodology for accurate EPM diagnosis.[82] Moreover, many EPM cases have antibody titers in CSF that far exceed that which would be present due to passive transfer across the BBB. Two studies examining an extensive collection of horses with neurologic disease demonstrated that a simple ratio of serum:CSF *S. neurona* titers was sufficient to reveal intrathecal antibody production and an accurate diagnosis of EPM caused by *S. neurona*.[83,84] Therefore, the use of the more expensive and laborious C-value or AI can be limited to cases that have uncompelling ELISA titer results (ie, the serum:CSF ratio equals the cut-off) and/or abnormally high CSF albumin concentration (including conditions associated with a "leaky" BBB).

Although the use of serum:CSF titer ratios has not been investigated for *N. hughesi* infection, it is likely that this serodiagnostic approach will be valuable for the diagnosis of EPM caused by this parasite.

Several serologic assays are available to measure antibodies against *S. neurona* or *N. hughesi* and can be used to assess intrathecal antibody production. Enzyme-linked immunosorbent assays (ELISAs) have been developed based on parasite antigens expressed as recombinant proteins in *E. coli*.[40,85–88] Specifically, the SnSAG and NhSAG surface antigens from *S. neurona* or *N. hughesi*, respectively, have been used as the serologic targets for ELISAs since these surface proteins are abundant and typically elicit robust antibody responses in horses that have been infected with either of these two parasite species.[89–91] ELISAs based on the SnSAG2, SnSAG3, and SnSAG4 surface antigens have been validated extensively and were used to demonstrate the value of specific intrathecal antibody detection.[83,84] These assays are currently offered commercially for EPM diagnostic testing (Equine Diagnostic Solutions, LLC).

The *S. neurona* indirect fluorescent antibody test (IFAT) uses whole, culture-derived *S. neurona* merozoites as the antigen source. Like ELISA, this assay yields an endpoint antibody titer and can be used to detect intrathecal antibody production. The *S. neurona* IFAT was optimized and validated at the University of California-Davis[92,93] and is currently offered by their Veterinary Diagnostic Laboratory. Additionally, the UC-Davis facility offers an IFAT based on *N. hughesi* tachyzoites to detect antibodies against this alternative EPM parasite.

An ELISA based on the SnSAG1 surface protein has been described.[85] However, it has been found that this protein is not expressed by all strains of *S. neurona*,[62] thereby reducing its utility for antibody detection[86] and EPM diagnosis.[94] Assays that combine SnSAG1 with 2 additional SnSAGs (SnSAG5 and SnSAG6) are currently offered commercially (Pathogenes, Inc.; Prota, LLC). However, there are no published reports describing the validation of the assays so their reliability remains uncertain.

For immunodiagnosis of EPM caused by *N. hughesi,* an ELISA based on the NhSAG1 surface protein yields high sensitivity and specificity when compared with the gold standard (Western blot) for detecting antibodies against this parasite.[46] The NhSAG1 ELISA is offered commercially by Equine Diagnostic Solutions, LLC.

Although serum antibody titers have been used to estimate the probability of EPM,[93] seemingly obviating the need for CSF collection and testing, studies that have used diverse collections of neurologic disease cases have shown that a serum titer alone is a poor predictor of EPM.[83,84]

The use of several different biomarkers to aid EPM diagnosis has been investigated, with mixed results. Concentrations of heavy-chain phosphorylated neurofilaments[95] and soluble CD14[96] were found to be elevated in EPM horses, suggesting that these might be useful adjuncts for diagnosis. The acute phase proteins C-reactive protein and serum amyloid A were similarly investigated,[97] but neither was found to be helpful for identifying EPM horses. A recent study examining the use of a real-time PCR assay to detect parasite DNA in CSF samples suggests that this approach might improve the accuracy of diagnostic testing for EPM (**Box 2**).[98]

TREATMENT
Folate-inhibiting Drugs

A combination of sulfadiazine and pyrimethamine (SDZ/PYR), which block successive steps in protozoal folate synthesis, was one of the initial therapies for the treatment of EPM. A dosage regimen of PYR, 1 mg/kg, and SDZ, 20 mg/kg, administered once daily by mouth for at least 6 months has been considered the "standard" treatment of EPM. Because dietary folate can interfere with the uptake of diaminopyrimidine drugs such as PYR,[99] hay should not be fed for 2 hours before or after treatment. PYR given orally to horses at 1 mg/kg/d achieves a concentration of approximately 0.02 to 0.1 µg/mL in the CSF 4 to 6 h after administration.[100] Interestingly, these horses were allowed free access to prairie hay during this study, potentially reducing the bioavailability of the drug.[99] Additionally, as PYR is concentrated in CNS tissue relative to plasma,[101] the concentration at the desired site of action may be >0.1 µg/mL. Mean peak CSF concentrations of sulfonamide after single or multiple dosing (22–44 mg/kg) have been reported to be approximately 2 to 8 µg/mL.[102,103] The combination of sulfadiazine and pyrimethamine is available as an FDA-approved product for the treatment of EPM (ReBalance; PRN Pharmacal).

Pyrimethamine has significant adverse side effects, especially when used at a high nonstandard dose rate. Toxicity reflects both direct effects and inhibition of host folate synthesis. Serious side effects fortunately are rare but may include potentially fatal convulsions and recumbency, reproductive and neonatal disorders, oral ulcers, and signs of bone marrow suppression including leukopenia, neutropenia, anemia, and thrombocytopenia in decreasing frequency.[104–106] Pyrimethamine is considered teratogenic and causes both abortions and birth of malformed pups in treated rats.[107] At least 4 cases of a fatal syndrome have been observed in neonatal foals born to mares that were given these drugs during the latter stages of pregnancy.(R. MacKay,

---

Box 2
Achieving an accurate diagnosis of EPM

- Confirm the presence of clinical signs consistent with EPM by conducting a thorough neurologic examination
- Rule out other potential causes using available tools (eg, cervical radiography)
- Use immunodiagnostic testing to assess intrathecal antibody production against *S. neurona* or *N. hughesi*

unpublished observations, 1978-81)[106] Three of the mares had been supplemented with folic acid. Evidence from other species would suggest that supplementation with folic acid (a synthetic nonreduced form of folate) either won't prevent PYR-induced toxicity[108] or may even exacerbate it.[107] In light of these observations, the supplemental use of folic acid in SDZ/PYR treated horses cannot be justified. Most cases of bone marrow suppression resolve if treatment is suspended for 1 to 2 weeks. Folic acid (100 mg daily) is appropriate for the treatment of folate deficiency once PYR is discontinued. If signs are severe, treatment with folinic acid (100 mg IV or PO daily for 5 days) is indicated.

Triazines

Over the past 20+ years, 2 members of the triazine group of coccidiostats, diclazuril, and ponazuril (toltrazuril sulfone), have been approved by the FDA for the treatment of EPM. These drugs have been shown to have broad-spectrum anticoccidial activity in many avian and mammalian species and are thought to target the parasite's apicoplast organelle and mitochondrion.[109] The activity of triazine compounds against *S. neurona* was initially shown *in vitro*.[110,111] In horses, pharmacokinetic studies have established that therapeutic steady-state concentrations of both diclazuril and ponazuril are achieved by day 7 using labeled doses.[112,113] Moreover, use of a loading dose of ponazuril at 15 mg/kg (ie, 3 times the standard treatment dose rate) resulted in steady-state concentrations in blood and CSF by day 2.[114] Coadministration of corn oil has also been found to increase serum and CSF concentrations of ponazuril.[115]

An initial study using horses experimentally challenged with *S. neurona* showed that weekly treatment with ponazuril in paste formulation reduced antibody production against the parasite.[116] Subsequent work demonstrated that half doses of diclazuril (ie, 0.5 mg/kg), given daily as a pelleted top-dressing on feed, reached therapeutically effective levels in serum and CSF[117] and reduced seroconversion rates and antibody titers in naturally exposed foals and adult horses.[118,119] Collectively, these studies suggest that intermittent treatment with low doses of the triazine drugs might be an effective prophylactic for reducing parasite infection and the risk of EPM.

The formulations of these drugs adapted for clinical use in horses are Protazil (1.56% diclazuril; Merck Animal Health, Kansas City, KS) and Marquis (15% ponazuril; Boehringer Ingelheim Animal Health, Duluth, GA).

Another drug used commonly as an anticoccidial in calves, decoquinate, was evaluated in horses with presumptive EPM, at a dosage of 0.5 mg/kg daily for 10 days, in combination with the immunomodulator levamisole, 1 mg/kg daily.[120] Success rates of 93.6% and 89.3% were reported on the basis of improved neurologic gait score at the end of treatment and reversion of serum snSAG1,5,6 titers, respectively. Decoquinate was also shown to have potent inhibitory and cidal activity in vitro against 2 different isolates of *S. neurona*.[121] If this drug combination continues to perform well in wider use, it will obviously become an important treatment option. Additional antiprotozoal drugs are currently under investigation for use against *S. neurona* infection and treatment of EPM. Bumped kinase inhibitors (BKIs) that specifically target parasite calcium-dependent protein kinases have shown promise for the treatment of a variety of diseases caused by apicomplexan pathogens.[122] Growth of *S. neurona* is inhibited by BKIs at low nanomolar concentrations and proved effective for treating *S. neurona* in a murine infection model.[123] Use of transgenic *S. neurona* expressing firefly luciferase in a high throughput screen of an NIH clinical collection library of compounds identified 18 compounds that inhibited parasite growth.[124] While the BKIs and these newly identified compounds are promising antiprotozoal drugs that might prove effective for EPM treatment, significant work remains to be conducted before they will be ready for clinical use.

Antiinflammatory Therapy

Nonsteroidal antiinflammatory drugs such as flunixin meglumine are frequently given to moderately or severely affected horses during the first 3 to 7 days of antiprotozoal therapy. In the case of horses that are in danger of falling down or exhibit signs of brain involvement, the additional use of corticosteroids (0.1 mg/kg of dexamethasone twice daily) and dimethyl sulfoxide (1 g/kg as a 10% solution IV or by nasogastric tube twice daily) for the first several days may control the inflammatory response and associated clinical signs. Because the damaged CNS is susceptible to oxidant injury, it has become common practice to use pharmacologic doses of the antioxidant vitamin E (eg, 20 IU/kg daily per os) throughout the treatment period of horses. Although vitamin E therapy may not significantly alter the course of recovery, it is unlikely to cause harm.

Biological Response Modifiers

On the basis of the assumption that horses that develop EPM may be immune-compromised, immunomodulators have been included by some in the treatment of the disease. The drugs used include levamisole (1 mg/kg orally BID for the first 2 weeks of antiprotozoal therapy and for the first week of each month thereafter), killed P acnes (Eqstim; Neogen, Lansing, MI), mycobacterial wall extract (Equimune IV; Bioniche Animal Health Vetoquinol, Belville, Ontario, Canada), and transfer factor (4Life Transfer Factor, 4LifeResearch, Sandy, UT). No study has been published to date to evaluate the efficacy of these ancillary treatments in horses with EPM (**Box 3**).

PREVENTION

The prevention of EPM is difficult due to the widespread distribution of the etiologic agents in many parts of the US. Methods for effective control of this disease have not been delineated; however, it is prudent to attempt to eliminate known risk factors.

Access to opossums and other wildlife or pests to feed and water should be eliminated. Cereal grains should be kept in rodent-proof containers and forages should be protected from wildlife access by use of enclosed facilities. Although it remains unconfirmed whether insects such as flies and cockroaches can serve as biological vectors that transport S. neurona sporocysts, controlling the insect population on farms is advisable.

The case histories of EPM-affected horses frequently indicate previous adverse health events.[54] Close monitoring is warranted of heavily pregnant or lactating mares and of horses that have recently experienced a major illness, injury, or been transported a considerable distance or under arduous conditions.

Box 3
Treatment of EPM

- Use one of the FDA-approved anticoccidial drugs to eliminate CNS infection
  - Ponazuril (Marquis, Boehringer Ingelheim Animal Health
  - Diclazuril (Protazil, Merck Animal Health)
  - Sulfadiazine/Pyrimethamine (eg, ReBalance, PRN Pharmacal)
- Give supportive antiinflammatory therapy, as needed

Protective immunization against *S. neurona* and *N. hughesi* would be the ideal approach to prevent EPM. However, difficulties experienced in developing vaccines against other protozoan pathogens suggest that this approach may take many years to achieve. A conditional license was given for a killed *S. neurona* vaccine, but this product has been withdrawn as efficacy was not demonstrated.[125]

Perhaps of more immediate value would be the use of antiprotozoal drugs given according to a protocol that would allow initial infection and short-term immunity (ie, metaphylaxis) but prevent spread to the CNS. Any of the therapeutic drugs that are thought to kill *S. neurona* (eg, the triazine compounds) would be logical candidates for this intermittent preventative approach.

SUMMARY

Since EPM was initially described in the 1960s, diagnosis, treatment, and prevention have improved through advances in the understanding of the parasite and the disease. Epidemiologic studies have identified numerous risk factors associated with the development of the disease. Despite generally high seroprevalence of *S. neurona* in horses in the Americas, the annual incidence of EPM is less than 1%, thus demonstrating that infection does not equate with disease. Therefore, further studies are needed to gain a better understanding of the pathogenesis of parasite infection and the occurrence of EPM. Moreover, questions remain about the mode(s) of transmission and the contribution of *N. hughesi* to EPM incidence, so additional work is needed in this area. Challenge studies have confirmed that horses can be experimentally infected with *S. neurona*. However, severe and persistent clinical signs and abnormal CNS histology are not seen consistently. Several FDA-approved EPM treatments are now available. The development of an effective EPM vaccine remains a long-term goal, while prophylactic treatment with an antiprotozoal drug may be a viable preventative.

DISCLOSURE

D.K. Howe is the inventor listed on patents covering the assays offered for EPM diagnosis by Equine Diagnostic Solutions, LLC.

REFERENCES

1. Rooney JR, Prickett ME, Delaney FM, et al. Focal myelitis-encephalitis in horses. Cornell Vet 1970;60:494–501.
2. Prickett ME. Equine spinal ataxia. Paper presented at: 14th Annual Convention of the American Association of Equine Practitioners1968; Philadelphia, PA.
3. Cusick PK, Sells DM, Hamilton DP, et al. Toxoplasmosis in two horses. J Am Vet Med Assoc 1974;164(1):77–80.
4. Mayhew IG, De Lahunta A, Whitlock RH, et al. Equine protozoal myeloencephalitis. Proc Annu Conv Am Assoc Equine Pract 1977;22d:107–14.
5. Dubey JP, Davis SW, Speer CA, et al. *Sarcocystis neurona* n. sp. (Protozoa: Apicomplexa), the etiologic agent of equine protozoal myeloencephalitis. J Parasitol 1991;77(2):212–8.
6. Cheadle MA, Lindsay DS, Rowe S, et al. Prevalence of antibodies to *Neospora* sp. in horses from Alabama and characterisation of an isolate recovered from a naturally infected horse [corrected]. Int J Parasitol 1999;29(10):1537–43.
7. Dubey JP, Liddell S, Mattson D, et al. Characterization of the Oregon isolate of *Neospora hughesi* from a horse. J Parasitol 2001;87(2):345–53.

8. Hamir AN, Tornquist SJ, Gerros TC, et al. *Neospora caninum*-associated equine protozoal myeloencephalitis. Vet Parasitol 1998;79(4):269–74.
9. Marsh AE, Barr BC, Madigan J, et al. Neosporosis as a cause of equine protozoal myeloencephalitis. J Am Vet Med Assoc 1996;209(11):1907–13.
10. Lindsay DS, Steinberg H, Dubielzig RR, et al. Central nervous system neosporosis in a foal. J Vet Diagn Invest 1996;8(4):507–10.
11. Fenger CK, Granstrom DE, Langemeier JL, et al. Identification of opossums (*Didelphis virginiana*) as the putative definitive host of *Sarcocystis neurona*. J Parasitol 1995;81(6):916–9.
12. Dubey JP, Lindsay DS, Kerber CE, et al. First isolation of *Sarcocystis neurona* from the South American opossum, *Didelphis albiventris*, from Brazil. Vet Parasitol 2001;95(2–4):295–304.
13. Cheadle MA, Yowell CA, Sellon DC, et al. The striped skunk (*Mephitis mephitis*) is an intermediate host for *Sarcocystis neurona*. Int J Parasitol 2001;31(8):843–9.
14. Dubey JP, Saville WJ, Stanek JF, et al. *Sarcocystis neurona* infections in raccoons (*Procyon lotor*): evidence for natural infection with sarcocysts, transmission of infection to opossums (*Didelphis virginiana*), and experimental induction of neurologic disease in raccoons. Vet Parasitol 2001;100(3–4): 117–29.
15. Cheadle MA, Tanhauser SM, Dame JB, et al. The nine-banded armadillo (*Dasypus novemcinctus*) is an intermediate host for *Sarcocystis neurona*. Int J Parasitol 2001;31(4):330–5.
16. Dubey JP, Saville WJ, Lindsay DS, et al. Completion of the life cycle of *Sarcocystis neurona*. J Parasitol 2000;86(6):1276–80.
17. Barbosa L, Johnson CK, Lambourn DM, et al. A novel Sarcocystis neurona genotype XIII is associated with severe encephalitis in an unexpectedly broad range of marine mammals from the northeastern Pacific Ocean. Int J Parasitol 2015;45(9–10):595–603.
18. Dubey JP. Prevalence of *Sarcocystis* species sporocysts in wild-caught opossums (*Didelphis virginiana*). J Parasitol 2000;86(4):705–10.
19. Mullaney T, Murphy AJ, Kiupel M, et al. Evidence to support horses as natural intermediate hosts for *Sarcocystis neurona*. Vet Parasitol 2005;133(1):27–36.
20. Pivoto FL, de Macedo AG Jr, da Silva MV, et al. Serological status of mares in parturition and the levels of antibodies (IgG) against protozoan family Sarcocystidae from their pre colostral foals. Vet Parasitol 2014;199(1–2):107–11.
21. Pusterla N, Mackie S, Packham A, et al. Serological investigation of transplacental infection with *Neospora hughesi* and *Sarcocystis neurona* in broodmares. Vet J 2014;202(3):649–50.
22. McAllister MM, Dubey JP, Lindsay DS, et al. Dogs are definitive hosts of *Neospora caninum*. Int J Parasitol 1998;28(9):1473–8.
23. Antonello AM, Pivoto FL, Camillo G, et al. The importance of vertical transmission of *Neospora* sp. in naturally infected horses. Vet Parasitol 2012;187(3–4): 367–70.
24. Pusterla N, Conrad PA, Packham AE, et al. Endogenous transplacental transmission of *Neospora hughesi* in naturally infected horses. J Parasitol 2011; 97(2):281–5.
25. Anderson JA, Alves DA, Cerqueira-Cézar CK, et al. Histologically, immunohistochemically, ultrastructurally, and molecularly confirmed neosporosis abortion in an aborted equine fetus. Vet Parasitol 2019;270:20–4.
26. Leszkowicz Mazuz M, Mimoun L, Schvartz G, et al. Detection of *Neospora caninum* Infection in Aborted Equine Fetuses in Israel. Pathogens 2020;9(11):962.

27. Ruppert S, Lee JK, Marsh AE. Equine Protozoal Myeloencephalitis associated with Neospora caninum in a USA captive bred zebra (Equus zebra). Vet Parasitol Reg Stud Rep 2021;26:100620.
28. Fayer R, Mayhew IG, Baird JD, et al. Epidemiology of equine protozoal myeloencephalitis in North America based on histologically confirmed cases. J Vet Intern Med 1990;4(2):54–7.
29. Boy MG, Galligan DT, Divers TJ. Protozoal encephalomyelitis in horses: 82 cases (1972-1986). J Am Vet Med Assoc 1990;196(4):632–4.
30. Bentz BG, Granstrom DE, Stamper S. Seroprevalence of antibodies to Sarcocystis neurona in horses residing in a county of southeastern Pennsylvania. J Am Vet Med Assoc 1997;210(4):517–8.
31. Bentz BG, Ealey KA, Morrow J, et al. Seroprevalence of antibodies to Sarcocystis neurona in equids residing in Oklahoma. J Vet Diagn Invest 2003;15: 597–600.
32. Blythe LL, Granstrom DE, Hansen DE, et al. Seroprevalence of antibodies to Sarcocystis neurona in horses residing in Oregon. J Am Vet Med Assoc 1997; 210(4):525–7.
33. Saville WJ, Reed SM, Granstrom DE, et al. Seroprevalence of antibodies to Sarcocystis neurona in horses residing in Ohio. J Am Vet Med Assoc 1997;210(4): 519–24.
34. Tillotson K, McCue PM, Granstrom DE, et al. Seroprevalence of antibodies to Sarcocystis neurona in horses residing in northern Colorado. J Equine Vet Sci 1999;19(2):122–6.
35. James KE, Smith WA, Conrad PA, et al. Seroprevalences of anti-Sarcocystis neurona and anti-Neospora hughesi antibodies among healthy equids in the United States. J Am Vet Med Assoc 2017;250(11):1291–301.
36. Dubey JP, Kerber CE, Granstrom DE. Serologic prevalence of Sarcocystis neurona, Toxoplasma gondii, and Neospora caninum in horses in Brazil. J Am Vet Med Assoc 1999;215(7):970–2.
37. Dubey JP, Venturini MC, Venturini L, et al. Prevalence of antibodies to Sarcocystis neurona, Toxoplasma gondii and Neospora caninum in horses from Argentina. Vet Parasitol 1999;86(1):59–62.
38. Dangoudoubiyam S, Oliveira JB, Viquez C, et al. Detection of antibodies against Sarcocystis neurona, Neospora spp., and Toxoplasma gondii in horses from Costa Rica. J Parasitol 2011;97(3):522–4.
39. Hoane JS, Gennari SM, Dubey JP, et al. Prevalence of Sarcocystis neurona and Neospora spp. infection in horses from Brazil based on presence of serum antibodies to parasite surface antigen. Vet Parasitol 2006;136(2):155–9.
40. Bartova E, Sedlak K, Syrova M, et al. Neospora spp. and Toxoplasma gondii antibodies in horses in the Czech Republic. Parasitol Res 2010;107(4):783–5.
41. Dubey JP, Mitchell SM, Morrow JK, et al. Prevalence of antibodies to Neospora caninum, Sarcocystis neurona, and Toxoplasma gondii in wild horses from central Wyoming. J Parasitol 2003;89(4):716–20.
42. Pitel PH, Pronost S, Romand S, et al. Prevalence of antibodies to Neospora caninum in horses in France. Equine Vet J 2001;33(2):205–7.
43. Vardeleon D, Marsh AE, Thorne JG, et al. Prevalence of Neospora hughesi and Sarcocystis neurona antibodies in horses from various geographical locations. Vet Parasitol 2001;95(2–4):273–82.
44. Villalobos EM, Furman KE, Lara Mdo C, et al. Detection of Neospora sp. antibodies in cart horses from urban areas of Curitiba, Southern Brazil. Rev Bras Parasitol 2012;21(1):68–70.

45. Gupta GD, Lakritz J, Kim JH, et al. Seroprevalence of *Neospora, Toxoplasma gondii* and *Sarcocystis neurona* antibodies in horses from Jeju island, South Korea. Vet Parasitol 2002;106(3):193–201.

46. Hoane JS, Yeargan MR, Stamper S, et al. Recombinant NhSAG1 ELISA: a sensitive and specific assay for detecting antibodies against *Neospora hughesi* in equine serum. J Parasitol 2005;91(2):446–52.

47. Javanmardi E, Majidiani H, Shariatzadeh SA, et al. Global seroprevalence of Neospora spp. in horses and donkeys: A systematic review and meta-analysis. Vet Parasitol 2020;288:109299.

48. Gondim LF, Lindsay DS, McAllister MM. Canine and bovine *Neospora caninum* control sera examined for cross-reactivity using *Neospora caninum* and *Neospora hughesi* indirect fluorescent antibody tests. J Parasitol 2009;95(1):86–8.

49. Packham AE, Conrad PA, Wilson WD, et al. Qualitative evaluation of selective tests for detection of *Neospora hughesi* antibodies in serum and cerebrospinal fluid of experimentally infected horses. J Parasitol 2002;88(6):1239–46.

50. NAHMS. Equine Protozoal Myeloencephalitis (EPM) in the U.S. In: USDA:APHIS:VS. Fort Collins, CO: Centers for Epidemiology and Animal Health; 2001. p. 1–46.

51. MacKay RJ, Davis SW, Dubey JP. Equine protozoal myeloencephalitis. Compend Contin Educ Pract Vet 1992;14(10):1359–67.

52. Fenger CK, Granstrom DE, Langemeier JL, et al. Epizootic of equine protozoal myeloencephalitis on a farm. J Am Vet Med Assoc 1997;210(7):923–7.

53. Granstrom DE, Alvarez O Jr, Dubey JP, et al. Equine protozoal myelitis in Panamanian horses and isolation of *Sarcocystis neurona*. J Parasitol 1992;78(5):909–12.

54. Saville WJ, Reed SM, Morley PS, et al. Analysis of risk factors for the development of equine protozoal myeloencephalitis in horses. J Am Vet Med Assoc 2000;217(8):1174–80.

55. Saville WJ, Morley PS, Reed SM, et al. Evaluation of risk factors associated with clinical improvement and survival of horses with equine protozoal myeloencephalitis. J Am Vet Med Assoc 2000;217(8):1181–5.

56. Saville WJ, Stich RW, Reed SM, et al. Utilization of stress in the development of an equine model for equine protozoal myeloencephalitis. Vet Parasitol 2001;95(2–4):211–22.

57. Sofaly CD, Reed SM, Gordon JC, et al. Experimental induction of equine protozoan myeloencephalitis (EPM) in the horse: effect of *Sarcocystis neurona* sporocyst inoculation dose on the development of clinical neurologic disease. J Parasitol 2002;88(6):1164–70.

58. Cutler TJ, MacKay RJ, Ginn PE, et al. Immunoconversion against *Sarcocystis neurona* in normal and dexamethasone-treated horses challenged with S. neurona sporocysts. Vet Parasitol 2001;95(2–4):197–210.

59. Saville WJ, Sofaly CD, Reed SM, et al. An equine protozoal myeloencephalitis challenge model testing a second transport after inoculation with *Sarcocystis neurona* sporocysts. J Parasitol 2004;90(6):1406–10.

60. Asmundsson IM, Dubey JP, Rosenthal BM. A genetically diverse but distinct North American population of *Sarcocystis neurona* includes an overrepresented clone described by 12 microsatellite alleles. Infect Genet Evol 2006;6(5):352–60.

61. Elsheikha HM, Schott HC 2nd, Mansfield LS. Genetic variation among isolates of *Sarcocystis neurona*, the agent of protozoal myeloencephalitis, as revealed by

amplified fragment length polymorphism markers. Infect Immun 2006;74(6): 3448–54.

62. Howe DK, Gaji RY, Marsh AE, et al. Strains of *Sarcocystis neurona* exhibit differences in their surface antigens, including the absence of the major surface antigen SnSAG1. Int J Parasitol 2008;38(6):623–31.

63. Wendte JM, Miller MA, Lambourn DM, et al. Self-mating in the definitive host potentiates clonal outbreaks of the apicomplexan parasites *Sarcocystis neurona* and *Toxoplasma gondii*. PLoS Genet 2010;6(12):e1001261.

64. James KE, Smith WA, Packham AE, et al. *Toxoplasma gondii* seroprevalence and association with equine protozoal myeloencephalitis: A case-control study of Californian horses. Vet J 2017;224:38–43.

65. Schale S, Howe D, Yeargan M, et al. Protozoal coinfection in horses with equine protozoal myeloencephalitis in the eastern United States. J Vet Intern Med 2018; 32(3):1210–4.

66. Dubey JP, Murata FHA, Cerqueira-Cézar CK, et al. *Toxoplasma gondii* infections in horses, donkeys, and other equids: The last decade. Res Vet Sci 2020;132: 492–9.

67. Kimble KM, Gomez G, Szule JA, et al. Systemic Toxoplasmosis in a Horse. J Comp Pathol 2021;182:27–31.

68. Dubey JP, Lindsay DS. Isolation in immunodeficient mice of *Sarcocystis neurona* from opossum (*Didelphis virginiana*) faeces, and its differentiation from *Sarcocystis falcatula*. Int J Parasitol 1998;28(12):1823–8.

69. Marsh AE, Barr BC, Lakritz J, et al. Experimental infection of nude mice as a model for *Sarcocystis neurona*-associated encephalitis. Parasitol Res 1997; 83(7):706–11.

70. Witonsky SG, Gogal RM Jr, Duncan RB Jr, et al. Prevention of meningo/encephalomyelitis due to *Sarcocystis neurona* infection in mice is mediated by CD8 cells. Int J Parasitol 2005;35(1):113–23.

71. Sellon DC, Knowles DP, Greiner EC, et al. Depletion of natural killer cells does not result in neurologic disease due to *Sarcocystis neurona* in mice with severe combined immunodeficiency. J Parasitol 2004;90(4):782–8.

72. Hay AN, Potter A, Lindsay D, et al. Interferon gamma protective against *Sarcocystis neurona* encephalitis in susceptible murine model. Vet Immunol Immunopathol 2021;240:110319.

73. Spencer JA, Ellison SE, Guarino AJ, et al. Cell-mediated immune responses in horses with equine protozoal myeloencephalitis. J Parasitol 2004;90(2):428–30.

74. Fenger CK, Granstrom DE, Gajadhar AA, et al. Experimental induction of equine protozoal myeloencephalitis in horses using *Sarcocystis* sp. sporocysts from the opossum (*Didelphis virginiana*). Vet Parasitol 1997;68(3):199–213.

75. Tanhauser SM, Yowell CA, Cutler TJ, et al. Multiple DNA markers differentiate *Sarcocystis neurona* and *Sarcocystis falcatula*. J Parasitol 1999;85(2):221–8.

76. Ellison SP, Greiner E, Brown KK, et al. Experimental infection of horses with culture-derived *Sarcocystis neurona* merozoites as a model for equine protozoal myeloencephalitis. Int J App Res Vet Med 2004;2(2):79–89.

77. Dunigan CE, Oglesbee MJ, Podell M, et al. Seizure Activity Associated with Equine Protozoal Myeloencephalitis. Prog Vet Neurol 1995;6(2):50–4.

78. Reed SM, Granstrom DE. Equine protozoal encephalomyelitis. Paper presented at: 13th Annual Veterinary Medical Forum of the American College of Veterinary Internal Medicine, May 18-21,1995, Lake Buena Vista, FL.

79. Mayhew IG, deLahunta A, Whitlock RH, et al. Spinal cord disease in the horse. Cornell Vet 1978;68(Suppl 6):1–207.

80. Hamir AN, Moser G, Galligan DT, et al. Immunohistochemical study to demonstrate *Sarcocystis neurona* in equine protozoal myeloencephalitis. J Vet Diagn Invest 1993;5(3):418–22.

81. Furr M. Antigen-specific antibodies in cerebrospinal fluid after intramuscular injection of ovalbumin in horses. J Vet Intern Med 2002;16(5):588–92.

82. Furr M, Howe D, Reed S, et al. Antibody coefficients for the diagnosis of equine protozoal myeloencephalitis. J Vet Intern Med 2011;25(1):138–42.

83. Johnson AL, Morrow JK, Sweeney RW. Indirect Fluorescent Antibody Test and Surface Antigen ELISAs for Antemortem Diagnosis of Equine Protozoal Myeloencephalitis. J Vet Intern Med 2013;27(3):596–9.

84. Reed SM, Howe DK, Morrow JK, et al. Accurate antemortem diagnosis of equine protozoal myeloencephalitis (EPM) based on detecting intrathecal antibodies against *Sarcocystis neurona* using the SnSAG2 and SnSAG4/3 ELISAs. J Vet Intern Med 2013;27(5):1193–200.

85. Ellison SP, Kennedy T, Brown KK. Development of an ELISA to Detect Antibodies to rSAG1 in the Horse. J Appl Res Vet Med 2003;1(4):318–27.

86. Hoane JS, Morrow J, Saville WJ, et al. Enzyme-Linked Immunosorbent Assays for Detection of Equine Antibodies Specific to *Sarcocystis neurona* Surface Antigens. Clin Diagn Lab Immunol 2005;12(9):1050–6.

87. Yeargan MR, Howe DK. Improved detection of equine antibodies against *Sarcocystis neurona* using polyvalent ELISAs based on the parasite SnSAG surface antigens. Vet Parasitol 2011;176(1):16–22.

88. Yeargan M, de Assis Rocha I, Morrow J, et al. A new trivalent SnSAG surface antigen chimera for efficient detection of antibodies against *Sarcocystis neurona* and diagnosis of equine protozoal myeloencephalitis. J Vet Diagn Invest 2015;27(3):377–81.

89. Ellison SP, Omara-Opyene AL, Yowell CA, et al. Molecular characterisation of a major 29 kDa surface antigen of *Sarcocystis neurona*. Int J Parasitol 2002;32(2):217–25.

90. Howe DK, Gaji RY, Mroz-Barrett M, et al. *Sarcocystis neurona* merozoites express a family of immunogenic surface antigens that are orthologues of the *Toxoplasma gondii* surface antigens (SAGs) and SAG-related sequences. Infect Immun 2005;73(2):1023–33.

91. Marsh AE, Howe DK, Wang G, et al. Differentiation of *Neospora hughesi* from *Neospora caninum* based on their immunodominant surface antigen, SAG1 and SRS2. Int J Parasitol 1999;29(10):1575–82.

92. Duarte PC, Daft BM, Conrad PA, et al. Comparison of serum indirect fluorescent antibody test with two Western blot tests for the diagnosis of equine protozoal myeloencephalitis. J Vet Diagn Invest 2003;15(1):8–13.

93. Duarte PC, Daft BM, Conrad PA, et al. Evaluation and comparison of an indirect fluorescent antibody test for detection of antibodies to *Sarcocystis neurona*, using serum and cerebrospinal fluid of naturally and experimentally infected, and vaccinated horses. J Parasitol 2004;90(2):379–86.

94. Johnson AL, Burton AJ, Sweeney RW. Utility of 2 immunological tests for antemortem diagnosis of equine protozoal myeloencephalitis (*Sarcocystis neurona* infection) in naturally occurring cases. J Vet Intern Med 2010;24(5):1184–9.

95. Morales Gomez AM, Zhu S, Palmer S, et al. Analysis of neurofilament concentration in healthy adult horses and utility in the diagnosis of equine protozoal myeloencephalitis and equine motor neuron disease. Res Vet Sci 2019;125:1–6.

96. Hay AN, Wagner B, Leeth CM, et al. Horses affected by EPM have increased sCD14 compared to healthy horses. Vet Immunol Immunopathol 2021;242: 110338.
97. Mittelman NS, Stefanovski D, Johnson AL. Utility of C-reactive protein and serum amyloid A in the diagnosis of equine protozoal myeloencephalitis. J Vet Intern Med 2018;32(5):1726–30.
98. Bernardino PN, Smith WA, Conrad PA, et al. Molecular detection of *Sarcocystis neurona* in cerebrospinal fluid from 210 horses with suspected neurologic disease. Vet Parasitol 2021;291:109372.
99. Bogan JA, Galbraith A, Baxter P, et al. Effect of feeding on the fate of orally administered phenylbutazone, trimethoprim and sulphadiazine in the horse. Vet Rec 1984;115(23):599–600.
100. Clarke CR, MacAllister CG, Burrows GE, et al. Pharmacokinetics, penetration into cerebrospinal fluid, and hematologic effects after multiple oral administrations of pyrimethamine to horses. Am J Vet Res 1992;53(12):2296–9.
101. Cavallito JC, Nichol CA, Brenckman WD Jr, et al. Lipid-soluble inhibitors of dihydrofolate reductase. I. Kinetics, tissue distribution, and extent of metabolism of pyrimethamine, metoprine, and etoprine in the rat, dog, and man. Drug Metab Dispos 1978;6(3):329–37.
102. Brown CM, Morrow JK, Carleton CL, et al. Persistence of serum antibodies to *Sarcocystis neurona* in horses moved from North America to India. J Vet Intern Med 2006;20(4):994–7.
103. Green SL, Mayhew IG, Brown MP, et al. Concentrations of trimethoprim and sulfamethoxazole in cerebrospinal fluid and serum in mares with and without a dimethyl sulfoxide pretreatment. Can J Vet Res 1990;54(2):215–22.
104. MacKay RJ, McLellan J, Mallicote M. Pyrimethamine toxicosis in horses given a compounded medication. Equine Vet Ed 2017;30(12):e468–71.
105. Piercy RJ, Hinchcliff KW, Reed SM. Folate deficiency during treatment with orally administered folic acid, sulphadiazine and pyrimethamine in a horse with suspected equine protozoal myeloencephalitis (EPM). Equine Vet J 2002;34(3): 311–6.
106. Toribio RE, Bain FT, Mrad DR, et al. Congenital defects in newborn foals of mares treated for equine protozoal myeloencephalitis during pregnancy. J Am Vet Med Assoc 1998;212(5):697–701.
107. Chung MK, Han SS, Roh JK. Synergistic embryotoxicity of combination pyrimethamine and folic acid in rats. Reprod Toxicol 1993;7(5):463–8.
108. Castles TR, Kintner LD, Lee CC. The effects of folic or folinic acid on the toxicity of pyrimethamine in dogs. Toxicol Appl Pharmacol 1971;20(4):447–59.
109. Hackstein JH, Mackenstedt U, Mehlhorn H, et al. Parasitic apicomplexans harbor a chlorophyll a-D1 complex, the potential target for therapeutic triazines. Parasitol Res 1995;81(3):207–16.
110. Lindsay DS, Dubey JP. Determination of the activity of diclazuril against *Sarcocystis neurona* and *Sarcocystis falcatula* in cell cultures. J Parasitol 2000;86(1): 164–6.
111. Lindsay DS, Dubey JP, Kennedy TJ. Determination of the activity of ponazuril against *Sarcocystis neurona* in cell cultures. Vet Parasitol 2000;92(2):165–9.
112. Dirikolu L, Lehner F, Nattrass C, et al. Diclazuril in the horse: its identification and detection and preliminary pharmacokinetics. J Vet Pharmacol Ther 1999;22(6): 374–9.
113. Furr M, Kennedy T. Cerebrospinal fluid and serum concentrations of ponazuril in horses. Vet Ther 2001;2(3):232–7.

114. Reed SM, Wendel M, King S, et al. Pharmacokinetics of Ponazuril in Horses. Paper presented at: 58th Annual Convention of the American Association of Equine Practitioners, December 1-5, 2012; Anaheim, CA.

115. Furr M, Kennedy T. Effects of coadministration of corn oil and ponazuril on serum and cerebrospinal fluid concentrations of ponazuril in horses. J Vet Intern Med 2020;34(3):1321–4.

116. Mackay RJ, Tanhauser ST, Gillis KD, et al. Effect of intermittent oral administration of ponazuril on experimental *Sarcocystis neurona* infection of horses. Am J Vet Res 2008;69(3):396–402.

117. Hunyadi L, Papich MG, Pusterla N. Diclazuril nonlinear mixed-effects pharmacokinetic modelling of plasma concentrations after oral administration to adult horses every 3-4 days. Vet J 2018;242:74–6.

118. Pusterla N, James K, Bain F, et al. Investigation of the Bi-Weekly Administration of Diclazuril on the Antibody Kinetics to *Sarcocystis neurona* in Healthy Horses. J Equine Vet Sci 2021;104:103713.

119. Pusterla N, Packham A, Mackie S, et al. Daily feeding of diclazuril top dress pellets in foals reduces seroconversion to *Sarcocystis neurona*. Vet J 2015;206(2):236–8.

120. Ellison SP, Lindsay DS. Decoquinate Combined with Levamisole Reduce the Clinical Signs and Serum SAG 1, 5, 6 Antibodies in Horses with Suspected Equine Protozoal Myeloencephalitis. Int J App Res Vet Med 2012;10(1):1–7.

121. Lindsay DS, Nazir MM, Maqbool A, et al. Efficacy of decoquinate against *Sarcocystis neurona* in cell cultures. Vet Parasitol 2013;196(1–2):21–3.

122. Van Voorhis WC, Doggett JS, Parsons M, et al. Extended-spectrum antiprotozoal bumped kinase inhibitors: A review. Exp Parasitol 2017;180:71–83.

123. Ojo KK, Dangoudoubiyam S, Verma SK, et al. Selective inhibition of *Sarcocystis neurona* calcium-dependent protein kinase 1 for equine protozoal myeloencephalitis therapy. Int J Parasitol 2016;46(13–14):871–80.

124. Bowden GD, Land KM, O'Connor RM, et al. High-throughput screen of drug repurposing library identifies inhibitors of *Sarcocystis neurona* growth. Int J Parasitol Drugs Drug Resist 2018;8(1):137–44.

125. Saville WJA, Dubey JP, Marsh AE, et al. Testing the *Sarcocystis neurona* vaccine using an equine protozoal myeloencephalitis challenge model. Vet Parasitol 2017;247:37–41.

Clostridial Diseases (Botulism and Tetanus)

Jacob M. Swink, DVM, MS, DACVIM (LAIM)[a], William F. Gilsenan, VMD, DACVIM (LAIM)[b],*

KEYWORDS

- Botulism • Clostridium • Equine • Neurologic • Neurotoxin • Tetanus • Vaccine

KEY POINTS

- Classic clinical presentations of both disease processes allow for presumptive diagnosis in most cases.
- Progression of disease can occur rapidly, so therapeutic intervention must be prompt to maximize the patient's chance of survival.
- Antimicrobial and antitoxin therapy is crucial to halt progression of disease.
- Recovery from both diseases requires several weeks of nursing care, but full recovery usually occurs in horses that survive disease.
- Highly effective vaccines are available against both botulism and tetanus and are critical in preventative approaches to control.

INTRODUCTION

A sudden onset of neurologic disease in horses can pose challenges to both veterinarians and horse owners. Swift and appropriate therapeutic intervention might have a profound influence on a patient's outcome, but advanced diagnostics are frequently necessary to achieve a definitive or presumptive diagnosis. Moreover, neurologic disease has the potential to affect multiple horses on the same premises and can cause rapid deterioration of an affected horse's status. It is critical for the equine practitioner to be familiar with neurologic assessment and the process of neurolocalization. Possession of these skills can facilitate timely recognition of common equine neurologic diseases and an appropriate list of differential diagnoses.

Tetanus and botulism are 2 common and potentially fatal equine neurologic diseases that result in starkly different clinical signs. However, they are frequently described alongside one another because they are both caused by toxins produced by clostridial organisms. In addition, tetanus and botulism produce characteristic neurologic deficits that usually allow for a provisional diagnosis based on a thorough

[a] Brown Equine Hospital, 876 Stoystown Road, Somerset, PA 15501, USA; [b] Rood and Riddle Equine Hospital, 2150 Georgetown Road, Lexington, KY 40511, USA
* Corresponding author.
E-mail address: bgilsenan@roodandriddle.com

Vet Clin Equine 38 (2022) 269–282
https://doi.org/10.1016/j.cveq.2022.05.004
0749-0739/22/© 2022 Elsevier Inc. All rights reserved.

vetequine.theclinics.com

physical examination. When either tetanus or botulism is suspected, timely therapeutic intervention and administration of antidotes are essential to maximize a horse's chances of recovery. Highly effective vaccines have been fortunately developed against both botulism and tetanus. Consequently, with proper client education and preventive medicine, clinical disease and subsequent losses can often be avoided altogether.

The objective of this article is to present the most recent information on pathophysiology, clinical signs, diagnosis, therapy, and prevention of tetanus and botulism.

TETANUS

Tetanus is a neurologic disease of people and animals caused by exotoxins of *Clostridium tetani*. *C tetani* is a gram-positive obligate anaerobic bacterium. It is ubiquitous in soil but has also been isolated from dust and air samples, human hair, and wounds.[1] It can be found in the gastrointestinal tract of healthy herbivorous animals.[2,3] Wilkins and colleagues[2] reported recovery of *C tetani* in 5.9% (7/118) of fecal samples in Durban, South Africa. Seasonal variation of tetanus has been reported in humans and dogs,[4–6] but the effect of season appears to vary considerably based on geography. Horses should be considered susceptible to disease year-round, as they are more sensitive to tetanus toxin than other herbivorous domestic animals.[7]

Like other clostridial species, *C tetani* is a spore-forming organism. Spores are characteristically described as "drumstick-shaped."[8] The ability of the bacterium to produce spores enables it to survive in aerobic environments while remaining resistant to intense heat and most disinfectants.[9] Spores will survive boiling but can be eliminated by autoclaving at 115°C (239°F) for 20 minutes.[9] When environmental conditions become suitable, spores can germinate, allowing the vegetative bacterium to produce toxins (**Box 1**).[8]

Pathophysiology

As *C tetani* spores do not actively produce toxins, the organism must be in its vegetative state to induce disease. Most commonly, deep penetrating wounds provide ideal anaerobic conditions that enable *C tetani* spores to germinate. Lesions that result in a compromised vascular supply or local tissue necrosis are more likely to facilitate an anaerobic environment. Green and colleagues[10] reported in a review of 20 equine tetanus cases that puncture wounds and lacerations to the distal limbs were the most common sites of initial infection. Other sites of injury leading to tetanus included lacerations to the face and tail docking.[10] Postparturient mares with reproductive injuries or retained fetal membranes and neonatal foals with umbilical infections are at a heightened risk of developing tetanus. Because the dose required to induce tetanus in the horse is so low, small wounds might act as a site of infection. Moreover, spores can survive in tissues for several months.[7] In up to 50% of cases, the site of initial infection might have healed by the onset of clinical signs.[6]

Box 1
Conditions that favor germination of *C tetani* spores

Anaerobic or low oxygen tension environment

Temperatures near 37°C

Neutral pH (~7.0)

Once *C tetani* spores germinate, the bacteria are motile via flagella. *C tetani* induces disease via 2 primary toxins: tetanolysin and tetanospasmin. Tetanolysin is a hemolysin toxin that induces local tissue damage and cell lysis, facilitating an environment for anaerobic infection.[3] Tetanospasmin is a 150-kDa polypeptide molecule that becomes immediately cleaved by host proteases into a heavy chain and a light chain.[11] The 2 chains remain joined by a disulfide bond. Tetanospasmin diffuses into the vasculature and spreads hematogenously before binding to ganglia (autonomic nervous system) and neuromuscular junctions (somatic nervous system). Once bound, the toxin becomes internalized by endocytosis and is carried along the axon in a retrograde fashion at a pace of 75 to 250 mm per day.[12] The toxin eventually enters the central nervous system, reaching the neuronal cell body. It then crosses the synaptic cleft and enters the inhibitory interneuron (Renshaw) cells. The active light chain acts on synaptobrevin (vesicle-associated membrane protein) in the Renshaw cells to irreversibly impede the release of 2 inhibitory neurotransmitters: glycine and gamma-aminobutyric acid (GABA).[13–15] This toxic action results in a release from inhibition, leading to spastic muscle contractions, muscular rigidity, and the clinical signs typically associated with tetanus.

Clinical Signs

Clinical signs develop approximately 7 to 21 days following inoculation.[7,10] The incubation period can be shortened or prolonged depending on several factors. The duration of incubation period and rate of disease progression are inversely proportional to the inoculation dose and the extent of necrotic tissue. Increasing distance of the site of inoculation to the central nervous system may prolong the incubation time. The earliest clinical signs can be subtle. Affected horses may be hesitant to lower their necks owing to pain and stiffness. In a recent retrospective study by van Galen and colleagues,[16] stiffness was the most commonly identified clinical sign of affected horses being presented to a referral hospital. As disease progresses, the horse's gait becomes stilted, and evidence of sustained facial muscle contraction results in retraction of the lips, flaring of nostrils, and an inability to open the mouth (trismus). These facial features are commonly referred to as *risus sardonicus* ("sardonic grin"). Prolapse of the nictitating membranes (third eyelid) is frequently noted and results from retraction of the globe within the orbit. Urine retention can result secondary to increased urethral sphincter tone. Fecal and gas retention, leading to constipation and bloat, can occur in the gastrointestinal tract owing to increased anal sphincter tone and decreased gastrointestinal motility. Tachycardia has been described as a common feature of tetanus in people owing to the toxin's effect on the sympathetic nervous system.[17] This effect is less clear in horses, as both tachycardia and bradycardia have been described.[16,18] Tachycardia observed in horses may be more likely related to pain, stress, and dehydration. In advanced stages of tetanus, affected horses ultimately become recumbent. Horses are prone to muscular convulsions, or tetanic spasms, which can be mistaken for seizures, although a horse's consciousness during these episodes should exclude this possibility.[18] Mortality is high, and affected horses usually die from respiratory paralysis if they are not euthanized first. Other severe, and potentially fatal, complications can occur, including aspiration pneumonia secondary to regurgitation, decubital ulceration, and colic. A clinical scoring system has been described to facilitate objective classification of infected horses (**Table 1**).[19]

Diagnosis

Definitive antemortem diagnosis is difficult if not impossible. The small infective dose required to induce clinical disease in horses heightens the difficulty in isolating

Table 1 Proposed clinical scoring system for horses and donkeys affected by tetanus[19]	
Clinical Score	Clinical Signs
1	Mild signs: Nictitating membrane flashing, ears pulled caudally, stiff gait but able to walk and eat without difficulty
2	Moderate signs: Nictitating membrane flashing, ears pulled caudally, limbs still and walking with difficulty, trismus and generalized muscle spasm, still capable of eating and drinking but with some difficulty
3	Severe signs: Capable of standing but unable to walk, severe trismus, difficulty with prehension, mastication, and swallowing food
4	Terminal signs: Unable to stand, walk, or eat

neurotoxins. Successful culture of C tetani from wounds in affected horses has been reported, but anaerobic culture methods did not yield growth of C tetani in 46% to 70% of cases in people.[16,20,21] Gram-stain smears of infected wounds can be attempted, but spores have been reported in only a minority of cases. Moreover, the similar morphologic appearance of other clostridial spores lessens the utility of this diagnostic technique. A real-time polymerase chain reaction (PCR) assay has been developed for detection of the C tetani neurotoxin gene, facilitating rapid diagnosis in people.[22] This assay is not readily available in veterinary medicine. Antemortem diagnosis is typically presumptive based on history, physical examination findings, and clinical signs. Identification of a penetrating or infected wound, especially in an unvaccinated horse, should increase clinical suspicion of tetanus. Because tetanus is identified as a diagnosis of exclusion, efforts to rule out differential diagnoses should be made. Disease states that might result in a similar clinical picture include rabies, strychnine intoxication, exertional rhabdomyolysis, and myositis.

Clinicopathologic findings in patients with tetanus are generally nonspecific unless secondary disease is present. Increases in inflammatory markers (white blood cell count, fibrinogen, serum amyloid A) may be present secondary to wound infection or concurrent pneumonia. Increases in muscle enzymes (creatine kinase, aspartate aminotransferase) can be observed secondary to damage caused by wound infection or recumbency. Cerebrospinal fluid analysis and advanced imaging techniques (computed tomography, MRI) are expected to yield normal findings.

On postmortem examination, abnormal findings are associated with secondary complications, including pneumonia, intramuscular (IM) hemorrhage, and decubital ulceration. Again, identification of tetanus toxins is hampered by the small amount of toxin needed to induce disease. Of 28 adult horses and foals with presumed tetanus, definitive diagnosis via postmortem examination was not achieved in any of the cases in one retrospective study.[16]

Treatment

There are several important pillars that comprise a therapeutic plan for the equine patient with tetanus: elimination of the infectious agent, neutralization of circulating neurotoxin, control of muscular spasms, establishment of active immunity against neurotoxins, and provision of high-quality supportive care.

Elimination of the infectious agent is critical to minimize the amount of C tetani exotoxin produced once the horse's condition has been assessed. Antimicrobial therapy with potassium penicillin (22,000 IU/kg intravenously [IV] every 6 hours) is generally accepted as the first line of therapy; some clinicians prefer to treat with doses as high as 50,000 IU/kg IV every 6 hours during the first 48 hours of treatment. Recently, evidence has emerged indicating that penicillin has the capacity to augment inhibitory effects on the neurotransmitter GABA, potentially exacerbating the toxic effects of tetanospasmin.[23] Moreover, penicillin has been studied as a means of triggering epileptic seizures in laboratory animals, prompting investigation for alternative therapies for affected people.[24,25] Therapy with metronidazole has been compared with penicillin for treatment of tetanus in people; results suggest that metronidazole yields superior results.[26] Based on these data, metronidazole (25 mg/kg orally [PO] every 12 hours or 10–20 mg/kg IV every 6 to 8 hours) could be considered an alternative to penicillin in treatment of equine patients.[7] The expense of IV metronidazole formulation may limit its clinical utility to the treatment of foals. Metronidazole may also be administered per rectum (50 mg/kg every 12 hours) if the affected patient is unable to swallow.[7] The limited antimicrobial spectrum of both penicillin and metronidazole should be considered in recumbent horses at risk for developing aspiration pneumonia. Broadspectrum antimicrobial drugs that might be effective for the treatment of both tetanus and resultant aspiration pneumonia in recumbent horses include ceftiofur sodium and oxytetracycline.[27,28] The clinician should consider risks of antimicrobial-associated colitis when formulating a treatment plan, particularly as these risks can vary geographically.

Administration of tetanus antitoxin (TAT) is critical to halting progression of clinical disease. Treatment allows binding and inactivation of any tetanus toxin that is circulating in the vascular system. A variety of doses and routes of administration have been described (**Box 2**). The optimal course of TAT therapy is not known. Intrathecal administration of TAT was described and reported to be successful in upward of 75% of cases by Muylle and colleagues.[29] More recent reports have indicated success rates between 0% and 33%.[10,30] A prospective study in Ghana investigated the efficacy of intrathecal TAT in human neonates with tetanus, but no benefit from this route of administration could be demonstrated.[31] It is of major importance to recognize that, once internalized into a neural body, tetanus toxin cannot be inactivated by TAT. For this reason, it should be anticipated that clinical disease associated with tetanus will continue to worsen for 1 to 2 days before signs begin to improve.[7]

The use of TAT has been implicated in the pathogenesis of an acute and often fatal form of hepatitis (Theiler disease) 45 to 90 days after administration.[32] Despite the risk of Theiler disease, therapy with TAT is absolutely indicated in horses that have developed signs of tetanus. The cause of Theiler disease and its relation to TAT have been a longstanding topic of speculation. Divers and colleagues[33] have demonstrated that Equine Parvovirus (EqPV-H) is the likely cause of Theiler disease. TAT is an equine biologic agent via which EqPV-H can be transmitted from infected donors to recipients.[33] Given this critical advancement in the understanding of Theiler disease, and the newly

---

Box 2
Reported tetanus antitoxin doses for adult horses

5000 to 30,000 IU IV or IM once[10]

2500 IU subcutaneous every 24 hours for 5 days after initial dose[10]

5000 to 2,500,000 IU IV or IM once[19]

30,000 IU IV once[19]

20,000 IU IM once 24 hours after initial dose[19]

30,000 to 50,000 IU intrathecal once[29]

achieved ability to screen equine plasma donors for EqPV-H, the risk of severe hepatitis associated with TAT is expected to lessen in the future.

The release from inhibition that occurs in the Renshaw cells leads to sustained muscle contraction and spasm. Consequences of uncontrolled muscular spasm include pain, stress, and respiratory paralysis. Promotion of muscle relaxation is an integral component to the tetanus patient's comfort and healing process. A multimodal approach is recommended, and a variety of strategies might be successful. Phenothiazine tranquilizers, such as acepromazine maleate (0.03–0.05 mg/kg, IV or IM, up to every 4 hours), and methocarbamol (10–20 mg/kg PO every 8 hours), a centrally acting skeletal muscle relaxant, provide muscle relaxation, are inexpensive, and are readily accessible. For these reasons, they are commonly used in the management of tetanus but are likely insufficient as monotherapy in more severe cases (**Box 3**).

Convalescence from tetanus is expected to take days to weeks following the irreversible binding of tetanospasmin to the inhibitory interneurons. Clients should be informed early in the treatment process that the recovery is usually protracted and costly. During this period, it is necessary to manage pain, dysphagia, and sometimes recumbency. Patients must be kept in a dark, padded, and quiet room, as stimulation may promote severe muscle spasms and even respiratory paralysis. The importance of supportive nursing care cannot be overstated. For horses that are unable to swallow, an indwelling nasogastric tube can be placed to allow administration of feed. Complete enteral supplements (Well-Gel, Purina Animal Nutrition, Shoreview, MN, USA; Platinum Enteral Immunonutrition Formula, Platinum Performance, Buellton, CA, USA) are available to ensure patients receive an appropriate complement of nutrients. Repeated nasogastric intubation should be avoided to minimize stress to the patient. For patients that cannot tolerate enteral feedings, provision of partial or total parenteral nutrition should be pursued.

In addition to administration of TAT, it is recommended to treat affected horses with tetanus toxoid at the onset of treatment. The dose of tetanus toxin that is required to induce disease is so low that it is insufficient to initiate an anamnestic response on its own, rendering recovered, unvaccinated horses susceptible to reinfection once TAT antibodies have been bound or cleared from the body.

Prognosis

Prognosis for horses affected with tetanus is guarded to poor, especially for recumbent animals. Horses that are able to stand, drink, and eat voluntarily before therapeutic intervention have a significantly better prognosis for survival.[34] Mortality is

---

Box 3
Therapeutics used to mitigate muscular spasms

Acepromazine maleate

Methocarbamol

Diazepam

Dantrolene

Xylazine

Magnesium sulfate

Phenobarbital

Sodium Phenobarbital

estimated at 54% to 80%.[7,10,19,35] In one retrospective study, mortality increased to 94% for horses with severe or terminal signs of disease.[19] Another study found that, of horses that were presented with dysphagia, 87% did not survive.[35] Green and colleagues[10] reported a significant association between survival and prophylactic vaccination within the prior 12 months. van Galen and colleagues[34] reported 75% survival in affected horses that had been vaccinated against tetanus; in this study, clinical disease in vaccinated horses was mild or moderate. The same study reported similar mortalities between affected foals (66.7%) and adults (68.4%).[34] Evidence is conflicting on whether the dose of TAT affects survival rate.[34,35] Importantly, most equids that do survive treatment have the potential to fully recover.[19] In one retrospective study, 93.8% of surviving horses had recovered completely.[34] Reported sequelae included ataxia and unspecified lameness.[34]

Prevention

A tetanus toxoid vaccine for horses is available (Tetanus Toxoid, Zoetis Animal Health, Parsippany NJ, USA). Naïve adults should initially receive 2 doses 4 to 6 weeks apart with annual vaccinations following.[36] Broodmares should be vaccinated as normal adults and boostered 4 to 6 weeks prepartum. Foals born to vaccinated mares should undergo a 3-dose series: once at 4 to 6 months of age; once 4 to 6 weeks after the first dose; and once at 10 to 12 months of age.[36] Foals from unvaccinated mares should have a similar schedule, but with the first dose at 3 to 4 months of age.[36] An additional booster around incidents that could lead to a clinical case (eg, puncture wound, surgery) is recommended as well. Kendall and colleagues[37] studied a population of horses in Sweden that were treated with a tetanus toxoid (Equilis Pretenza Te, Intervet AB, Stockholm, Sweden) once at 5 to 11 months of age, again 4 weeks after the initial dose, and then a third dose 15 to 17 months after the second dose. Antibody titers against tetanus remained above detectable levels in nearly all studied horses after 3 years. Although the study's findings suggest that vaccine recommendations can be revised, the American Association of Equine Practitioners (AAEP) currently recommends that adults be vaccinated annually.

BOTULISM

Botulism is a neuromuscular disease caused by intoxication with the botulinum neurotoxin (BoNT) produced by clostridial species. Of those that produce BoNTs, *Clostridium botulinum* is the most clinically significant in equine medicine, especially in North America and Europe, as it produces 3 of the most common neurotoxins (types A, B, and C). There are 8 different BoNTs (A, B, Ca, Cb, D, E, F, and G). In general, type A is found west of the Rocky Mountains, type B in the Mid-Atlantic United States and Kentucky, and type C in Europe. Eighty-five percent of cases in North America are caused by type B.[38] Type D was recently reported to cause 12 cases in Israel.[39]

C botulinum spores are highly resistant to environmental stressors and vegetate until ideal conditions occur. These bacteria prefer anaerobic and alkaline or neutral conditions. When exposed to acidic or oxygenated conditions, the bacteria sporulate.[40] Once germinated and growing, BoNT production ensues. Decaying organic matter provides ideal growth conditions for BoNT-producing organisms and is involved in the pathogenesis of many clinical cases.

There are 3 different routes by which an equid can acquire botulism. One means of infection involves ingestion of preformed BoNT. This typically occurs when the animal ingests feed, soil, or carrion in which clostridial organisms have produced the BoNT. An alternative route is absorption of BoNT through a wound that is infected with toxin-producing clostridial organisms (wound botulism). A third possible route occurs when

BoNT-producing organisms inhabit the gastrointestinal tract and produce toxins (toxicoinfectious botulism). This form of intoxication occurs most commonly in foals and is also known as "shaker foal syndrome" owing to the clinical signs.

Pathophysiology
The botulism toxin is a single polypeptide chain that is cleaved into a 100-kDa heavy and 50-kDa light chain connected by a disulfide bond.[41] The sequence of BoNT is 35% homologous with that of tetanospasmin.[13] At the site of absorption, BoNTs cross epithelial barriers and enter the vasculature. The systemic circulation carries BoNTs to peripheral nerve terminals, where they enter the presynaptic nerve. BoNTs are unable to cross the blood-brain barrier and thus only affect peripheral nerves.

At the peripheral nerve, the heavy chain binds and facilitates endocytosis into the neuron.[41] The BoNT is internalized into the presynaptic nerve via the endosome, where it experiences a pH change.[13] An acidic environment encourages dissociation of the heavy and light chains, which frees the light chain to diffuse into the cytosol.[13] The light chain has metalloprotease activity, which targets neuronal soluble N-ethylmaleimide-sensitive factor attachment protein (SNAP) receptor (SNARE) proteins; these proteins normally function in neurotransmitter exocytosis.[41] The specific SNARE protein targeted may vary based on the toxin type. BoNT types A and E act on SNAP-25 (synaptosomal associated protein), whereas types B, D, F, and G cleave VAMP-2 (synaptobrevin/vesicle-associated membrane protein).[41] Type C cleaves syntaxin 1 in addition to SNAP-25.[41] Ultimately, protein cleavage prevents release of acetylcholine and results in neuroparalysis. Clinical signs seem to be dose dependent and will persist until new synapses are formed; the type of toxin may play a role in the duration of neuroparalysis as well.[28]

Clinical signs
Because of the mechanism of toxicity, the clinical signs of botulism can be described as diffuse, symmetric, flaccid paralysis and loss of muscle strength. Although it has been suspected that different toxins may have slight differences in clinical manifestations, this has been unproven in the horse. Clinical signs are the same despite different routes of intoxication as well.

Clinical signs can appear from 12 hours to 17 days following exposure to the toxin.[18,28] The rapidity of progression may indicate the degree of intoxication, as more severe disease and shorter incubations usually result from higher levels of BoNT exposure. Thus, the severity of initial signs of botulism can vary widely from weakness, dysphagia, and poor muscle tone to acute death. Other signs of the disease can include increased time lying down, inability to rise, colic, muscle fasciculations, low head carriage, and a shuffling gait.[18] It is important to note that although affected horses may be profoundly weak, they are not expected to have proprioceptive deficits. Muscle groups with relatively high requirements for acetylcholine tend to become affected earlier than other groups. These muscle groups include those of the tongue, eyelids, tail, and anal sphincter. In the very acute or mild case, owners may note that the animal takes longer than "normal" to consume its concentrate. Muscle fasciculations may start focally and progress to affect the entire body. The equid may tire and become recumbent. Some horses may regain their strength and stand for a period before tiring and lying down once again. This cycle may repeat until recumbency can no longer be overcome. Such horses may die secondary to respiratory failure owing to progressive weakening of the diaphragm.

Clinical signs in foals may appear first as muscle fasciculations, which may become coarse and involve the entire body. These clinical signs are responsible for the common name "shaker foal syndrome." These foals can tire and lay down, only to regain their strength and stand again like affected adults. They too can cycle through standing and recumbency.

Affected horses may be dehydrated, as some lose the ability to consume water. Heart rate can be normal or elevated if dehydration or stress is present. Respiratory rate can be normal but may be decreased as the diaphragm weakens. Tachypnea can be found in horses with concurrent respiratory disease, such as aspiration pneumonia, which is a common sequela to dysphagia.

Diagnosis

Definitive diagnosis of botulism can be difficult, and diagnosis is usually a clinical one. Few other diseases can cause acute-onset diffuse muscle weakness and flaccid paralysis in horses. An easy "diagnostic test" to institute in the field would be to offer the affected equid 250 mL of concentrate; affected horses will generally take longer than 2 minutes to consume this amount, whereas normal counterparts could consume this with ease, often in less than 1 minute.[18]

Ancillary diagnostics should be performed to evaluate the patient and to rule out other differential diseases. Complete blood count is usually within normal limits, although concurrent infection (eg, aspiration pneumonia) may cause changes within the leukogram. Serum biochemistry analysis (SBA) may yield normal findings. However, in some cases of botulism, SBA abnormalities can develop because of secondary disease. Elevations in muscle enzymes are expected if the equid has been recumbent, has had difficulty standing, or is showing signs of colic. Electrolyte disturbances and/or azotemia may be present if the horse has been dysphagic or unable to drink for an extended period. Endoscopic examination should be performed in horses with dysphagia to rule out abnormalities within the nasopharynx. Examination of the oral cavity is recommended to rule out dental disease, oral foreign bodies, or tongue abscessation as causes of dysphagia. Cerebrospinal fluid analysis is expected to yield normal results in horses with botulism.

Additional laboratory diagnostics can be used to support the clinical diagnosis of botulism through finding the preformed BoNT or BoNT-producing clostridial organisms in foodstuffs, serum, gastrointestinal tract, or wounds of an affected animal, or detection of serum antibodies against the causative clostridial organisms. A mouse bioassay is currently considered the gold-standard diagnostic for detection of botulism; the assay has a high specificity (97% in one study).[42] In this test, serum from the affected patient is injected into naïve and vaccinated mice, and they are monitored for clinical disease. However, because horses are much more sensitive to BoNT than mice, false-negative results can occur if concentrations are less than the threshold of disease. The low sensitivity (32%) presented by Johnson and colleagues[43] reflects the challenges associated with the mouse bioassay technique. Enrichment cultures can improve the sensitivity of the assay.[32] Unfortunately, the mouse bioassay can take several weeks to yield results.

Detection of BoNT via enzyme-linked immunosorbent assay is possible, but these assays have not yet been validated in the horse.[27] Quantitative real-time PCR for BoNT genes has been developed and offers a sensitivity of greater than 88% and specificity of greater than 98% for BoNT types A, B, and C.[42] In the United States, fecal or feed samples should be submitted to the National Veterinary Services Laboratory in Ames, Iowa. Botulism spores are rarely found in fecal samples from normal horses, and their detection in feces from suspect cases may be useful.[38] Spores were found in 70% of "shaker foal" fecal samples in one study.[38]

Differentials for botulism can be found in **Box 4**.

| Box 4 |
| Differential diagnoses for botulism |
| White muscle disease |
| Hyperkalemic periodic paralysis (HYPP) |
| Hypocalcemia |
| White snakeroot toxicity |
| Ionophore toxicity |
| Lead toxicity |
| Organophosphate toxicity |

Treatment

The most important and time-sensitive treatment for botulism is neutralization of circulating BoNT. Through administration of botulism antitoxin, circulating BoNT can be bound and eliminated before translocation into cells. Thirty-thousand IU for a foal or 70,000 IU for an adult can provide protection for 60 days.[38] As the antitoxin only binds free BoNT, that which has entered cells can cause clinical signs to worsen for the following 12 to 24 hours.[18] Although expensive, currently available antitoxins include polyvalent (bivalent for types A and B; Sanofi Pasteur Ltd, Toronto, Ontario, Canada; trivalent for types A, B, and C; Lake Immunogenics, Ontario, NY, USA) and monovalent (type B; EquiPlas, PlasVacc, Templeton, CA, USA; ImmunoGlo, Mg Biologics, Ames, IA, USA).

Elimination of causative organisms is important in cases of toxicoinfectious and wound botulism. Some medications can potentiate neuromuscular weakness (aminoglycosides, procaine penicillin, tetracyclines) and should therefore be avoided.[28] Potassium penicillin or a cephalosporin may therefore be the best antimicrobial option for treatment in these horses.

Concurrent diseases should also be managed in botulism cases. Broad-spectrum antibiotics are indicated for aspiration pneumonia. Mineral oil and/or cathartics may prevent impactions or can be treatments in actively colicking horses. Nutrition and hydration are essential factors to consider in botulism cases, as most become dysphagic and are unable to adequately eat or drink. Feeding tubes can be used to provide sufficient amounts of water and complete enteral nutrition products (Well-Gel; Purina Animal Nutrition; Platinum Enteral Immunonutrition Formula; Platinum Performance). IV fluids and/or parenteral nutrition may need to be used in patients that cannot tolerate enteral feeding owing to ileus or lateral recumbency.

Supportive nursing care for equids that become recumbent can be time-consuming, expensive, and labor intensive, but is critical. Provision of supportive nursing care includes moving the equid to prevent decubital ulceration and compartment syndrome, alternating recumbency every 3 to 4 hours to minimize lung consolidation, and sedation to control excessive thrashing. This may be difficult to achieve in many horses but can be successful in foals. A sling might be necessary to lift some affected horses but should not be used to maintain the horse in the standing position, as this can hasten exhaustion and can also impede respiration. Severely affected horses may experience such profound respiratory depression that mechanical ventilation becomes necessary.

Prognosis

The course of disease and prognosis ultimately depend on the amount of toxin absorbed or ingested. Toxin type may affect prognosis, but the exact difference in horses remains to be demonstrated.

Recovery takes at least 7 to 14 days and is dependent on construction of new neuromuscular endplates. The time until full-muscle recovery may be 1 month.[44]

Johnson[45] most recently reported that horses that arrived standing had a 67% rate of survival; those that remained standing during hospitalization had a 95% rate of survival. Dysphagia may take 2 to 14 days to resolve.[45]

Overall survival rates in outbreak situations and hospitalized cases have varied (10%–48%),[34] and rates have been variable between types. Complications of botulism, including pneumonia, diarrhea, and decubital ulceration, occurred in 62% of affected horses in one study, but these complications were not associated with nonsurvival.[45]

Treatment of foals has been reported to be more successful, with one report publishing a survival rate of 96% of treated cases and 90% overall.[46] In the same study, 30% of foals required mechanical ventilation.[46] Wilkins and Palmer[47] reported that 7 of 8 (87.5%) mechanically ventilated foals with botulism survived to discharge. Mechanical ventilation of an adult horse with presumed botulism has been described.[48] Although the horse was successfully weaned off mechanical ventilation after 2 weeks of therapy, euthanasia became necessary when large colon volvulus developed several days later.

Prevention

A BoNT type B toxoid vaccine is available (BotVax B; Neogen, Lansing, MI, USA). The AAEP recommends annual vaccination of adult horses.[36] Unvaccinated adults need a 3-dose series, each 1 month apart. Broodmares should receive a booster 4 to 6 weeks before parturition. Foals born from vaccinated mares should be given the 3-dose series at 4-week intervals starting at 2 to 3 months of age and then boostered annually. Foals from unvaccinated mares should receive the same initial 3-dose series, but at 1 to 3 months of age. As the vaccine targets type B, cross-protection against other types is not guaranteed. Foals who suffer from failure of transfer of passive immunity should be treated accordingly to ensure that they acquire an adequate serum immunoglobulin G concentration.[49]

Eliminating possible exposures is also key in prevention. This can be completed via ensuring that hay and feed are of good quality and free of contamination from decaying debris; storing foodstuffs appropriately; and inspection of water sources and pastures for dead animals.

CLINICS CARE POINTS

- Diagnosis of tetanus often occurs based on history and unique clinical signs (sardonic grin, sawhorse stance, and third eyelid prolapse) due to the high degree of sensitivity of the horse to the neurotoxin as well as the difficulties in detecting circulating neurotoxin.

- Treatment is often targeted at neutralizing circulting neurotoxins (tetanus antitoxin), eliminating the source of neurotoxins (infection or ingestion), and providing supportive care to the affected individual.

- The prognosis is generally poor for affected anmials. Vaccination is a key tool in prevention of disease.

DISCLOSURE

The authors have no financial interests to disclose.

REFERENCES

1. Bytchenko B. In: Veronesi R, editor. Microbiology of tetanus. tetanus: important new concepts. Amsterdam (the Netherlands: Excerpta Medica; 1981. p. 28–39.
2. Wilkins CA, Richter MB, Hobbs WB, et al. Occurrence of Clostridium tetani in soil and horses. S Afr Med J 1988;73(12):718–20.
3. Cook TM, Protheroe RT, Handel JM. Tetanus: a review of the literature. Br J Anaesth 2001;87(3):477–87.
4. Starybrat D, Burkitt-Creedon JM, Ellis J, et al. Retrospective evaluation of the seasonality of canine tetanus in England (2006–2017): 49 dogs. J Vet Emerg Crit Care 2021;31(4):541–4.
5. Bansal J, Jain R, Gaur K. Seasonal variation in non neonatal tetanus: 7 years retrospective record based study. IMJ Health 2015;1(4):31–5.
6. Ashley MJ, Bell JS. Tetanus in Ontario: a review of the epidemiological and clinical features of 102 cases occurring in the 10-year period 1958-1967. Can Med Assoc J 1969;100(17):798–805.
7. MacKay R. Tetanus. large animal internal medicine. 6th edition. St. Louis, MO: Elsevier; 2018. p. 1097–9.
8. Popoff MR. Tetanus in animals. J Vet Diagn Invest 2020;32(2):184–91.
9. Timoney J, Gillespie J, Scott F, et al. The genus Clostridium. Hagan and Bruner's microbiology and infectious diseases of domestic animals. Ithaca (NY): Comstock Publishing Associates; 1988. p. 214–22.
10. Green SL, Little CB, Baird JD, et al. Tetanus in the horse: a review of 20 cases (1970 to 1990). J Vet Intern Med 1994;8(2):128–32.
11. Helting TB, Parschat S, Engelhardt H. Structure of tetanus toxin. Demonstration and separation of a specific enzyme converting intracellular tetanus toxin to the extracellular form. J Biol Chem 1979;254(21):10728–33.
12. Erdmann G, Wiegand H, Wellhöner HH. Intraaxonal and extraaxonal transport of 125I-tetanus toxin in early local tetanus. Naunyn Schmiedebergs Arch Pharmacol 1975;290(4):357–73.
13. Turton K, Chaddock JA, Acharya KR. Botulinum and tetanus neurotoxins: structure, function and therapeutic utility. Trends Biochem Sci 2002;27(11):552–8.
14. Poulain B. [Molecular mechanism of action of tetanus toxin and botulinum neurotoxins]. Pathol Biol (Paris) 1994;42(2):173–82.
15. Pellizzari R, Rossetto O, Lozzi L, et al. Structural determinants of the specificity for synaptic vesicle-associated membrane protein/synaptobrevin of tetanus and botulinum type b and g neurotoxins. J Biol Chem 1996;271(34):20353–8.
16. Galen G van, Saegerman C, Rijckaert J, et al. Retrospective evaluation of 155 adult equids and 21 foals with tetanus in Western, Northern, and Central Europe (2000–2014). Part 1: description of history and clinical evolution. J Vet Emerg Crit Care 2017;27(6):684–96.
17. Goonetilleke A, Harris JB. Clostridial neurotoxins. J Neurol Neurosurg Psychiatr 2004;75(suppl 3):iii35–9.
18. Furr M. Disorders associated with clostridial neurotoxins: botulism and tetanus. equine neurology. Hoboken (NJ): John Wiley & Sons, Inc; 2015. p. 319–27.
19. Kay G, Knottenbelt DC. Tetanus in equids: a report of 56 cases. Equine Vet Educ 2007;19(2):107–12.
20. Ansari M, Matros L. Tetanus. Compend Contin Educ Vet 1982;4:473–6.
21. Campbell Ji, Lam Tm, Huynh Tl, et al. Microbiologic characterization and antimicrobial susceptibility of Clostridium tetani isolated from wounds of patients with clinically diagnosed tetanus. Am J Trop Med Hyg 2009;80(5):827–31.

22. Akbulut D, Grant KA, McLauchlin J. Improvement in laboratory diagnosis of wound botulism and tetanus among injecting illicit-drug users by use of real-time PCR assays for neurotoxin gene fragments. J Clin Microbiol 2005;43(9): 4342–8.

23. Rossokhin AV, Sharonova IN, Bukanova JV, et al. Block of GABAA receptor ion channel by penicillin: Electrophysiological and modeling insights toward the mechanism. Mol Cell Neurosci 2014;63:72–82.

24. Kozan R, Ayyildiz M, Agar E. The effects of intracerebroventricular AM-251, a CB1-receptor antagonist, and ACEA, a CB1-receptor agonist, on penicillin-induced epileptiform activity in rats. Epilepsia 2009;50(7):1760–7.

25. Purpura DP, Penry J, Tower D. Experimental models of epilepsy. New York: Raven Press; 1972.

26. Farrar JJ, Yen LM, Cook T, et al. Tetanus. J Neurol Neurosurg Psychiatr 2000; 69(3):292–301.

27. Ribeiro MG, Nardi Júnior G de, Megid J, et al. Tetanus in horses: an overview of 70 cases. Pesqui Veterinária Bras 2018;38:285–93.

28. Nout-Lomas YS, Reed SM. Botulism. Equine internal medicine. St. Louis, MO: Elsevier; 2018. p. 672–6.

29. Muylle E, Oyaert W, Ooms L, et al. Treatment of tetanus in the horse by injections of tetanus antitoxin into the subarachnoid space. J Am Vet Med Assoc 1975; 167(1):47–8.

30. Steinman A, Haik R, Elad D, et al. Intrathecal administration of tetanus antitoxin to three cases of tetanus in horses. Equine Vet Educ 2000;12(5):237–40.

31. Neequaye J, Nkrumah FK. Failure of intrathecal antitetanus serum to improve survival in neonatal tetanus. Arch Dis Child 1983;58(4):276–8.

32. Guglick MA, MacAllister CG, Ely RW, et al. Hepatic disease associated with administration of tetanus antitoxin in eight horses. J Am Vet Med Assoc 1995; 206(11):1737–40.

33. Divers TJ, Tennant BC, Kumar A, et al. New parvovirus associated with serum hepatitis in horses after inoculation of common biological product. Emerg Infect Dis 2018;24(2):303–10.

34. van Galen G, Rijckaert J, Mair T, et al. Retrospective evaluation of 155 adult equids and 21 foals with tetanus from Western, Northern, and Central Europe (2000-2014). Part 2: prognostic assessment. J Vet Emerg Crit Care San Antonio 2017;27(6):697–706.

35. Reichmann P, Lisboa JAN, Araujo RG. Tetanus in equids: a review of 76 cases. J Equine Vet Sci 2008;28(9):518–23.

36. Vaccination guidelines | AAEP. Available at: https://aaep.org/guidelines/vaccination-guidelines. Accessed October 20, 2019.

37. Kendall A, Anagrius K, Gånheim A, et al. Duration of tetanus immunoglobulin G titres following basic immunisation of horses. Equine Vet J 2016;48(6):710–3.

38. Whitlock RH, Buckley C. Botulism. Vet Clin North Am Equine Pract 1997;13(1): 107–28.

39. Shnaiderman-Torban A, Elad D, Kelmer G, et al. An outbreak of equine botulism type D in Israel. Equine Vet Educ 2018;30(11):594–7.

40. Rossetto O, Pirazzini M, Montecucco C. Botulinum neurotoxins: genetic, structural and mechanistic insights. Nat Rev Microbiol 2014;12(8):535–49.

41. Li B, Peet NP, Butler MM, et al. Small molecule inhibitors as countermeasures for botulinum neurotoxin intoxication. Molecules 2011;16(1):202–20.

42. Johnson AL, McAdams-Gallagher SC, Sweeney RW. Quantitative real-time PCR for detection of neurotoxin genes of Clostridium botulinum types A, B and C in equine samples. Vet J 2014;199(1):157–61.
43. Johnson AL, McAdams-Gallagher SC, Aceto H. Accuracy of a mouse bioassay for the diagnosis of botulism in horses. J Vet Intern Med 2016;30(4):1293–9.
44. MacKay R. Botulism. large animal internal medicine. 6th edition. St. Louis (MO): Elsevier; 2018. p. 1101–4.
45. Johnson Al, McAdams-Gallagher Sc, Aceto H. Outcome of adult horses with botulism treated at a veterinary hospital: 92 cases (1989–2013). J Vet Intern Med 2015;29(1):311–9.
46. Wilkins PA, Palmer JE. Botulism in foals less than 6 months of age: 30 cases (1989–2002). J Vet Intern Med 2003;17(5):702–7.
47. Wilkins PA, Palmer JE. Mechanical ventilation in foals with botulism: 9 cases (1989–2002). J Vet Intern Med 2003;17(5):708–12.
48. Taylor SD, Toth B, Townsend WM, et al. Mechanical ventilation and management of an adult horse with presumptive botulism. J Vet Emerg Crit Care 2014;24(5):594–601.
49. Liepman RS, Dembek KA, Slovis NM, et al. Validation of IgG cut-off values and their association with survival in neonatal foals: IgG cut-off values and association with survival in neonatal foals. Equine Vet J 2015;47(5):526–30.

Neurologic Disorders of the Foal

Martin O. Furr, DVM, DIP ACVIM, PhD, MA Ed

KEYWORDS

- Neonate • Neonatal encephalopathy • Neurology • Equine

KEY POINTS

- Neonatal encephalopathy is the most common neurologic abnormality found in equine neonates.
- Neonatal encephalopathy causes a wide range of neurologic abnormalities.
- Clinical signs primarily reflect brain and brainstem injury.
- There are at least 3 broad etiologic categories resulting in clinical signs of neonatal encephalopathy.
- Careful classification of disease etiology is warranted to further our understanding of risk factors, effects of treatment, and expected outcomes.

The incidence of neonatal neurologic disease is difficult to determine from available data due to the issues of disease definition and confounding conditions. The literature is dominated by studies of noninfectious neonatal encephalitic disease, and there are many fewer descriptions of other neonatal neurologic conditions. Hypoxic-ischemic encephalopathy (HIE) was identified as the cause of death in 14% of foals less than 7 days of age in one study[1] and another study estimated the incidence of occurrence of neonatal maladjustment of about 1% of all neonates.[2] Among sick hospitalized foals an incidence of 2.6%–10% has been reported for neonatal neurologic disease.[3–6]

In addition to neonatal encephalopathy (NE), bacterial meningitis, traumatic injury, and developmental or congenital defects among others occur and substantively affect equine neonatal health. Of these conditions, bacterial infection of the nervous system has been reported by various authors. One large scale postmortem study found an incidence of bacterial infection of the nervous system of 9.6% (52/543 cases of neurologic disease), of which "roughly half" were foals, although the ages were not detailed.[7] Sanchez *and colleagues*[8] (2008) reported bacterial meningitis in 11 of 423

The author has no commercial or financial conflicts of interest regarding the production of this article.
Department of Physiological Sciences, College of Veterinary Medicine, Oklahoma State University, Room 264 McElroy Hall, Stillwater, Ok, USA
E-mail address: martin.furr@okstate.edu

Abbreviations	
NE	Neonatal encephalopathy
CNS	Central nervous system
CSF	Cerebrospinal fluid
NMS	Neonatal maladjustment syndrome
HIE	Hypoxic - ischemic encephalopathy
HPAA	Hyothalamic-pituitary adrenal axis
GABA	Gamma-amino butyric acid
NMDA	N-methyl-D - aspartate
DHEA	dihydroepiandrosterone
ATP	adenosine triphosphate
IP3	inositol-3-phosphate
SAE	sepsis associated encephalopathy
NI	neonatal isoerythrolysis
SIRS	systemic inflammatory response syndrome

septic foals (2.6%) while other authors reported an incidence of 5.2%[3] although this report was based on a very small sample.

Congenital and developmental malformations occur in the foal; however, these seem to be rare, except for cervical vertebral stenotic malformation which is typically expressed later in life. Abnormalities described include abnormalities of the brain (eg, hydrocephalus, Dandy –Walker syndrome, cerebellar hypoplasia), and spine/spinal cord (eg, occipitoatlantoaxial malformations, lordosis, kyphosis, spina bifida, hemi- or transitional vertebrae, meningomyelocele). In one study reporting the findings of 608 foals with congenital defects which resulted in death, hydrocephalus was found in 3%, and cleft cranium with meningomyelocele was found in 1.6%.[9] The incidence of traumatic nervous system injury in foals is unknown. Based on the predominance of noninfectious NE, this review will focus on that disorder.

NEONATAL ENCEPHALOPATHY

Neonatal encephalopathy (NE) describes a syndrome of noninfectious central nervous system (CNS) disease in newborn foals (birth to 72 hours of age) expressed as behavioral changes, altered consciousness, lack of affinity for the dam, disorientation, wandering, and loss of suckling ability. Signs may progress to blindness, abnormal phonation, seizures, and dysphagia.

The terminology used over the years has changed in relation to this disorder, further confusing careful classification and understanding of neonatal neurologic illness. Lay terms reflecting the clinical signs such as "dummies," "barkers," and "wanderers" have been used for many years, and early literature used the term neonatal maladjustment syndrome (NMS), reflecting the concept that the disorder arose from a maladaptation to extrauterine life.[10] Later work, extrapolating from human medicine, applied the term hypoxic/ischemic encephalopathy (HIE), on the assumption that this was most likely a common etiology in such cases.[11] While this is certainly true in many cases, it is clearly not true in every foal, hence the more generic term "Neonatal Encephalopathy" has gained favor in recent years.

Much of our understanding over the last many years has been compromised by the discussion of foals with NE as if it were one disease with a single pathophysiological mechanism. Some early descriptions of the syndrome reported that the pathophysiology of the disease was the result of hypoxia and ischemia of the brain occurring before, during, or shortly after parturition resulting in cellular energy failure and neuronal cell death.

Table 1
Classification of putative causes for equine neonatal encephalopathy

Neonatal Encephalopathy		
Maladaptation to Extra-uterine Life	Perinatal Asphyxia	Metabolic Abnormalities
Altered neurosteroid concentrations	Dystocia	Sepsis
Abnormal progesterone concentrations	Umbilical cord abnormalities (torsion, compression)	Kernicterus
Altered HPAA function (?)	Severe maternal disease	Electrolyte abnormalities (sodium, hypoglycemia, hypocalcemia, etc,)
	Placental disease	Uremic encephalopathy

Findings over the recent years, however, have suggested that NE may arise due to several different mechanisms, each with unique clinical and pathologic changes. Our terminology and description of the diseases must become more refined if we are to make pro gress in understanding the incidence and most effective methods of treatment.

It is worthwhile to think of NE as a "syndrome" encompassing many different conditions with a variety of causes each resulting in a similar clinical presentation, but with very different potential outcomes and optimal treatments. Like other tissues, when there is brain dysfunction the body has only limited ways in which it can respond, hence the clinical expression of the neurologic abnormalities is often not useful in distinguishing between the different causes of that dysfunction. The major difference may be only a matter of severity, timing, or rate of progress–features that are often of insufficient sensitivity to determine differences in etiology.

Careful evaluation of clinical reports and recent research suggest that there are likely 3 different pathophysiological mechanisms giving rise to NE: (1) maladaptation to extrauterine life mediated by physiologic and endocrine responses, (2) perinatal asphyxia, and (3) metabolic derangements (systemic illness, sepsis, electrolyte disorders, and so forth). While these different mechanisms may give rise to similar clinical neurologic presentation, the outcome and treatment approaches are vastly different (Table 1).

Maladaptation

Some of the earliest descriptions of NE are were considered to reflect a maladaptation to extrauterine life.[10] While this concept somewhat fell out of favor in preference to a consideration of perinatal asphyxia as the cause, recent research has demonstrated that the concept of maladaptation most likely plays a role in some cases of equine NE.

The fetus exists in a specific physiologic state appropriate to the support of healthy growth and differentiation. Data suggest that fetal foals, which are neurologically mature in late gestation, are maintained in a sleep-like, semi-conscious state. A number of specific physiologic mechanisms exist which contribute to this environment, including high concentrations of adenosine (produced from a low oxygen environment), neurosteroids (allopregnanolone, pregnanolone, and androstane), warmth, and minimization of tactile stimulation due to buoyancy in fetal fluids.[12–14]

Neuroactive steroids have multiple functions including the promotion of neurogenesis, synaptogenesis, myelinogenesis, altering neuronal excitability, modulation of neuronal circuits (involved in maternal behavior and fetal brain programming), are neuroprotective, and modulate the hypothalamic–pituitary–adrenal axis (HPAA) and the stress response.[15–17] The neurosteroids interact with gamma-aminobutyric acid (GABA) and N-methyl-D-aspartate (NMDA) receptors in the CNS. A particularly important component of their action is CNS depression, leading to the semi-comatose condition of the equine fetus. The most important of these compounds are progesterone and allopregnanolone. Progesterone is produced in large quantities from the placenta and is metabolized to allopregnanolone by 5 alpha-reductase in the CNS.[17]

At the time of parturition, these inhibiting influences are reduced or eliminated and specific stimulatory mechanisms engage leading to conscious arousal necessary for extrauterine life. With the severance of the umbilical cord, fetal production of allopregnanolone is abruptly reduced due to the reduced concentration of the progesterone precursor; this results in increased mental alertness and awareness due to the reduced depressive effects of the neurosteroids. In addition, allopregnanolone is thought to have anticonvulsant activities, associated with its cerebral suppressive properties.[18] An additional specific mechanism initiated at parturition is the reflex stimulation of the locus coeruleus (by a currently unknown mechanism), leading to increased concentration of norepinephrine, stimulating the transition to consciousness at birth.[19] Additional activation occurs via a variety of stimulatory modalities such as cold, tactile stimulation, and hypoxia.

The role of neurosteroids in equine NE has been investigated in a variety of settings.

The steroid progestogen concentrations are normally high at the time of birth and decrease rapidly during the first day of life; early research has demonstrated persistent high concentrations of progestogens in sick foals.[20,21] The concentration of allopregnanolone and progestogens are influenced by a number of factors. Cerebral hypoxia stimulates the production of neurosteroids, and both allopregnanolone and progestogens protect the CNS from hypoxic-mediated cellular injury; allopregnanolone also has antiinflammatory properties in the CNS[15]

A single normal neonatal foal was infused with allopregnanolone resulting in altered consciousness and other signs consistent with NE while in one study of 54 foals (32 with a clinical diagnosis of NMS, 12 with other neurologic disorders, and 10 normal foals) higher concentrations of neurosteroids were found in sick foals during the first 48 hours of life compared with normal or foals suffering from other neurologic disorders.[22]

In addition to the influence of neurosteroids on the development of NE, altered concentrations of other hormones which may influence consciousness have been reported. In a group of sick foals the concentration of the androgens androstenedione and dehydroepiandrosterone (DHEA) were increased in foals with NMS compared with healthy foals or sick non-NMS foals.[23] Androgens do interact with GABA$_a$ receptors on neurons and glial cells; however, it is an antagonist, while progesterone and allopregnanolone are agonists.[24,25] DHEA also interacts with the NMDR receptor, mediating excitotoxicity.[23] The role of androgens in the development of NE is difficult to deduce from this study, however, as many NMS affected foals were also considered septic, which leads to the encephalopathy of sepsis.[26,27] These findings demonstrate the web of interactions associated with critical neonatal disease.

Alterations in the HPAA have been demonstrated in critically ill foals, and higher concentrations of progesterone, aldosterone, and ACTH were found to be associated with reduced survival[28]; the effects on NE were not specifically examined, however. Previous studies have demonstrated the presence of increased concentration of progesterone in foals with a variety of critical illnesses.[20,21] The association of critical neonatal illness and NE is well recognized and further investigation of these relationships in foals with NE is needed. Hence, accumulating evidence suggests a role for the alteration of the endocrine responses associated with mediating consciousness and preparing the foal for extra-uterine life; however, a great deal remains to be learned about these mechanisms, and treatments that might be used to influence their progression.

Perinatal Asphyxia

Neonatal Encephalopathy is observed in many clinical settings in which fetal/perinatal asphyxia is likely, such as intrauterine umbilical cord occlusion, decreased placental blood flow from systemic illness or shock, premature placental separation, or dystocia. Regardless of the precise mechanism, asphyxia results in a cascade of events in the CNS which result in cerebral dysfunction. The key components include cellular energy failure, altered calcium metabolism, and alterations in cerebral blood flow; it is important to recognize that many of these events have not been specifically confirmed to occur in neonatal foals, although these universal cellular processes are likely to bridge species.

Once present from any mechanism, asphyxia creates a cellular oxygen deficit leading to a decreased brain glycogen and increased brain lactate which is observed within 2 minutes in experimental animals. High energy phosphate compounds also begin to decrease after 2 minutes of hypoxia, being reduced by 30% after only 6 minutes.[29,30] Neonates of several species are somewhat resistant to the effects of hypoxia compared with adults of the same species, due to a lower rate of energy metabolism, and a lower rate of lactate accumulation.[30] Further, in laboratory rodents, cardiovascular function is maintained in neonates compared with adults in the face of hypoxia.[31] These observations have NOT been confirmed in foals at the present time. The reduced concentration of cellular high-energy phosphate is a key linchpin in the cascade of events that follow, which include altered neurotransmitter metabolism, altered calcium metabolism, and altered blood flow. Of particular importance is the observation that low ATP concentrations persist for up to 72 hours following the correction of a hypoxic event.[32] This potentially has important implications for the progression of clinical recovery.

One important consequence of CNS cellular energy failure is the impact on neurotransmitter metabolism. Glutamate is released from the axon terminus and it interacts with 2 major types of receptors, the ionotropic (NMDA, AMPA mediating sodium, potassium, and calcium flux) and metabotropic (phosphoinositide hydrolysis and protein C activation).[30] Excessive glutamate from the synaptic cleft is absorbed by astrocytes which, via an energy requiring process convert the glutamate to glutamine. In the condition of cellular energy failure, there is reduced recycling of glutamate, which subsequently accumulates in the tissue at concentrations that are toxic to neurons. Further, secondary effects include persistent depolarization leading to increased intracellular calcium via persistent activation of the metabotropic receptors and production of IP3, as well as the failure of intracellular mechanisms to sequester calcium. Increased cytosolic calcium activates intracellular phospholipids, nucleases, proteases, and uncouples oxidative phosphorylation. The end result of the perturbations is cellular death either via rapid cell death due to massive sodium influx and cellular swelling, or delayed mechanisms associated with increased intracellular calcium.[30] In the context of perinatal asphyxia, similar events occur in other organs leading to multisystemic clinical abnormalities. This is in contrast to the clinical presentation associated with maladaptation.

Metabolic Derangements

A final etiologic category for NE includes a variety of metabolic abnormalities. The precise role of these changes is often difficult to ascertain as they may be both a cause and result of the NE. They are related due to their role in causing clinical abnormalities of NE, for which the CNS is secondarily affected.

Sepsis

The association of sepsis and altered mental status is well described in human medicine and is referred to as Sepsis Associated Encephalopathy (SAE).[26,27] This describes noninfectious diffuse abnormalities of cerebral function and includes altered mental status and conscious awareness, behavioral changes, and altered cognition.[26] Electroencephalographic abnormalities and increased biomarkers of brain injury such as S-11b and neuron-specific enolase are associated.[26] The pathophysiology is complex involving neuronal responses to systemic inflammation, oxidative stress and mitochondrial dysfunction leading to neuronal apoptosis, inflammatory signaling and blood–brain barrier breakdown which may facilitate passage of neurotoxic factors into the CNS parenchyma.[26,27] Systemic inflammation initiates physiologic changes in brain signaling via influence on the vagus nerve, initiating cerebral responses via its connection to brainstem nuclei primarily through the nucleus tractus solitarius which have direct effects on blood pressure, vasopressin secretion and the adrenal axis; these will also influence the amygdala and hippocampus which are responsible for behavior.[27,33,34]

Sepsis-induced encephalopathy has not been formally described in neonatal foals, but clinical experience indicates an association and clearly systemic inflammation can lead to clinical neurologic abnormalities which either mimic or contribute to morbidity of NE. Increased concentrations of the biomarker ubiquitin C-terminal hydrolase 1 (UCHL1) have been demonstrated in the plasma of foals with a putative diagnosis of HIE.[35]

Kernicterus

Kernicterus, also known as bilirubin encephalopathy, seems to be rare in the neonatal foal. In 72 foals with neonatal isoerythrolysis (NI) 6 (8.3%) had kernicterus.[36] The odds of developing kernicterus increased by 1.13 for each 1 mg/dL increase in maximum total bilirubin concentration.[36] The bilirubin concentration necessary for the development of kernicterus is not clear, but the total maximum serum bilirubin associated with confirmed cases was at least 19 mg/dL.[36–38] All reported cases of kernicterus in the veterinary literature are secondary to NI, although a number of factors are risk factors in human infants, including sepsis, polycythemia, prematurity, hypothyroidism, low serum albumin concentration, presence of acidosis, and hypoxia leading to increased neuronal sensitivity.[39] Similar factors likely exist in foals, but remain unexamined at the present time.

Clinical signs of kernicterus are nonspecific and include altered mentation and seizures; a full description of clinical signs is usually complicated by the presence of signs associated with severe anemia and hypoxia in foals with NI. Antemortem diagnosis is achieved by the presence of appropriate clinical signs in the presence of total bilirubin concentrations greater than 19 mg/dL. Icteric cerebrospinal fluid (CSF) is usually present, but it must be recognized that a very slight yellow discoloration of CSF has been reported in normal neonatal foals up to 10 days of age.[40] In human infants magnetic resonance imaging of the brain has shown value in confirming the diagnosis of bilirubin encephalopathy,[39] and would likely be of value in foals as well; however, this has not been described to date. Treatment is nonspecific as described later in discussion, and the practice of photodynamic therapy as used in human infants has not been applied to foals.

Electrolyte abnormalities

Electrolyte abnormalities including hyper- or hyponatremia and hypocalcemia can lead to NE.[41] Plasma sodium concentrations less than 120 meq/L are associated with neurologic abnormalities which include altered mentation, ataxia, abnormal stance, or seizures; concentrations greater than 170 meq/L may lead to similar clinical signs.[42–44] Hypocalcemia is not uncommon in critically ill neonatal foals and has been associated with seizure activity.

Diffuse encephalopathy secondary to renal failure (uremic encephalopathy) has been described in a variety of species, yet seems to be rare in horses and foals, particularly given the frequency with which renal insufficiency occurs in critical neonates.[45,46] It is possible, however, that the disorder is overlooked and signs are attributed to HIE or NMS rather than being secondary to renal disease. Of 332 horses with renal failure, 40 had some form of neurologic abnormality; however, only 5 had conclusive evidence that the abnormalities were not related to endotoxemia or electrolyte abnormalities.[46]

CLINICAL FINDINGS IN NEONATAL ENCEPHALOPATHY

The clinical findings associated with NE are extensive and have been widely described over many years, beginning with the first clear description in the veterinary medical literature in 1930.[47] Clinical abnormalities reported in association with a diagnosis of NE, NMS or perinatal asphyxia include altered consciousness and disorientation, wandering, lack of affinity for the dam, lack of suckle, ataxia, tremors, star-gazing, blindness, recumbency, seizures, abnormal phonation, and dysphagia. Signs can be present from birth or may develop several hours later. Abnormalities of other body systems have also been associated with foals with NE, such as gastrointestinal ileus, retained meconium, enteritis, colitis and diarrhea, cardiac dysrhythmias, renal failure, and hepatic disease. It is likely that many of these clinical abnormalities are complications associated with impaired nursing, malnutrition, failure of passive transfer, or perinatal asphyxia as a primary organ-specific event. There is likely to be substantial interaction among these different clinical abnormalities, with a primary cause leading to secondary effects (**Fig. 1**).

Treatment

Treatment of NE is dictated by the clinical presentation and abnormalities present, rather than a proscriptive approach based on a putative diagnosis, due to the wide range of abnormalities that might be present as well as differences in severity. High-quality supportive care is needed to mitigate the effects of impaired nursing, thermoregulation, respiratory abnormalities, seizures, and impaired ambulation. Specific laboratory abnormalities must be corrected, and attention to the prevention of complications is important.

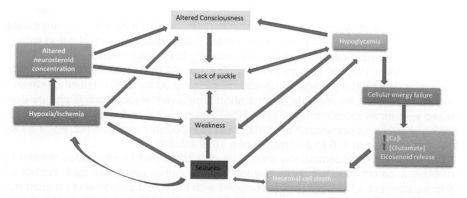

Fig. 1. Interactions of multiple factors in the development of seizures associated with neonatal encephalopathy. Altered consciousness is a key central component, as a cause and result of numerous complex interactions.

As with the care of any ill neonate, the foal should be housed in an environment that enhances the caretaker's ability to deliver care and mitigates the development of complications. This should include housing in a stall which will allow for frequent observation as well as external heating to either prevent or correct hypothermia and allows the foal to stay dry and avoid the development of decubiti if it is down. An environment that provides the ability to restrain the mare and administer fluids or other medications as needed is also important.

In foals with uncomplicated maladjustment, that is no signs of asphyxia or metabolic derangements, in addition to supportive care one can attempt to accelerate the adaption to extrauterine life by using the "Madigan Squeeze" procedure.[19] The purpose of this procedure is to simulate the pressure induced by parturition, thus resetting the HPA axis, although the precise endocrine changes induced by the procedure, if any, are currently unknown. The procedure is performed using a large diameter soft cotton rope which is looped around the chest in a surcingle fashion, then pressure is applied for up to 20 minutes. In one reported study in which 195 foals with NMS were treated with either conventional medical therapy or the squeeze technique, the overall outcome was equivalent (87% success for medical treatment vs 86% for the squeeze technique); however, foals treated using the squeeze technique had a faster recovery, with 4% versus 37% success (medical treatment vs squeeze treatment; $P < .001$) at 1 hour after treatment, and 35% success versus 68% success (medical treatment vs squeeze treatment) at 24 hours or less.[19] Treatment failure at 72 hours was equivalent between treatment groups (13% vs 14%).[19] Some foals treated using this thoracic compression procedure also received medical treatment, and some foals also received the squeeze treatment multiple times. Hence, the true effects of the "squeeze technique" are unclear at the present time.

The procedure seems to be safe to perform in foals in which respiratory depression is not present and there are no fractured ribs; thoracic compression in these foals might worsen respiratory compromise or cause serious intrathoracic injury. Further, foals should not have abdominal distention, as thoracic compression in these patients might lead to pain, diaphragmatic compression, or reflux of gastric contents with the risk of aspiration.

The thoracic compression procedure seems to reduce the duration of illness in some patients, is easy to apply, and is associated with very little risk or expense; however, it is important to recognize that it is unlikely to have any effect in foals with perinatal asphyxia or other metabolic compromises; patient selection is, therefore, important.

Dehydration and hypoglycemia are common in foals with NE arising from any cause due to impaired nursing. Polyionic replacement fluids should be administered to correct dehydration and expand fluid volume; warming the fluids is helpful in cold environments or when the foal is hypothermic. The normal maintenance fluid rate for a neonate is 100 to 120 mg/kg/d (210–250 mLs/h for a 50 kg foal). If failure of passive transfer is present, intravenous plasma should be given. Hypoglycemia can be corrected with intravenous dextrose (5%–10%) at a rate of 4 to 8 mg/kg minute; bolus dosing should be discouraged as it may lead to rebound hypoglycemia. For a 50 kg foal, this equates to 120 to 240 mLs/h of a 10% solution.

Serum glucose concentrations should be monitored and infusion rates titrated to maintain a serum glucose concentration in the normal range, as tight control of glucose concentration has been associated with improved outcomes in critical human patients.[48] Persistent hypoglycemia has been associated with nonsurvival in foals; however, the impact of blood glucose concentrations on outcome in NE specifically has not been investigated.[49] Given the importance of neuronal energy failure in the pathophysiology of some forms of NE, maintaining blood glucose is of particular importance in affected foals. The evidence for the effects of abnormal glucose concentrations in NE in other species is conflicting, with both hypo- and hyperglycemia associated with worse outcomes.[50–52] In human infants hyperglycemia was temporally associated with increased frequency of seizures.[53] Some evidence exists indicating hypoglycemia is neuroprotective in experimental animals with perinatal asphyxia; however, this is not a consistent finding. In horses hypoglycemia was highly associated with neurologic disorders including seizures, subclinical EEG abnormalities, alterations in consciousness disorientation, blindness, and deafness.[54] Hypoglycemia has been reported to be a leading cause of neurologic abnormalities in human infants with metabolic or infectious diseases.[55] Hemorrhage of cortical white matter and infarction have been documented in up to 94% of human newborns.[56] Similar lesions have been observed in neonatal foals diagnosed with NMS; however, they were attributed to hypoxia.[11,57,58] The relationship between these events and brain pathology is complex and cannot be elucidated in foals with currently available data; however, substantial overlap between these 2 pathologic events seems likely.

In foals that do not have ileus or enteritis, enteral feeding is often an effective method to maintain hydration status and provide nutritional support and is most easily achieved with an indwelling nasogastric tube. Milk or milk replacer at 15%–20% of the foal's body weight/d should be administered divided into feedings every 1 to 2 hrs for those foals which will tolerate enteral feeding.

In ill neonatal foals, hypothermia is a common finding due to the combined effects of minimal body stores of fat, hypoglycemia, weakness leading to recumbency on cold ground, poor mechanisms of heat generation (perhaps associated with maladaptation), or sepsis. Previous studies have documented a reduced survival in hypothermic foals.[59] In human infants suffering from HIE, however, therapeutic hypothermia has become a routine standard of care, either as a whole body or selective (head) cooling, to a temperature range of 33.5° to 35.0° C.[60] Studies of therapeutic hypothermia have demonstrated a reduced risk of death or major neurodevelopmental disabilities in human infants with moderate or severe HIE.[61] The role of hypothermia in equine neonates with perinatal asphyxia and HIE is unknown at the current time; however, it would seem that intentional permissive hypothermia in the care of critical equine neonates is premature until more is known about optimum temperatures, protocols, and affects on other body systems.

Given the association of electrolyte abnormalities in critical neonatal illness correcting all electrolyte disorders is very important. Intravenous magnesium has been investigated and advocated for the treatment of NE in humans and foals. Magnesium has several effects at the cellular level which may be beneficial in ameliorating the effects of cellular hypoxia. Magnesium blocks the NMDA receptor, reducing the release of glutamate; secondary effects are to block calcium entry into the cell–both neurotoxic events in the pathophysiology of hypoxia.[62] For these reasons, magnesium has been advocated for the treatment of NE in foals[63] and for HIE in human infants.[62,64] Results regarding the effectiveness of this approach are conflicting. In a model of hypoxia in newborn rats magnesium treatment was associated with recovery;[65] however, other studies have revealed worse damage associated with postasphyxial magnesium treatment.[66] Such results indicate that the age of the subject and the timing of treatment related to injury have a substantial influence on the effects of the treatment. A meta-analysis of human clinical intervention studies found that magnesium treatment had no effect on survival or severe neurodevelopmental outcomes, or the incidence of seizures in human infants with HIE.[62] Short-term composite outcome (survival with abnormal neurodevelopmental examination) was improved, however.[62] An additional study investigating the effects of magnesium treatment on the CSF concentrations of glutamate and aspartate found that the concentration of the excitatory amino acids increased proportionately to the severity of clinical illness and that the postnatal administration of magnesium sulfate did not alter the concentrations observed.[64] Hence, there seems to be little justification at the present time for the administration of magnesium sulfate to foals with NE.

As described above, perinatal asphyxia is a multi-systemic illness and successful treatment requires a multi-pronged approach, based on a full and complete assessment of the foal's condition including the assessment of metabolic status, blood pressure, and tissue perfusion. Correction of both hypoxia and impaired tissue perfusion must be achieved. Hypoxemia is usually best corrected by the administration of humidified nasal oxygen (5–10 L/min). Maintaining the foal in sternal recumbency will optimize oxygenation, but if hypoventilation is present oxygen supplementation is unlikely to be effective. In cases of hypoventilation due to CNS respiratory depression treatment with doxapram as a continuous rate infusion seems to be the most effective[67]; alternatively theophylline can be used, but dosage and blood concentration must be carefully monitored to limit toxicity. Caffeine seems to have little effect and its use is not recommended.[67] Mechanical ventilation is required for those foals which do not respond to respiratory stimulants.

Seizures are common in foals with NE; in one study of full-term foals with NE in a hospital setting 48/246 foals (19.5%) experience seizures during hospitalization.[68] Those that had seizures were 8 times more likely to be hospitalized for more than 10 days, and 5.4 times more likely to require cardiovascular support compared with those that did not have seizures.[68] Overall survival rate did not differ between groups, however.[68] In another study examining 94 foals with NE, seizures were identified in 22% of affected foals, and the presence of seizures did not have an effect on survival.[69] Another study, however, found that the presence of seizures in hospitalized equine neonates in the first 24 hours increased the odds of nonsurvival (odds ratio (OR): 21.5, 95% confidence interval (CI): 2.26–352.88) compared with those that do not experience seizures.[70] These studies reported only clinically apparent seizures. In human neonates subclinical seizures (aka electrographic seizures), that is electrophysiological seizures without observable clinical expression, are reported to occur more commonly than electroclinical seizures.[71] Electrographic seizures have been documented by the author (unpublished data), but remain unreported in the equine neonatal literature at the present time.

Seizure activity contributes to foal morbidity because seizure activity increases cerebral oxygen consumption and contributes to ongoing injury.[72] The consequences of seizures in the neonate include a drop in cerebral ATP and phosphocreatine concentration and a secondary increase in pyruvate, of which a large proportion is then metabolized to lactate.[73] This cerebral hyperlactatemia leads to local vasodilation, which in concert with hypertension associated with seizures results in an increased cerebral blood flow and delivery of energy substrate.[74] Despite these protective effects, in experimental neonatal animals seizures result in a drastic decrease in brain glucose concentrations (within minutes), an effect observed even in the presence of increased blood glucose concentrations.[73,75] The decreased brain glucose and increased brain lactate mimic the effects of asphyxia, and exacerbate the energy failure which is a central component of the pathophysiology of asphyxia. Further, seizures are associated with a substantial increase in mean systemic blood pressure, hypoventilation, and apnea, all of which may contribute to CNS injury.[30]

Hypoxia of only 20 minutes duration has been found to impair cerebral autoregulation, resulting in a reduction of cerebral arterial oxygen concentration up to 50% of normal.[76]

Seizure activity also results in excessive release of glutamate. Clearly, seizures are both a cause and result of cerebral hypoxia, and control of seizures is important in the overall management of affected foals.

For the reasons described above, seizures should be treated immediately and not allowed to progress. Diazepam (0.11–0.44 mg/kg IV) is frequently used, although an effective alternative is midazolam (0.04–0.1 mg/kg IV).[77] Both agents are fairly short-acting, and if seizures persist or recur then longer-acting alternatives such as phenobarbital (2–10 mg/kg IV BID) can be used. Alternatively, midazolam can be administered by CRI (0.02–0.06 mg/kg/h) for persistent seizure activity.[77]

An attractive drug for the control of seizures is levetiracetam, which is widely used in human and small animal medicine. Pharmacokinetic studies have found a half-life of 7.7 ± 0.5 hrs, and a dose of 32 mg/kg IV or orally BID results in plasma concentrations that are similar to target concentrations for seizure control in humans.[78] Studies on the clinical use of levetiracetam in neonatal foals are not currently available.

Outcome and Prognosis

In the authors' experience as well as published literature, most foals (85%) with uncomplicated maladjustment will survive with appropriate treatment. Those foals which have perinatal asphyxia, however, have a poorer prognosis which depends in large part on the severity and duration of the hypoxia, which is usually unknown and is difficult to quantify. These patients often also tend to have complications such as systemic inflammatory response syndrome (SIRS), joint infections, or respiratory disease (aspiration pneumonia, meconium aspiration, and so forth) which make the prognosis much less favorable. Foals that have signs of cerebral necrosis as suggested by high CSF protein, intracranial bleeding or increased intracranial pressure have a guarded to poor prognosis. Poor outcomes likely result from comorbidities or acquired complications such as sepsis, prematurity.[69]

CLINICS CARE POINTS

- When treating foals with foals with NE it is critical to: Maintain energy balance with nutritional support.
- Establish and maintain proper hydration and electrolyte balance Control seizures aggresively Provide a warm and dry treatment space.

REFERENCES

1. Cohen ND. Causes of and farm management factors associated with disease and death in foals. J Am Vet Med Assoc 1994;204:1644-51.
2. Bernard WV, Reimer JM, Cudd T. Historical features, clinicopathologic findings, clinical features, and outcome of equine neonates presenting with or developing signs of central nervous system disease. Proc Amer Assoc Eq Pract 1995;41: 222–4.
3. Viu J, Monreal L, Jose-Cunlleras E, et al. Clinical findings in 10 foals with bacterial meningoencephalitis. Equine Vet J 2012;44:100–4.
4. Sanchez LC, Lester GD. Equine neonatal sepsis: microbial isolates, antimicrobial resistance, and short and long-term outcomes. In: Davenport D, Patrdis M, editors. 18th Annual Veterinary Medical Forum 2000:223 - 224. Seattle, WA.

5. Koterba AM, Brewer BD, Tarplee FA. Clinical and clinicopathological characteristics of the septicaemic neonatal foal: Review of 38 cases. Equine Vet J 1984;16: 376–83.

6. Platt H. Septicaemia in the foal. A review of 61 cases. Br Vet J 1973;129:221–9.

7. Laugier C, Tapprest J, Foucher N, et al. A necropsy survey of neurologic diseases in 4,319 horses examined in Normandy (France) from 1986 - 2006. J Eq Vet Sci 2009;29:561–8.

8. Sanchez LC, Giguere S, Lester GD. Factors associated with survival of neonatal foals with bacteremia and racing performance of surviving Throughbred: 423 cases (1982 - 2007. J Am Vet Med Assoc 2008;233:1446–52.

9. Crowe MW, Swerczek TW. Equine congenital defects. Am J Vet Res 1985;46: 353–8.

10. Rossdale PD. Modern concepts of neonatal disease in foals. Equine Vet J 1972;4: 117–28.

11. Palmer A, Rossdale PD. Neuropathology of the convulsive foal syndrome. J Reprod Fertil 1975;23:691–4.

12. Diesch TJ, Mellor DJ. Birth transitions: Pathophysiology, the onset of consciousness and possible implications for neonatal maladjustment syndrome in the foal. Equine Vet J 2013;45:656–60.

13. Mellor DJ, Diesch TJ. Birth and hatching: key events in the onset of awareness in the lamb and chick. NZ Vet J 2007;55:51–60.

14. Mellor DJ, Diesch TJ. The importance of 'awareness' for understanding fetal pain. Brain Res Rev 2005;49:455–71.

15. Hirst JJ, Kelleher MA, Walker DW, et al. Neuroactive steroids in pregnancy: key regulatory and protective roles in the foetal brain. Steroid Biochem Mol Biol 2014;139:144–53.

16. Brunton PJ. Programming the brain and behaviour by Early-Life Stress: a focus on neuroactive steroids. J Neuroendocrinol 2015;27:468–80.

17. Toribio RE. Equine Neonatal Encephalopathy. Vet Clin North Am Equine Pract 2019;35:363–78.

18. Mellon SH, Griffin LD. Neurosteroids: biochemistry and clinical significance. Trends Endocrinol Metab 2002;13:35–43.

19. Aleman M, Weich KM, Madigan JE. Survey of veterinarians using a novel physical compression squeeze procedure in the management of neonatal maladjustement syndrome in foals. Animals (Basel) 2017;7:69.

20. Houghton E, Holtan D, Grainger L, et al. Plasma progestagen concentrations in the normal and dysmature newborn foal. J Reprod Fertil Suppl 1991;44:609–17.

21. Rossdale PD, Ousey JC, Mcgladdery AJ, et al. A retrospective study of increased plasma progestagen concentrations in compromized neonatal foals. Reprod Fertil Dev 1995;7:567–75.

22. Aleman M, Pickles KJ, Conley AJ, et al. Abnormal plasma neuroactive progestagen derivatives in ill, neonatal foals presented to the neonatal intensive care unit. Equine Vet J 2013;45:661–5.

23. Swink JM, Rings LM, Snyder HA, et al. Dynamics of androgens in healthy and hospitalized newborn foals. J Vet Intern Med 2021;35:538–49.

24. Majewska MD. Neuronal actions of dehydroepiandrosterone possible roles in brain development, aging, memory, and affect. Ann NY Acad Sci 1995;774: 111–20.

25. Stárka L, Dušková M, Hill M. Dehydroepiandrosterone: a neuroactive steroid. J Steroid Biochem Mol Biol 2015;145:254–60.

26. Lacobone E, Bailly-Salin J, Polito A, et al. Sepsis-associated encephalopathy and its differential diagnosis. Crit Care Med 2009;37:S331–6.
27. Chaudhry A, Duggal AK. Sepsis Associated Encephalopathy. Adv Med 2014. https://doi.org/10.1155/2014/762320.
28. Dembek KA, Timko KJ, Johnson LM, et al. Steroids, steroid precursors, and neuroactive steroids in critically ill neonates. Vet J 2017;225:42–9.
29. Vannucci RC, Duffy TE. Cerebral metabolism in fetal and neonatal rat brain during anoxia and recovery. Am J Phys 1977;230:1269–75.
30. Volpe JJ. Hypoxic-Ischemic Encephalopathy. In: Volpe JJ, editor. Neurology of the newborn. Philadelphia, PA: W. B. Saunders; 1995. p. 211–59.
31. Holowach-Thurston J, McDougal DB. Effect of ischemia on metabolism of the brain of the newborn mouse. Am J Phys 1969;216:348–52.
32. Palmer C, Brucklacher RM, Cristensen ME, et al. Carbohydrate and energy metabolism during the evolution of hypoxic-ischemic brain damage in the immature rat. J Cereb Blood Flow Metab 1990;10:227–35.
33. Ebersoldt M, Sharshar T, Annane D. Sepsis-associated delirium. Intensive Care Med 2007;33:941–50.
34. Siami S, Annane D, Sharshar T. The encephalopathy in sepsis. Crit Care Clin 2008;24:67–82.
35. Ringger NC, Giguere S, Morresey PR, et al. Biomarkers of brain injury in foals with hypoxic-ischemic encephalopathy. J Vet Intern Med 2011;25:132–7.
36. Polkes AC, Giguere S, Lester GD, et al. Factors associated with outcome in foals with neonatal isoerythrolysis (72 cases, 1988-2003). J Vet Intern Med 2008;22:1216–22.
37. David JB, Byars TD, Braniecki A, et al. Kernicterus in a foal with neonatal isoerythrolysis. Comp Contln Educ Pract Vet 1998;20:517–20.
38. Loynachan AT, Williams NM, Freestone JF. Kernicterus in a neonatal foal. J Vet Diagn Invest 2007;19:209–12.
39. Perlman JM, Volpe JJ. Bilirubin. In: Volpe JJ, editor. Volpe's neurology of the newborn. 6th edition. Philadelphia, PA: Elsevier; 2018. p. 730–62.
40. Furr M, Bender H. Cerebrospinal fluid variables in clinically normal foals from birth to 42 days of age. Am J Vet Res 1994;55:781–4.
41. Johnson AL, Gilsenan WF, Palmer JE. Metabolic encephalopathies in foals - pay attention to the serum biochemistry panel. Equine Vet Educ 2012;24:233–5.
42. Lakritz J, Madigan J, Carlson GP. Hypovolemic hyponatremia and signs of neurologic disease associated with diarrhea in a foal. J Am Vet Med Assoc 1992;200:1114–6.
43. Collins NM, Axon JE, Carrick JB, et al. Severe hyponatraemia in foals: clinical findings, primary diagnosis and outcome. Aust Vet J 2016;94:186–91.
44. Hardefeldt LY. Hyponatraemic encephalopathy in azotaemic neonatal foals: four cases. Aust Vet J 2014;92:488–91.
45. Bouchard PR, Weldon AD, Lewis RM, et al. Uremic encephalopathy in a horse. Vet Pathol 1994;31:111–5.
46. Frye MA, Johnson JS, Traub-Dagartz JL, et al. Putative uremic encephalopathy in horses: five cases (1978-1998). J Am Vet Med Assoc 2001;218:560–6.
47. Reynolds EB. Clinical notes on some conditions met within the mare following parturition and in the newly born foal. Vet Rec 1930;10:277–80.
48. Bagshaw SM, Egi M, George C, et al. Early blood glucose control and mortality in critically ill patients. Aust Crit Care Med 2009;37:463–70.
49. Hollis AR, Furr MO, Magdesian KG, et al. Blood glucose concentrations in critically ill neonatal foals. J Vet Intern Med 2008;22:1223–7.

50. Spies EE, Lababidi SL, McBride MC. Early hypoglycemia is associated with poor gross motor outcome in asphyxiated term newborns. Pediatr Neurol 2014;50: 586–90.
51. Tam EWY, Haeusslein LA, Bonifacio SL, et al. Hypoglycemia is associated with increased risk for braininjury and adverse neurodevelopmental outcome in neonates at risk for encephalopathy. J Pediatr 2012;161:88–93.
52. Basu SK, Kaiser JR, Guffey D, et al. Hypoglycaemia and hyperglycaemia are associated with unfavourable outcome in infants with hypoxic ischaemic encephalopathy: a post hoc analysis of the CoolCap Study. Arch Dis Child Fetal Neonatal Ed 2016;101:F149–55.
53. Pinchefsky EF, Hahn CD, Kamino D, et al. Hyperglycemia and glucose variability are associated with worse brain function and seizures in neonatal encephalopathy: a prospective cohort study. J Pediatr 2019;209:23–32.
54. Aleman M, Costa LRR, Crowe C, et al. Presumed neuroglycopenia caused by severe hypoglycemia in horses. J Vet Intern Med 2018;32:1731–9.
55. Montassir H, Maegaki Y, Ogura K, et al. Associated factors in neonatal hypoglyemic brain injury. Brain Devel 2009;31:649–56.
56. Burns CM, Rutherford MA, Boardman JP, et al. Patterns of cerebral injury and neurodevelopmental outcomes after symptomatic neonatal hypoglycemia. Pediatrician 2008;122:65–74.
57. Palmer A, Rossdale PD. Neuropathological changes assocated with the neonatal maladjustment syndrome in the thoroughbred foal. Res Vet Sci 1976;20:267–75.
58. Palmer AC, Leadon DP, Rossdale PD, et al. Intracranial haemorrhage in previable, premature, and full term foals. Equine Vet J 1984;16:383–9.
59. Furr M, Tinker MK, Edens L. Prognosis for neonatal foals in an intensive care unit. J Vet Intern Med 1997;11:183–8.
60. Douglas-Escobar M, Weiss MD. Hypoxic-Ischemic Encephalopathy: a review for clinicians. J Amer Med Assoc Pediatr 2015;169:397–403.
61. Tagin MA, Wollcot CG, VIncer MJ, et al. Hypothermia for neonatal hypoxic eschemic encephalopathy: an updated systemic review and meta-analysis. Arch Pediatr Adolesc Med 2012;166:558–66.
62. Tagin M, Shah PS, Lee K-S. Magnesium for newborns with hypoxic-ischemic encephalopathy: a systematic review and meta-analysis. J Perinatol 2013;33:663–9.
63. Wilkins P. Magnesium infusion in hypoxic-ischemic encephalopathy. Proc Annu Meet Am Coll Vet Intern Med 2001;19:242–3.
64. Khashaba MT, Shouman BO, Shlout AA, et al. Excitatory amino acids and magnesium sulfate in neonatal asphyxia. Brain Devel 2006;28:375–9.
65. Seimkowicz E. Magnesium sulfate dramatically improves immediate recovery of rats from hypoxia. Resuscitation 1997;35:53–9.
66. Sameshima H, Ota A, Ikenoue T. Pretreatent with magnesium sulfate protects against hypoxic-ischemic brain injury but post-asphyxial treatment worsens braininjury in 7 day old rats. Am J Obstet Gynecol 1999;180:725–30.
67. Giguere S, Slade JK, Sancehz LC. Retrospective comparison of caffeine and doxopram for the treatment of hypercapnia in foals with hypoxic-ischemic encephalopathy. J Vet Intern Med 2008;22:401–5.
68. Savage VL, Collins NM, Axon JE, et al. The effect of generalized seizures on outcome of foals with neonatal encephalopathy: 246 cases. Aust Eq Vet 2015; 34:40.
69. Lyle-Dugas J, Giguere S, Mallicote MF, et al. Factors associated with outcome in 94 hospitalized foals diagnosed with neonatal encephalopathy. Equine Vet J 2017;49:207–10.

70. Gold J, Chaffin MK, Burgess BA, et al. Factors associated with non-survival in foals diagnosed with perinatal asphyxia syndrome. J Eq Vet Sci 2016;38:82–6.
71. Scher MS, Aso K, Beggarly ME, et al. Electrographic seizures in preterm and full-term neonates: Clinical correlates, associated brain lesions, and risk for neurological sequelae. Pediatr 1993;91:128–34.
72. Perlman JM. Intervention strategies for neonatal hypoxic-ischemic cerebral injury. Clin Therap 2006;28:1353–65.
73. Fujikawa DG, Vannuci RC, Dwyer BE, et al. Generalized seizures deplete brain energy reserve in normoxemic newborn monkeys. Brain Res 1988;454:51–9.
74. Young RS, Osbakken MD, Briggs W, et al. ^{31}P NMR study of cerebral metabolism during prolonged seizures in the neonatal dog. Ann Neurol 1985;18:14–20.
75. Fujikawa DG, Dwyer BE, Lake RR, et al. Local cerebral glucose utilization during status epilepticus in newborn primates. Am J Phys 1989;256:C1160–7.
76. Tweed A, Cote J, Lou H, et al. Impairment of cerebral blood flow autoregulation in the newborn lamb by hypoxia. Pediatr Res 1986;20:516–9.
77. Wilkins P. How to use midazolam to control equine neonatal seizures. Proc 51st Ann Conv Amer Assoc Eq Pract 2005;51:279–80.
78. Macdonald KD, Hart KA, Davis JL, et al. Pharmacokinetics of the anticonvulsant levetiracetam in neonatal foals Equine. Vet J 2018;50:532–6.

Arboviral Equine Encephalitides

Ramiro E. Toribio, DVM, MS, PhD

KEYWORDS

- Alphavirus • Flavivirus • Encephalitis • Encephalomyelitis • Horse • West Nile
- Eastern • Western • Venezuelan

KEY POINTS

- Increasing number of human and equine cases of Eastern equine encephalitis (EEE) and Venezuelan equine encephalitis (VEE) in the Americas as well as West Nile virus encephalitis (WNVE) lineage 2 in Europe is raising concerns on these arboviral diseases. Western equine encephalitis (WEE) is rarely diagnosed in people or horses.
- Weather changes affecting vector emergence and bird migration patterns could be contributing to the increasing cases of arboviral infections in horses and humans.
- Evolutionary strategies allow these viruses to reach the central nervous system by breaching the blood brain barrier or direct access through the olfactory epithelium.
- Despite medical treatment, EEE, VEE, and WEE have higher equine mortality rates (50–90%) compared with WNVE (<40%).
- Vaccination against these viruses is highly effective and is the best measure to prevent them.

INTRODUCTION

A number of viruses transmitted by biological vectors or through direct contact, air, or ingestion cause neurologic disease in equids. Of interest are viruses of the *Togaviridae*, *Flaviviridae*, *Rhabdoviridae*, *Herpesviridae*, *Bornaviridae*, and *Bunyaviridae* families. Many are classified as arboviruses because they use arthropod vectors, whereas others are transmitted directly via ingestion, inhalation, or integument damage. They reach the central nervous system (CNS) through blood, carried by mononuclear cells, or via retrograde axonal transport to the spinal cord or directly to the brain via the olfactory and nasopharyngeal epithelium. Lesions and clinical signs are the result of vascular damage, hemorrhage, thrombosis, edema, inflammation, neuronal and glial cell degeneration and dysfunction, apoptosis, and necrosis. Variable degree of inflammation is present with these viruses but lack of an inflammatory response

College of Veterinary Medicine, The Ohio State University, 601 Vernon Tharp Street, Columbus, OH 43210, USA
E-mail address: toribio.1@osu.edu

Vet Clin Equine 38 (2022) 299–321
https://doi.org/10.1016/j.cveq.2022.04.004
vetequine.theclinics.com
0749-0739/22/© 2022 Elsevier Inc. All rights reserved.

does not rule out their presence. The goal of this article is to provide an overview on pathophysiologic and clinical aspects of arboviruses of equine importance, including alphaviruses (*Togaviridae*) and flaviviruses (*Flaviviridae*). Information on the relevance of members of the *Bunyaviridae* family and equine disease is scarce.

Togaviral Encephalitis

Equine togaviral encephalitides (encephalomyelitis) are caused by viruses of the *Martellivirales* order, *Togaviridae* family, and *Alphavirus* genus that includes four viruses (Eastern equine encephalitis virus [EEEV], Madariaga virus [MV], Western equine encephalitis virus [WEEV], and Venezuelan equine encephalitis virus [VEEV]). Alphaviruses are small spherical viruses with a lipid bilayer and a positive-sense single-stranded RNA (Class IV). The RNA (11.4–11.7 kb) encodes structural (C, E1, E2, E3) and nonstructural (nsP1–P4) proteins.[1,2] Protein C is the core nucleocapsid, whereas E1–E3 will mature into glycoprotein spikes that facilitate receptor binding and cell membrane fusion.[2] E2 glycoprotein binds to heparan sulfate sites on the cell membrane to mediate viral attachment and entry.[3] Glycoproteins E1 and E2 are immunogenic and induce neutralizing antibodies. With the application of molecular techniques, these viruses have been reclassified and new types and subtypes will likely be included in the coming years.[2]

These togaviral encephalitides are restricted to the Americas.[1,4] Depending on the virus, the biological cycle includes mosquitoes, birds, small mammals (rodents, marsupials, bats), and equids. In temperate climates, neurologic disease is seasonal (spring to fall), whereas in warmer or tropical regions, it occurs throughout the year, with exacerbation during the rainy season. The distribution of these viruses is regional. They are not a problem in Europe, but recent studies classify them as potential emergent diseases for humans and horses.[4,5] Alphaviruses do not cause clinical disease in their natural reservoirs (birds, rodents). Most people and horses do not develop clinical signs and in those affected signs are mild and nonspecific. It is estimated that less than 10% of people with systemic signs will develop neurologic disease. EEEV and VEEV are more neuroinvasive. Young animals and children are more likely to develop signs that can be more severe. Incubation varies from 2 days to 3 weeks, depending on the virus (virulence) and immunity.

Eastern Equine Encephalitis/Madariaga Virus Encephalitis

Etiology

Eastern equine encephalitis (EEE) (encephalomyelitis) is a neurologic condition of equids and people caused by the EEEV and transmitted by mosquitoes. It is the deadliest alphavirus for humans and horses, with mortality rates up to 50% and 90%, respectively.[6,7] Four linages have been described.[2] Most strains in North America and the Caribbean comprise lineage I, whereas strains in Central and South America are from lineages II, III, and IV.[2] Differences in genetic conservation between North and South American lineages may be related to viral adaptations to different mosquito and vertebrate species.[2] Recent gene sequence analysis showed that North and South American lineages are different viruses within the EEE complex.[2] South American lineages II, III, and IV have been reclassified as the Madariaga virus (MV)[2,8] that typically causes neurologic disease in horses and donkeys.[2] Before 2010, MV was not associated with encephalitis in humans. However, this changed with an outbreak of neurologic disease in humans and horses in Panama.[9] MV is in the list of emerging pathogens causing neurologic signs in people in Latin America, particularly in children.[9–12] MV has been found in *Culex* spp. (*Melanoconion*), rodents, opossums, bats, birds, and snakes.[12] *Aedes* spp. and *Psorophora* spp. can transmit MV.[11]

Epidemiology

First cases of EEE in equids and humans were documented in Massachusetts (eastern) in 1831 and 1838, respectively. The virus was first isolated from a horse in 1933. The largest EEE outbreak in the United States occurred in New Jersey in 1959 with 32 human cases in 8 weeks.[6] Most cases in North America occur from late spring to early fall. The virus has a wide distribution, present in North, Central, and South America and the Caribbean. In North America, it is more common in northeastern, southeastern, and Gulf States from Maine to Texas.[6,7] Occasional cases occur in other states, in particular near the GREAT LAKES. Equine cases have been reported in Ontario and Quebec, Canada.[13] An increase in equine cases recently occurred in Michigan, Wisconsin, and New England states. Most affected horses and donkeys are not vaccinated, with no breed or sex predilection. In North America, human cases have been rare, but it is becoming an emergent pathogen, with 6 to 11 human cases per year, mainly in eastern and southeastern states.[6,14] Human cases may be preceded by equine cases. The increasing incidence of EEE in people and horses has been attributed in part to climate changes and environmental perturbations that improve mosquito proliferation and changes in bird migration patterns.[6] The human fatality rate is 30% or higher, with neurologic sequelae seen in 50% of survivors.[6,7] Equine mortality is much higher (up to 90%) despite aggressive medical treatment. The EEE is a notifiable disease, and cases in the United States are monitored via ArboNET,[15] the Centers for Disease Control and Prevention (CDC) arboviral disease surveillance system.

Biological cycle

In North America, EEEV persists in an enzootic (sylvatic) cycle between passerine birds and ornithophilic mosquitoes such as *Culiseta melanura*. In Central and South America, *Culex* spp. is the main vector and rodents, marsupials and bats are the important hosts in this region.[2,12] Reptiles and amphibian may be involved in the southern United States.[16] Native birds do not develop clinical disease but establish enough viremia to transmit the virus to mosquitoes. *Culiseta melanura* does not feed on mammals and apparently does not contribute to disease in these animals. However, escape from the enzootic to the epizootic cycle occurs with less discriminant "bridging" mosquitoes (*Culex* spp., *Aedes* spp., *Coquillettidia* spp., *Anopheles* spp., *Psorophora* spp., and *Ochlerotatus* spp.) that feed on mammals, birds, reptiles, and amphibians, infecting equids, humans, exotic birds, and other animals.[17] Vectors such as chicken mites (*Dermanyssidae*), chicken lice (*Menacanthus stramineus*), and assassin bugs (*Reduviidae*) may maintain EEEV in some bird populations.[17] Wide vector range in the tropics may contribute to viral diversity in South American lineages.[2] Factors that contribute to spillover include weather changes that impact mosquito populations and bird migration patterns, environmental disturbances, and changes in human behavior which increase the likelihood of viral exposure.[17] Equids and humans do not develop sufficient viremias to transmit the virus to mosquitoes and are terminal hosts. Few cases of aerosol transmission have been documented in animals and people.[18] Occasional cases have been reported in pigs, cattle, sheep, cervids, camelids, and nonnative birds.[19] During winter, the virus enters in diapause in vectors.

Western Equine Encephalitis

Etiology

Western equine encephalitis or encephalomyelitis (WEE) is a rare viral progressive neurologic condition of horses and humans in North, Central, and South America.[20]

Etiologic agents in the WEEV antigenic serocomplex include viruses from the Americas (WEEV, Highlands J [HJV], Fort Morgan, Buggy Creek, Aura), Europe/Africa (Sindbis, Ockelbo, Babanki), and Oceania (Whataroa). Equine disease by most of these viruses has not been documented. There are two variants of interest in the WEEV serocomplex (WEEV and HJV). Within the WEEV variant, there are two groups (A and B) and under group B there are three sublineages.[21] HJV has traditionally been classified as a subtype of WEEV, but serologic and genetic testing indicates that this is a distinct alphavirus. Both WEEV and HJV are related to the Sindbis virus that is prevalent in eastern Africa, the Middle East, Europe, and Australia.[22,23] There is evidence WEEV and HJV arouse from recombination between EEEV and a Sindbis-like virus.[22,24]

Epidemiology

WEE was first reported in 1930 in the San Joaquin Valley, California (western),[25] where approximately 6000 equids developed neurologic disease and 3000 died or were euthanized (50% mortality rate).[25] Since then many epizootics occurred in western states affecting thousands of equids with mortality rates of 20% to 50%. The virus also infects people, but mortality is lower. Human cases, including fatalities have been documented in locations where horses were affected.[26] In the 1930s, more cases were documented in Minnesota in a 3-year period than in other states, with 41,159 equids affected of which 9200 died. Aedes spp. was the responsible vector.[26] Human and equine cases of WEE have been documented in Latin America, as far south as Argentina.[27] In the United States, WEEV causes most infections in western states, although HJV is responsible for human and equine cases in eastern and southern states.[22] WEEV is less pathogenic than EEEV and VEEV. Prevalence in horses has decreased because of extensive vaccination and mosquito control practices.

The number of human and equine cases of WEE has been declining since the 1960s, and no cases have been documented in over 20 years in the United States, but sporadic human cases occur in South America.[20]

Biological cycle

In North America, *Culex tarsalis* is the main vector that maintains WEEV in a bird-mosquito cycle. Warm weather and humidity lead to a rapid increase in the *Culex tarsalis* population. Less discriminant mosquito species (eg, *Aedes* spp.) that feed on birds, rodents, and reptiles lead to viral spills into horses and people. Reptiles and amphibian can amplify WEEV and develop viremias. Rodents and small mammals are important in the wild cycle in the southern United States and Latin America.[28] Birds can develop viremia and clinical disease, which seldom is fatal, except exotic birds where the disease can be severe.[29] HJV has a transmission cycle similar to EEEV,[22] and HJV is maintained in birds near swampy areas and is transmitted by *Culiseta melanura*, the main vector for EEEV in North America. As such, HJV transmission to horses and humans uses "bridge" mosquitoes, including *Aedes* spp. and *Ochlerotatus* ssp. HJV is less pathogenic than WEEV to equids and people.[30] HJV can cause disease in some birds,[30] but most native birds are asymptomatic. In Central and South America, rodents, bats, and reptiles are reservoirs for HJV, resembling EEEV. In Latin America, *Aedes* spp. seems to be an important vector of WEEV, but the disease is rare. Ticks may contribute to the life cycle of WEEV.

Venezuelan Equine Encephalitis

Venezuelan equine encephalitis or encephalomyelitis (VEE) is a neurologic disease of humans and equidae mainly present in Latin America, but it has been documented in the southern United States.[31]

Etiology

The genome organization and protein encoding of VEEV are similar to EEEV and WEEV. This virus has six subtypes (I–VI) with antigenic variants within each subtype that display epizootic and enzootic patterns. Subtype I includes variants IAB (VEEV, epizootic), IC (VEEV, epizootic), ID (VEEV, enzootic), IE (VEEV, enzootic), and IF (Mosso das Pedras virus, enzootic); subtype II (Everglades virus, enzootic); subtype III includes IIIA (Mucambo virus A, enzootic), IIIB (Tonate virus B, enzootic), IIIC (Mucambo virus C, enzootic), and IIID (Mucambo virus D, enzootic); subtype IV (Pixuna virus, enzootic); subtype V (Cabassou virus, enzootic); and subtype VI (Rio Negro virus, enzootic).[31–34] Viral phylogenetic analysis suggests that this virus evolved recently.[31] Most VEEV encephalitis in equids and people are caused by variants IAB and IC (epizootic) that are efficiently amplified in the equid-mosquito cycle with high equine viremias that pass the virus to mosquitoes. Pathogenic variants can spread rapidly through susceptible equine populations.[35] Enzootic variants (ID, IE, and II–IV) have been considered minimally pathogenic to equids and people.[31,35] However, the 1993 (Chiapas) and 1996 (Oaxaca) outbreaks in Mexico were caused by subtype IE.[36] Enzootic strains circulate in rodents and wild animals, and indiscriminate vectors (eg, *Ochlerotatus* spp.) are responsible for spillover to people and equids. *Ochlerotatus taeniorhynchus* resides in salty marshes and coastal areas of South, Central, and North America and feeds on mammals, birds, and reptiles, explaining vector and outbreak colocalization.

Epidemiology

The first documented equine outbreak of VEE occurred in Colombia in 1935, although there is evidence of cases in previous years. By 1936, the outbreak spread to Venezuela and years later to Trinidad.[35] Donkeys served as efficient viral amplifiers and contributed to this outbreak.[31] The virus was first isolated from equine brains in Venezuela in 1938 leading to its name (the Venezuela virus; VEEV).[37] The connection between equine and human disease was made in 1950 in Colombia, and the virus was isolated from the brain of affected people in Venezuela.[31,38] The largest documented VEE outbreak occurred in Colombia in the 1960s,[32] where approximately 200,000 people became ill and over 100,000 equids died. Clinical signs in most affected people were nonspecific, whereas in equids signs were mainly neurologic, resulting in high mortality (over 90%). Human and equine outbreaks were also documented in Peru in the 1940s. One outbreak in Ecuador in 1969 affected 31,000 humans with 310 fatalities and around 20,000 equids died.[32]

Sporadic epidemics have occurred in Colombia, Venezuela, Peru, Ecuador, Central America, and Mexico.[31,32,34,39,40] A number of outbreaks in the 1960s–1970s were attributed to the incompletely inactivated vaccines.[31] The Middle America epizootic started in El Salvador and Guatemala in 1969 to rapidly spread to nearby countries, including Mexico.[31,32,39,40] The outbreak followed the Mexican Pacific coast to reach Texas in 1971,[31,32] where approximately 2000 horses were affected with a 75% mortality rate and 110 human cases, but fortunately no deaths.[31,32,39,40] This regional outbreak resulted in 50,000 human cases with 93 fatalities and 50,000 equine deaths.[32] The outbreak was contained after vector control and massive equine vaccination with TC-83 attenuated virus (tissue culture 83; this is a donkey-derived VEEV attenuated after 83 passages in tissue culture). After a 20-year quiescent period, the virus resurfaced in Venezuela in 1992 to lead in 1995 to the second largest outbreak in Venezuela and Colombia, with 100,000 human cases.[31,32,34,41] These outbreaks were caused by subtype IC.[34,41] The restriction of animal movement, vector control, and vaccination with TC-83 vaccine were successful in containing the virus.[31] Major human epidemics have not occurred in the absence of affected equidae.[31] Aerosol or non-equine amplifying hosts may be important in the transmission of certain VEEV subtypes because sporadic human cases have been documented in the absence of equine disease.[31] VEE is a reemerging disease and a potential public health threat.[42]

Biological cycle
Enzootic cycle (sylvatic). This cycle includes rodents, some birds, and mosquitoes. Main rodent reservoirs include *Sigmodon* spp., *Oryzomys* spp., *Zigodontomys* spp., *Heteromys* spp., *Peromyscus* spp., and *Proechimys* spp.[32] These animals develop sufficient viremia to infect vectors and maintain the cycle.[32] Opossums, bats, and other wild mammals may be involved.[12,32] Important enzootic mosquito vectors include *Culex (Melanoconion) cedecei, Culex iolambdis, Culex portesi, Culex ocossa, Culex panocossa, Culex taeniopus, Psorophora ferox, Mansonia titillans,* and *Coquillettidia venezuelensis.* Other mosquitoes species are potential vectors.[43,44] Ticks (*Amblyomma* spp., *Hyalomma* spp.), hematophagous mites (*Dermanyssus gallinae*), and black flies (*Simulium* spp.) can be potential vectors of VEEV.[45,46]

Epizootic cycle. This cycle includes equids and *Aedes* spp. as the bridge vector (eg, *Aedes [Ochlerotatus] taeniorhynchus*) and mainly variants IAB and IC. Other vectors involved in the transmission of epizootic variants include *Ochlerotatus* spp., *Psorophora* spp., *Mansonia indubitans,* and *Deinocerites pseudes.*[32] This cycle has high equine mortality and is the one mainly affecting humans. Efficient viral amplification of epizootic variants by equids has epidemiologic implications to other animals and people.[31,40] Humans, dogs, rabbits, and ruminants can develop sufficient viremias to transmit the virus to mosquitoes.[31,32,47] VEE mortality in people is much lower (<1%) than with EEEV and WEEV, but VEE mortality in equids is high (over 50%). Birds are not important amplifiers.

Pathogenesis
Pathogenic mechanisms between alphaviruses are similar with some unique differences. These viruses persist in infected mosquitoes for their entire life. Alphaviruses replicate in vector and host cells.[48] The disease process is divided into an extraneural phase, neural invasion, and neuropathogenicity. These viruses induce cytopathic effects in vertebrate cells characterized by apoptosis and necrosis in neural and extraneural tissues.

After a bite from an infected mosquito, the saliva carries the virus to dermal tissue where it affects dendritic cells that transport the virus to lymphoid tissue where viral replication takes place, mainly in macrophages.[14] Through E2 glycoprotein, alphaviruses bind to cell surface heparan sulfate to mediate viral entry. Affinity for heparan sulfate may in part be responsible for neurovirulence.[3] Replication in myeloid cells (macrophages and dendritic cells) is not very efficient for EEEV compared with VEEV, which contributes to differences in disease progression and clinical signs. However, EEEV replicates efficiently in fibroblasts, osteoblast, and smooth muscle cells.[49] Many cell types in different organs are permissive to EEEV replication, which is evident on histopathology.[50] Most features of WEEV are shared with EEEV. VEEV replicates in myeloid cells locally, lymphoid tissue, and osteoblasts and fibroblasts.[49] Viremia by WEEV is low in humans and horses. At least in the experimental setting, WEEV viremias in horses and donkeys could be sufficient to potentially infect mosquitoes.[51] WEEV is more neuroinvasive than HJV.

B and T cells are important in clearing alphaviruses. Natural killer T cells protect against VEEV.[52] In animals with antibody titers, the virus is usually eliminated. Alphaviruses induce type I and type II interferon (IFN) responses (IFN $\alpha/\beta/\gamma$) that could be detrimental to their replication and propagation.[53] VEEV is susceptible to the antiviral effects of IFN and as a defensive strategy the virus interferes with innate immunity by reducing IFN production, hampering adaptive immunity,[54] resulting in high viremias that facilitate neuroinvasion and neurologic disease.[31] If these defense mechanisms are infective, the virus disseminates to other organs resulting in viremia and fever. At this point, the virus reaches the CNS by breaching the blood brain barrier (BBB) or reaching nerve endings of the olfactory (rhinencephalon) or trigeminal nerves (brain stem). Intrathecally produced antibodies may reduce disease severity.[53] EEEV replicates in endothelial cells, neurons, and glial cells leading to neurologic signs. The production of IFN-γ by CD4+ T cells in CNS may be protective against VEEV.[53] However, for most virulent VEEV variants, peripheral influx of immune cells has little effect on restricting viral replication.[52] Moreover, an exaggerated immune response leading to neuronal death and inflammation may worsen the disease.[53]

Regardless the route of infection, subcutaneous or aerosol, VEEV mainly uses the olfactory neuroepithelium to enter the CNS.[52] Astrocytes are highly sensitive to VEEV.[52] VEEV can also use trigeminal nerve endings.[52] It can damage the BBB, contributing to inflammation, edema, and leukocyte infiltration (secondary viral invasion).[52] VEEV enters the CNS faster with aerosol exposure because of the direct invasion of the olfactory neuroepithelium and rhinencephalon compared with subcutaneous exposure that requires local replication and viremia to then reach the olfactory epithelium.[52] Therefore, VEEV has the higher risk for aerosol transmission. Most animals clear the virus within 1 week.[53] VEEV proliferation in nervous tissue is 10 to 100 times faster than EEEV and immunization against VEEV does not protect against EEEV and WEEV.[37]

The fact that N-methyl-D-aspartate (NMDA) receptor antagonists reduce neuronal injury in experimental infections with alphaviruses suggests that these viruses activate neurotoxic pathways leading to excitotoxicity.[55] EEEV, VEEV, and WEEV infections tend to be more severe in children, infants, and the elderly, but data on the effect of age on equine disease severity are scarce.

The incubation period for EEEV ranges from 3 to 15 days.[6,14] After inoculation of WEEV, horses develop fever in 2 to 4 days and neurologic signs 7 to 10 days later. Viremia in horses infected with VEEV can be detected as early as 1-day postinfection, peaks by day 3 and can last 4 to 5 days.[31,53]

Clinical signs

Horses, donkeys, and mules develop similar clinical signs with alphaviral infections. Initially, there is fever, anorexia, and lethargy that are nonspecific and associated with viremia. It progresses to obtundation (sleeping sickness), incoordination, hyperexcitability, dysphagia, muscle tremors, impaired vision, head pressing, circling, staggering, aimless wandering, leaning against walls, paresis, paralysis, recumbency, convulsions, comma, and death.[25] There could be pruritus, respiratory failure, diarrhea, and large colon impaction. Neurologic signs develop 4 to 10 days after infection depending on the virus. A second pyrexic event (biphasic fever) often develops with neurologic signs. Most of the infected people with alphaviruses will develop fever, chills, malaise, headache, vomiting, myalgia, and joint pain, which are nonspecific and reasoned these viral infections often go unnoticed.[20] Less than 5% of people infected with alphaviruses develop neurologic disease.[7,20] Horses could amplify EEEV, in particular MV , and equine infections may occur weeks before human cases, however, both are terminal hosts.[10] Horses with neurologic disease are less likely to be viremic. Incubation is longer and signs are less severe with WEE compared with EEE and VEE.

Alphaviral neurologic disease is more severe in horses and donkeys than in people. Most equids die or are euthanized within few days after neurologic signs develop and those that recover often have residual neurologic deficits.

In the 1930 California WEE outbreak, fever was followed by lethargy, somnolence, excitability, incoordination, teeth grinding, paresis, paralysis, dysphagia, and bladder paralysis. Horses with mild signs had good recovery and minimal sequelae, whereas half with severe neurologic disease died or were euthanized within 8 days.[25] In the Minnesota WEE outbreak, most of the horses survived (20%–50% mortality).[26] WEE disease is more severe in horses and donkeys than in people.[56]

Signs of VEEV are not different from other encephalitides. Multiple animals are often affected with VEE in the vicinity. Mortality rate in equids ranges from 50% to 90%.

Signs reported in dogs, pigs, ruminants, and camelids infected with EEEV include pyrexia, lethargy, ataxia, vestibular signs, nystagmus, circling, seizures, recumbency, and torticollis.

Older human adults, young children, and infants are more likely to develop alphaviral disease, including neurologic signs. Innate immunity is central in eliminating these viruses and developing neurons are more susceptible to alphaviruses because of reduced IFN production and NMDA receptor-mediated excitotoxicity.[57]

Many of the clinical signs in horses are shared with other conditions.

Diagnosis

Neurologic signs are nonspecific. Conditions to consider in the differential diagnoses include West Nile virus (WNV) encephalitis, rabies, equine protozoal myeloencephalitis (EPM), equine herpesvirus 1 (EHV-1) myeloencephalopathy (EHM), toxicities (eg, leukoencephalomalacia), metabolic disorders (eg, hepatic encephalopathy), aberrant parasite migration, and others (eg, tumors, abscessation). Cervical vertebral malformation (wobblers) and equine degenerative myelopathy (EDM)/neuroaxonal dystrophy (NAD) are unlikely based on clinical findings and disease progression. Borna disease has not been documented in the Americas. A definitive diagnosis may be reached at the postmortem examination. Geography, season, age, breed, and vaccination status could narrow the differential diagnoses. In temperate regions, seasonality reduces the list of causes. Obtundation and head pressing suggest viral encephalitides, toxicities, or hepatic encephalopathy.

Hematology and serum chemistry are not specific but could guide in the diagnosis, whether infectious, toxic, or metabolic in origin. Horses with alphavirus infection could have leukopenia and lymphopenia early on, but hematological abnormalities are not diagnostic. The evaluation of cerebrospinal fluid (CSF) reveals pleocytosis with increased protein concentrations. However, normal CSF does not rule out viral disease. Neutrophilic pleocytosis is a consistent and unique finding with EEE. Absence of neutrophilic pleocytosis makes EEE less likely but does not exclude this etiologic agent. VEE and WEE typically have increased CSF protein and mononuclear pleocytosis, but CSF can be unremarkable.

In addition to clinical signs, serology, molecular methods, virus isolation, and histopathology are complementary and confirmatory methods. The detection of IgM-specific antibodies with capture enzyme-linked immunosorbent assay (ELISA) can be valuable early in the disease. Disease progression leading to death is often rapid and the value of serology is mostly epidemiologic. The presence of IgG is not indicative of disease unless seroconversion is demonstrated with pair titers. Other serologic methods include complement fixation (CF), hemagglutination inhibition (HI), virus neutralization (VN), immunofluorescence (IF), and plaque reduction neutralization test (PRNT). Serologic tests on serum and CSF (CF, HI, PRNT, ELISA, IF) have proven useful with VEE. Antibodies against VEEV can be detected as early as 5 days after exposure. Vaccination history is important. The presence of IgM-specific to VEEV is considered diagnostic. The interpretation of seropositive animals in enzootic areas can be challenging, in particular for VEEV.

Reverse transcriptase polymerase chain reaction (RT-PCR) can be diagnostic or confirmatory. RT-PCR can detect viral genomic material in blood, nervous, and peripheral tissue. Viral isolation from neural and peripheral tissue should be attempted to further characterize the pathogen, which also has epidemiologic and public health implications.

Histopathology may indicate a viral infection but is not definitive. Immunohistochemistry and in situ hybridization are highly specific and sensitive to detect EEEV, VEEV, and WEEV in formalin-fixed equine brain tissue.[58]

Pathology

Gross pathologic findings in nervous and peripheral tissue are indistinguishable between EEE, VEE and WEE. In the brain, there is mild to severe congestion, necrosis, and malacia. Histologically, there could be polioencephalomyelitis, leptomeningitis, meningoencephalitis, vasculitis, perivascular lymphocytic cuffing, hemorrhage, thrombosis, gliosis, neuronophagia, and microabscessation.[50,59] Neurons and glial cells can be surrounded by neutrophils, lymphocytes, plasma cells, and macrophages.[50,59] Neutrophilic infiltration is a consistent finding with EEE, but not characteristic with VEE and WEE. Perivascular cuffing is evident in the white matter of the cerebral cortex. Similar lesions can be present in the spinal cord. Lesions are more evident in the cerebral cortex, thalamus, hypothalamus, and mesencephalon.[50] EEEV can be identified in neurons, astrocytes, oligodendrocytes, microglia, and leukocytes.[50] In extraneural tissue, EEEV causes necrosis and mononuclear inflammatory infiltration in the myocardium, gastrointestinal tract, bladder, spleen, liver, pancreas, and lymphoid tissue. EEEV can be identified in peripheral tissues.[50] Extraneural lesions indicate that many clinical signs of EEE are not neurologic in nature. Visceral lesions including gastrointestinal, hepatic, and pancreatic necrosis have been documented with VEEV.

Prognosis

For most horses with neurologic signs, the prognosis is guarded to poor, with 50% to 90% mortality rate. Prognosis is poor for EEE and VEE but better for WEE. Mortality is lower with WNV (<40%).

Public health/zoonosis

Alphaviruses are a zoonotic risk, in particular VEEV, and precautions should be taken when dealing with suspect cases, alive or dead. Aerosol transmission to people has been documented with EEEV and VEEV. In fact, EEEV and VEEV were evaluated as potential biological weapons by the United States and the Soviet Union during the Cold War.[14,35] Notification to public and animal health authorities is important when cases are documented.

Flaviviral Encephalitis

Flaviviruses causing equine neurologic disease are mainly restricted to WNV, which has worldwide distribution. In contrast, equine alphaviral neurologic disease is limited to the Americas. Alphaviruses and flaviviruses have similarities in their clinical presentation, seasonality, vectors, hosts, and basic pathogenic principles. The introduction of WNV to the New World initially resulted in epidemics with high morbidity and variable human, equine, and avian mortality to subsequently adapt and transition into a novel endemic cycle. The relevance of other flaviviruses (eg, Japanese encephalitis virus [JEV]) in equine neurologic disease remains unclear. Other *Flaviviriae* viruses (Hepacivirus, Pegivirus) have been recently linked to equine liver disease.

West Nile Virus Encephalomyelitis

Etiology

West Nile virus encephalitis or encephalomyelitis (WNVE) is an arboviral condition of worldwide distribution affecting horses, people, birds, and occasionally other species, with systemic and less frequently neurologic signs. WNV belongs to the *Amarillovirales* order, *flaviviridae* family, and *flavivirus* genus. As other members of the *flaviviridae* family, WNV is a 40 to 60 nm spherical enveloped virus with a protein nucleocapsid. It has a single-stranded positive-sense 11-kb RNA genome (Class IV) with a single open reading frame that is translated into a single polyprotein that is cleaved by host and viral proteases into three structural (capsid-C, pre-membrane [prM], envelop-E) and seven nonstructural proteins (NSPs).[60–62] The C protein has chaperone activity and contributes to nucleocapsid formation by associating with the RNA, which is crucial for viral assembly and replication.[60] This protein has been implicated with virus dissemination, cell apoptosis, and disruption of the BBB.[60] Cleavage of prM during final virus assembly yields M, a glycosylated protein. E is also a glycosylated protein involved in receptor binding, cell invasion, membrane fusion, viral entry, and neuroinvasiveness, and is very immunogenic.[60–63] This protein is also immunogenic in horses.[64] NSPs are central to viral replication, have enzymatic activity, and are required for particle assembly.[60–63]

WNV is a member of the JEV antigenic serogroup. Viruses in this serogroup cause similar disease across the world, including nonspecific systemic symptoms and less frequently, neurologic disease. These include the JEV (Asia), St. Louis encephalitis (Americas), Kunjin encephalitis (Oceania), Murray Valley encephalitis (MVEV; Australia/South Pacific), and WNV (Asia, Africa, Europe, Americas) viruses.[23,60,62,65–68] Other less studied members include Usutu, Koutango, Yaounde, Alfuy, and Cacipacore viruses.[64] Of these, JEV, WNV, and MVEV have been associated with neurologic disease in horses, donkeys, humans, birds, and occasionally other species.[4,23] As of 2021, nine WNV lineages and different clades that are not necessarily associated with geography have been described.[60,62] Lineage 1 (Africa, Europe, Asia, Americas, Oceania) produces severe neurologic disease in horses and people, and lineage 2 (Africa, Europe) causes subclinical to severe disease. Lineages 3–9 are distributed in Africa, Asia, and Europe.[60,62,69] Association between these lineages and equine disease is lacking, but they have been linked to human disease.[60] Lineage 1 has three clades (1a, 1b, 1c)[60,62]; clade 1a is the most distributed, including the United States, clade 1b (Kunjin virus) circulates in Australia, Borneo, and Papua New Guinea, and clade 1c occurs in India.[60] Lineage 2 has been identified as causing neurologic disease in people, horses, and birds in Africa and Europe, raising epidemiologic concerns.[5,70,71]

Epidemiology

Viruses in the JEV serogroup are arthropod-borne and circulate in avian and mammalian-mosquito cycles. WNV has a wide range of hosts; it replicates in birds, mammals, reptiles, amphibians, mosquitoes, and ticks.[60] The disease was first described in 1937 in the West Nile district in Uganda, where the virus was isolated from a febrile woman (West Nile fever).[72] The ecology of the virus was elucidated in the 1950s after several outbreaks in Egypt, where the virus was identified in children, birds, and vectors in the Nile delta and shown to be carried by mosquitoes.[72] The importance of birds as enzootic hosts was demonstrated in the 1960s.[72] Until 1997, WNV was not considered pathogenic to birds, but changed in Israel where a WNV outbreak caused encephalitis, paralysis, and death in different bird species.[72] First equine cases were documented in Egypt and France in the 1960s. It has been endemic in Africa, Asia, and Europe, with sporadic outbreaks.

Historically, WNV was restricted to Africa and the Middle East, however, it is currently also in Europe, Asia, Oceania, and the Americas. In 1999, WNV was introduced to the New World where it encountered naïve human and animal populations, resulting in high morbidity and mortality in birds, horses, and people. After first human, equine and avian cases were diagnosed in New York,[73–75] the virus spread rapidly across the United States, reaching peaks of equine (15,257) and human (9,862) cases in 2002 and 2003, respectively.[76,77] From 1999 to 2020, over 27,000 equine (all neurologic) and 52,000 human (25,290 with neurologic signs) cases have been documented in the United States.[76,77] WNV also resulted in massive mortality of exotic and native birds, including corvids, raptors, waterfowls, waterbirds, shorebirds, wading birds, parrots, doves, and chicken. The incidence of equine WNVE in the United States has dropped substantially (90 cases in 2019),[77] mainly due to massive vaccination, although most horses go undiagnosed because do not develop clinical disease, signs are nonspecific, and many developed immunity from natural exposure in a recently established endemic cycle. Most cases are unvaccinated horses.

In Europe, WNV resurfaced in 1996 to 2000, mainly lineage 1.[5] However, in recent years, there have been an increase of human and equine cases,[5] in particular in Central and Northern Europe.[5,70,71,78] Of interest, many of these have been caused by lineage 2, which is alarming.[5,71]

Lineage 2 was considered less pathogenic than lineage 1;[64] however, it has been shown that lineage 2 causes fatal neurologic disease in horses, people, and birds.[71,79,80] Immunization against lineage 1 protects animals against lineage 2.[60,67,81] Both lineages have strains with varying degrees of neuroinvasiveness.[71] Recent outbreaks in Europe, Africa, and Asia have been in part attributed to global warming altering bird migration patterns and early vector emergence.[69] WNV cases in the United States are monitored through the CDC ArboNET and the United States Department of Agriculture (USDA),[15,77] and in Europe by the European Centre for Disease Prevention and Control (ECDC).[78]

Unlike children, WNV rarely affects horses of less than 1 year of age. Horses $\geq$ 3 years of age are more likely to die than animals $\leq$ 2 year old.[82] In one study, females were more likely to die than males.[82] WNV seroprevalence in unvaccinated horses in Europe and the United States has been estimated at <10%,[83] which is lower than for Africa and Asia. In addition to horses, donkeys, mules, humans, and birds, WNVE has been documented in pigs, camelids, dogs, and cats. It may affect wild vertebrates.

WNVE is rarely diagnosed in Latin America despite abundance of permissive vectors and WNV being present in this region, from Mexico to Argentina and the Caribbean. Potential explanations include the lack of public and veterinary awareness, limited diagnostics, genetic drift leading to less virulent genotypes, and potential immune cross-protection from local flaviviruses.

Biologic cycle

The virus is maintained in an enzootic cycle involving culicine mosquitoes (*Culex* spp., *Aedes* spp.) and birds. In birds, WNV causes high viremias, which favor mosquito infection and viral dissemination to susceptible animals and people. In the enzootic cycle, birds develop high viremias but not clinical disease. Reptiles also develop high viremias and may contribute to dissemination in swampy areas.[84] Horses and humans are poor WNV amplifiers, and viremias are low and considered dead-end hosts. The disease is infectious but not contagious. In temperate climates, the disease is seasonal and follows vector emergence in the spring. In vectors, WNV virus uses horizontal and vertical transmission. During cold weather, WNV is maintained in avian reservoirs and hibernating vectors. Viral amplification is influenced by season, vector, type of host, immune status, and viral strain. In the tropics, there is no seasonal interruption of the cycle. Mosquitoes of the genus *Culex* spp. are the most effective at transmitting WNV because they feed on birds and are central to the enzootic cycle, but *Aedes* spp. contributes to spillovers because they are less discriminant feeders (birds, reptiles, mammals). Of importance are *Aedes albopictus*,[69] *Culex pipiens*, and *Culex tritaeniorhynchus*.[69] *Culex pipiens* was the main vector in the 1999 to 2002 North American outbreak.[85] *Aedes albopictus* has indiscriminate feeding habits and is a known zoonotic vector (eg, chikungunya virus, dengue virus, *Dirofilaria*). In fact, *Aedes albopictus* was shown to transmit WNV resulting in clinical disease in horses.[86]

The virus has been found in many species of *Aedes, Anopheles, Coquillettidia, Culex, Culiseta, Mansonia,* and *Ochlerotatus*.[60] The list of permissive vectors in North America is extensive, including *Culex pipiens, Culex quinquefasciatus, Culex nigripalpus, Culex tarsalis,* and *Culex restuans*. However, *Culex salinarius, Melanoconion* spp., *Aedes* spp., *Anopheles* spp., *Coquillettidia* spp., *Psorophora* spp., and *Ochlerotatus* spp. are bridge vectors that facilitate spillover and epizootics similar to alphaviruses. *Culex tritaeniorhynchus* and *Culex neavei* are ornithophilic and mammophilic mosquitoes, are bridge vectors for JEV complex viruses, and can transmit WNV to horses in Africa and Asia.[87] In Oceania, *Culex annulirostris* is the primary vector of WNV lineage 1 (clade 1b; Kunjin virus). WNV has been isolated from soft and hard ticks in Africa, Europe, and Asia, including *Argas* spp., *Ornithodoros* spp., *Hyalomma* spp., *Rhipicephalus* spp., *Amblyomma* spp., and *Dermacentor* spp. Experimental WNV transmission to animals with ticks has been reported.[69] Transstadial transfer of WNV occurs in ixodid ticks.[88] Limited diagnostic resources in developing countries has been a limitation to better understand the prevalence and biology of WNV.[69]

Pathogenesis

WNV causes a progressive and often severe meningoencephalomyelitis. After bitten by infected vectors, horses clear the virus or develop short-lasting low viremias,[79,86,89–91] may not show systemic signs, and only 10% develop neurologic disease.[86,89] Therefore, equids are not amplifying hosts. Mosquitoes that feed on infected horses remain negative for WNV and do not transmit the virus to other horses.[89] WNV enters cells via receptor-mediated endocytosis involving clathrin-coated pits.[60,61] Inside the endosome, the low pH triggers conformational changes on the E protein that result in its fusion with the endosomal membrane, releasing the nucleocapsid into the cytoplasm and uncoating the genome.[60,61] The fact that WNV replicates in mammalian, avian, reptile, amphibian, and insect cells suggests that the virus uses conserved receptors or different strategies depending on the cell type.[60] The virus will replicate in the endoplasmic reticulum and assemble into immature virions that will be transported through the Golgi apparatus to generate mature WNV that will be released via exocytosis.[60,61]

The virus enters the CNS through the disruption of BBB, transported by mononuclear cells that migrate into the CNS and retrograde axonal transport.[60,61] The hematogenous route seems important for WNV to cross the BBB and enter the CNS,[60] but the mechanisms remain unclear. Initial WNV entry is not associated with BBB damage, but using cell-associated virus transport (Trojan horse route) to induce an inflammatory response with cytokines and metalloproteinases that disrupt BBB integrity, favoring additional neuroinvasion and inflammation.[92] There is CNS immune cell infiltration, production of inflammatory cytokines, glial cell activation, neuronal dysfunction, apoptosis, and necrosis. Excitotoxicity with increased calcium flux leading to neuronal death seems to play a role in the pathogenesis of WNVE.[93]

Clinical signs

In equids, the incubation is 5 to 15 days.[82,86,89,91] Most of the people and horses are asymptomatic.[69,76,77] Less than 1% of people with systemic signs will develop neurologic disease.[69,76] Approximately, 10% to 15% of horses with experimental and natural infections develop neurologic signs.[69,79,86,89–91] Initial clinical signs are not specific and include pyrexia (up to 40°C [104°F]), anorexia, and lethargy. Fever is an inconsistent finding,[74,82,94,95] although biphasic fever has been reported.[74] Neurologic signs range from mild ataxia to fulminating encephalomyelitis. Musculoskeletal signs in general precede neurologic signs. Gait abnormalities are frequent. There could be symmetric or asymmetric lameness, weakness, toe dragging, and knuckling that will progress to ataxia, proprioceptive deficits, and muscle fasciculations that are more evident on the face and neck, tremors, somnolence, blindness, facial paralysis, bruxism, dysphagia, recumbency, and inability to rise.[74,82,91,94–97] Most affected horses maintain good mentation, but some are hyperexcitable. They can transition rapidly between hyperexcitable and quiet states. Animals with severe disease may go into coma. Compared with other viral diseases, muscle fasciculations, tremors, and behavioral changes are consistent findings in horses with WNVE.[74,82,91,94–96] Spinal cord signs are more evident with WNVE than with alphavirus encephalomyelitis. Hyperexcitability and aggressive behavior are not typical but may occur. In horses with neurologic disease, the mortality rate is 25% to 40%.[79,82,90] Recumbent animals are 60% to 80% likely to die or euthanized.[82,91,94,96] In South Africa, where most equine cases are caused from lineage 2, the severity of neurologic disease and fatality rate are similar to lineage 1.[69,79,80]

Diagnosis

The diagnosis of WNVE is based on clinical signs, vaccination history, season, geography, animal age, laboratory methods (serology, CSF evaluation, and molecular methods), pathology, and histopathology. Conditions to consider in the differential diagnosis include botulism, EPM, EHM, rabies, alphaviral encephalitides (EEE, VEE, WEE), cervicovertebral malformation (wobblers), EDM/NAD, intoxications, hepatic encephalopathy, parasite migration, Borna disease, leukoencephalomalacia, polyneuritis, and others less common disorders. Geography and season are valuable to narrow the diagnosis. In the Americas, botulism, rabies, alphaviral encephalitides, and EPM are at the top of the list, but not in other continents. Alphaviral encephalitides are seasonal and difficult to differentiate from WNVE, in particular early on or in animals with minimal cerebral signs. Rabies is not seasonal, is progressive, and difficult to differentiate due to its variable signs, and the diagnosis is postmortem. Therefore, knowing vaccination history is essential. Borna disease, rabies, and EHM are major differentials in Europe. Signs of EHM can overlap with WNVE, with season and history of disease (eg, respiratory disease, abortions) being important to differentiate. Wobblers should be easy to rule out.

Laboratory methods

Serologic methods used to detect antibodies against WNV include IgM antibody capture ELISA (MAC-ELISA), IgG ELISA, HI, CF, immunofluorescence assay, VN, PRNT, and microsphere immunoassay (MIA) to IgM.[5,23,60,64,66,73,74,79,86,90] IgG ELISAs are highly sensitive to detect antibodies but not very specific. The PRNT is a confirmatory test. In human medicine, MIA is becoming the preferred method because is faster than the MAC-ELISA and PRNT, and it has high sensitivity (>90%) and specificity (>90%). In vaccinated or naturally infected horses, MIA to the envelop protein showed excellent sensitivity and specificity.[64] The MAC-ELISA has been the preferred serologic method in horses. PRNT is used by some laboratories. In horses experimentally infected using *Aedes albopictus*, IgM can be detected as early as 7 days postinfection,[86] reaching high titers between days 10 to 13.[86] In that study, only one out of 12 horses developed neurologic signs, in line with reports that 10% of naturally or experimentally infected horses develop neurologic signs.[86,99] The IgM response in vaccinated horses is not detectable or minimal compared with natural disease that develops high titers.[100] RT-PCR using blood, CSF, or nervous tissue can be diagnostic or confirmatory. Viral isolation from blood, CSF, and nervous tissue could be attempted for further viral characterization. Immunohistochemistry and in situ hybridization can be diagnostic.[101] CSF evaluation shows increased protein and mononuclear lymphocytic pleocytosis, however, a normal CSF does not rule out WNVE. Hematology and serum chemistry are nonspecific but could be helpful in ruling in/out some conditions.

Pathology

Humans, equids, and birds develop diffuse inflammation of the CNS, including the brain and spinal cord. Gross necropsy reveals congestion, hemorrhage and edema of the meninges, cortex, brainstem, thalamus, hypothalamus, medulla oblongata, and spinal cord. On histopathology, there is mild to severe multifocal hemorrhages, thrombosis, and nonsuppurative polioencephalomyelitis that are more evident in the gray matter of the medulla oblongata, reticular substance, and brainstem.[101,102] There is perivascular cuffing, mononuclear infiltration (monocytes, lymphocytes, plasma cells), gliosis, neuronal degeneration, necrosis, and neuronophagia.[100,101]There could neutrophilic infiltration.[101,102] In the spinal cord, lesions are more evident in the thoracolumbar ventral horns.[101–103] In contrast to alphaviruses where lesions are more severe in the cerebral cortex, limbic system, and thalamus, with WNV most lesions are in the brainstem, medulla oblongata, and spinal cord.[101,102] These differences could be attributed in part on the main route of CNS invasion for flaviviruses (BBB disruption, retrograde flow) compared with alphaviruses (olfactory, trigeminal nerve endings). Unlike birds, WNV antigen is rarely found in extraneural tissue in horses, suggesting that this virus is more neurotropic than alphaviruses. Most lesions in other organs are secondary. Immunohistochemistry demonstrates viral presence in neurons, which are often surrounded by glial cells.[101]

Public health

WNV is an infectious noncontagious virus of low zoonotic risk. However, good biosecurity measures must be taken. A case report of a veterinary student being infected with WNV during the necropsy of a WNV-positive horse was reported.[104]

Treatment

Treatment of alphaviral and flaviviral encephalitides is similar and described below under "Treatment of arboviral encephalitis."

Prevention

Prevention of alphaviral and flaviviral encephalitides is similar and described below under "Prevention of arboviral encephalitis."

Treatment of arboviral encephalitis. Treatment of horses with viral encephalitis is supportive and should be oriented at reducing cerebral and spinal cord inflammation, intracranial pressure, edema, and hemorrhage, controlling neurologic signs, and treating secondary infections. Nonsteroidal anti-inflammatory drugs (NSAIDs) are central to treatment. Flunixin meglumine (1.1 mg/kg, IV, twice daily) is the most commonly used NSAID, but others can be considered. Glucocorticoids (dexamethasone, methylprednisolone) may be beneficial at reducing inflammation, although their use is controversial due to the risk of increasing viremia. Methylprednisolone is occasionally used in people with alphaviral and flaviviral encephalitis. Dimethyl sulfoxide (0.1–1 g/kg, IV, 10% solution, once daily) is widely used for acute infectious and noninfectious equine neurologic disorders. Hypertonic saline solution (3%–7%) as a continuous rate infusion can be effective at reducing cerebral and spinal cord edema in horses with viral encephalomyelitis (R. Toribio, personal communication). Mannitol (0.25–2 g/kg, IV, 20% solution, over 20 minutes, once daily) is used by some clinicians although there is evidence that at least in other species hypertonic saline solution is superior, cheaper, and more practical than mannitol at reducing cerebral edema. Antioxidants (vitamin E, 5000–9000 IU, orally, twice daily, liquid formulation) can ameliorate neuronal oxidative injury. Fluid therapy may be indicated depending on the hydration, acid-base, and electrolyte status. Antimicrobials are often recommended to control secondary infections. Recumbent animals require caloric support as well as urinary and fecal evacuation. The prevention of self-trauma is often necessary. Sedatives (xylazine, detomidine), tranquilizers (acepromazine), and anticonvulsants (diazepam, midazolam) may be indicated. Antiviral drugs against alphaviruses and WNV have been evaluated in people, but information in horses is scarce and anecdotal. Given the importance of type I IFN and innate immunity in controlling viral encephalitis, one can speculate that IFN-α could be beneficial at reducing viral load, but equine data are lacking. Most (70%–80%) of the horses with WNVE improve with medical treatment, of which 20% will have long-term residual deficits, including weight loss, lethargy, ataxia, weakness, and cranial nerve dysfunction.[82] As previously mentioned, the prognosis is worse for alphaviral infections.

Prevention of arboviral encephalitis. Any horse with fever and neurologic signs should be handled under strict biosecurity protocols, including isolation, use of personal protective equipment, and thorough disinfection. Operators must assume that the condition could be contagious to other animals and people. VEEV has the highest zoonotic risk for direct aerosol transmission (biological weapon). Vector control and vaccination are at the center of preventing arboviral infections. Most of the horses and donkeys affected are not vaccinated.

The risk of alphaviral and flaviviral encephalitis is geographic and seasonal, and animals should be vaccinated annually, in early spring in temperate countries or before the vector peak season. Vaccination guidelines have been developed by the American Association of Equine Practitioners (AAEP).[105] Per AAEP guidelines, vaccines against EEE, WEE, WNV, and rabies (and tetanus) are core in North America and have been highly effective at reducing their incidence. Available alphavirus vaccines are multivalent, include inactivated EEEV and WEEV, but some also have VEEV. In addition, an assortment of encephalitis vaccines combining 4 to 8 antigens, including tetanus, WNV, influenza virus, EHV-1, EHV-4, and rabies viruses are available (Encevac, Merck Animal Health; Prestige, Merck Animal Health; Vetera, Boehringer Ingelheim; and INNOVATOR, Zoetis) (**Table 1**). There is some cross-protection between EEEV and VEEV, but not with VEEV.[37]

In foals, first vaccine should be given at 4 to 6 months followed by 1 to 2 boosters 1 month apart. In endemic or tropical areas, vaccinate pregnant mares 1 month before

Table 1 USDA-approved encephalitis vaccines for horses					
Name	Manufacturer	Dose	Age of Vaccination	Booster	Route
Prestige[a]	Merck	1 mL	6 mo	Annually	IM
Encevac[b]	Merck	1 mL	6 mo	Annually	IM
Vetera[c]	BI	1 mL	4 mo	Annually	IM
Equiloid Innovator[d]	Zoetis	1 mL	10 mo	Annually	IM
West Nile Innovator[e]	Zoetis	1 mL	10 mo	Annually	IM
Core Eq Innovator[f]	Zoetis	1 mL	3 mo	Annually	IM
Core Eq Innovator V[g]	Zoetis	1 mL	3 mo	Annually	IM

Abbreviations: EEEV, eastern equine encephalitis virus; EHV, equine herpesvirus; EIV, equine influenza virus; IM, intramuscular; VEEV, Venezuelan equine encephalitis virus; WEEV, western equine encephalitis virus; WNV, West Nile virus.
[a] Prestige is available in different formulations, with four to seven antigens (EEEV, WEEV, VEEV, WNV, EHV-1, EHV-4, EIV, and tetanus). Prestige 5 + WNV is the only one with WNV antigen.
[b] Encevac has three antigens (EEEV, WEEV, and tetanus).
[c] Vetera is available in different formulations, with four to eight antigens (EEEV, WEEV, VEEV, WNV, EIV, EHV-1, EHV-4, and tetanus). Some Vetera formulations do not have WNV.
[d] Equiloid Innovator has three antigens (EEEV, WEEV, and WNV).
[e] West Nile Innovator is available in different formulations, with three to five antigens (EEE, WEE, VEE, WNV, and tetanus).
[f] Rabies, tetanus, EEEV, WEEV, and WNV.
[g] Rabies, tetanus, EEEV, VEEV, WEEV, and WNV.

foaling. Horses younger than 4 years of age residing in endemic areas should be vaccinated 2 to 3 time per year.[91] Recently introduced horses should be vaccinated before or on arrival. The surveillance of equids and humans is important in endemic areas.

There is an attenuated VEEV subtype IAB strain vaccine (TC-83) that is restricted to control outbreaks. This vaccine derives from a VEEV isolated from the brain of a donkey in Trinidad (TrD strain), was developed by the US Army in 1961 for human use (laboratory personnel),[106] is not commercially available, and its strategic use has been effective at controlling equine VEE outbreaks in Latin America and Texas.[31]

Major advances in the development of vaccines against EEEV, WEEV, and VEEV have been made, including viral vector (vaccinia virus, alphavirus, adenovirus, flavivirus, canarypox, herpesvirus, lentivirus, vesiculovirus, and Sindbis virus), DNA, RNA, mRNA, plasmid, and protein subunit vaccines.[107] However, this has not been translated into field vaccines and traditional inactivated vaccines continue to be used. Genetically engineered attenuated vaccines against VEEV (eg, V3526) have proven effective in horses[108] but are not commercially available.

The introduction of WNV in North America in 1999 led to the rapid development of highly effective equine vaccines. WNV immunity in infected and vaccinated horses lasts 12 to 24 months.[99] There are three monovalent FDA-licensed WNV vaccines: two use inactivated virus (Vetera, Boehringer Ingelheim; INNOVATOR, Zoetis) and one is a chimera using E and prM proteins in a flavivirus vector (Prestige, Merck Animal Health) (see **Table 1**). A recombinant vaccine based on a canarypox virus vector (Recombitek WNV, Merial) was discontinued in the United States, but is available in Africa and Europe (Proteq, Boehringer Ingelheim). There are multiple polyvalent vaccines (see **Table 1**). In general foals should receive the first vaccine at 5 months of age, followed by 1 to 2 boosters, 1 month apart. First dose of some polyvalent vaccines are recommended at 10 months of age. In the United States, there are mono-valent WNV vaccines, but most vaccines currently used are polyvalent.

Vector control is central in the prevention of arboviral infections. Reducing mosquito breeding areas by eliminating standing water (eg, tires, buckets, cans, and ponds) is important. Approved insecticides should be considered to control adults and larvae. Biological pesticides (eg, *Bacillus thuringiensis*) are effective, widely used, are safe to animals, people, and plants, and friendly to the environment. Physical and chemical barriers between at-risk horses and mosquitoes, including blankets, repellants, nets, and fans should be considered during peak season.

Bunyaviridae

Sporadic cases of neurologic disease from viruses of the *Bunyaviridae* family (California encephalitis, Jamestown Canyon, La Crosse, Snowshoe hare, Shuni, and Argentinian Bunyamwera viruses) have been documented in horses.[91,109,110] These viruses use mosquito vectors including *Aedes* spp., *Culicoides* spp., *Culex* spp., and *Culiseta* spp. Their clinical and epidemiologic implications to equine neurologic disease remain unknown.

SUMMARY

Arboviruses are the main cause of viral encephalitis and encephalomyelitis in horses, donkeys, and mules. They are considered reemerging diseases, and climate change may contribute to the increasing number of human and equine cases. Neurologic signs from arboviruses are indistinguishable, and reaching a definitive diagnosis has clinical and epidemiologic implications. Strict biosecurity protocols should be followed due to the zoonotic potential of these conditions and overlap with other neurologic disorders (eg, rabies). Treatment is nonspecific, aimed at reducing neural inflammation, hemorrhage, edema, thrombosis, and neuronal death and controlling secondary complications. Most of the horses with alphavirus infections (EEE, VEE, and WEE) will die, whereas most horses with flavivirus infections (WNVE) will survive. Vaccination against equine arboviruses is highly effective.

REFERENCES

1. Arechiga-Ceballos N, Aguilar-Setien A. Alphaviral equine encephalomyelitis (Eastern, Western and Venezuelan). Rev Sci Tech 2015;34:491–501.
2. Arrigo NC, Adams AP, Weaver SC. Evolutionary patterns of eastern equine encephalitis virus in North versus South America suggest ecological differences and taxonomic revision. J Virol 2010;84:1014–25.
3. Gardner CL, Ebel GD, Ryman KD, et al. Heparan sulfate binding by natural eastern equine encephalitis viruses promotes neurovirulence. Proc Natl Acad Sci USA 2011;108:16026-31.
4. Chapman GE, Baylis M, Archer D, et al. The challenges posed by equine arboviruses. Equine Vet J 2018;50:436–45.
5. Lecollinet S, Pronost S, Coulpier M, et al. Viral equine encephalitis, a growing threat to the horse population in europe? Viruses 2019;12. https://doi.org/10.3390/v12010023.
6. Banda C, Samanta D. In: Eastern equine encephalitis. Treasure Island (FL: StatPearls; 2021.
7. Lindsey NP, Martin SW, Staples JE, et al. Notes from the field: multistate outbreak of eastern equine encephalitis virus - United States, 2019. MMWR Morb Mortal Wkly Rep 2020;69:50-1.

8. International Committee on Taxonomy of Viruses (ICTV). Virus taxonomy. 2020. Available at. https://talk.ictvonline.org/.

9. Carrera JP, Forrester N, Wang E, et al. Eastern equine encephalitis in Latin America. N Engl J Med 2013;369:732–44.

10. Blohm GM, Lednicky JA, White SK, et al. Madariaga virus: identification of a lineage iii strain in a venezuelan child with acute undifferentiated febrile illness, in the setting of a possible equine epizootic. Clin Infect Dis 2018;67:619–21.

11. Lednicky JA, White SK, Mavian CN, et al. Emergence of Madariaga virus as a cause of acute febrile illness in children, Haiti, 2015-2016. PLoS Negl Trop Dis 2019;13:e0006972.

12. Vittor AY, Armien B, Gonzalez P, et al. Epidemiology of emergent madariaga encephalitis in a region with endemic venezuelan equine encephalitis: initial host studies and human cross-sectional study in Darien, Panama. PLoS Negl Trop Dis 2016;10:e0004554.

13. Chenier S, Cote G, Vanderstock J, et al. An eastern equine encephalomyelitis (EEE) outbreak in Quebec in the fall of 2008. Can Vet J 2010;51:1011–5.

14. Morens DM, Folkers GK, Fauci AS. Eastern equine encephalitis virus - another emergent arbovirus in the United States. N Engl J Med 2019;381:1989–92.

15. Centers for Disease Control and Prevention (CDC). ArboNET. 2021. Available at. https://wwwn.cdc.gov/arbonet/maps/ADB_Diseases_Map/index.html.

16. Graham SP, Hassan HK, Chapman T, et al. Serosurveillance of eastern equine encephalitis virus in amphibians and reptiles from Alabama, USA. Am J Trop Med Hyg 2012;86:540–4.

17. Corrin T, Ackford R, Mascarenhas M, et al. Eastern equine encephalitis virus: a scoping review of the global evidence. Vector Borne Zoonotic Dis 2021;21: 305–20.

18. Reed DS, Lackemeyer MG, Garza NL, et al. Severe encephalitis in cynomolgus macaques exposed to aerosolized Eastern equine encephalitis virus. J Infect Dis 2007;196:441–50.

19. Nolen-Walston R, Bedenice D, Rodriguez C, et al. Eastern equine encephalitis in 9 South American camelids. J Vet Intern Med 2007;21:846–52.

20. Simon LV, Coffey R, Fischer MA. In: Western equine encephalitis. Treasure Island (FL: StatPearls; 2021.

21. Bergren NA, Auguste AJ, Forrester NL, et al. Western equine encephalitis virus: evolutionary analysis of a declining alphavirus based on complete genome sequences. J Virol 2014;88:9260–7.

22. Allison AB, Stallknecht DE. Genomic sequencing of Highlands J virus: a comparison to western and eastern equine encephalitis viruses. Virus Res 2009; 145:334–40.

23. Go YY, Balasuriya UB, Lee CK. Zoonotic encephalitides caused by arboviruses: transmission and epidemiology of alphaviruses and flaviviruses. Clin Exp Vaccin Res 2014;3:58–77.

24. Hahn CS, Lustig S, Strauss EG, et al. Western equine encephalitis virus is a recombinant virus. Proc Natl Acad Sci U S A 1988;85:5997–6001.

25. Meyer KF, Haring CM, Howitt B. The etiology of epizootic encephalomyelitis of horses in the San Joaquin Valley, 1930. Science 1931;74:227–8.

26. Eklund CM, Blumstein A. The relation of human encephalitis to encephalomyelitis EEEV WEEV in horses. JAVMA 1938;111:1734–5.

27. Mitchell CJ, Darsie RF Jr, Monath TP, et al. The use of an animal-baited net trap for collecting mosquitoes during western equine encephalitis investigations in Argentina. J Am Mosq Control Assoc 1985;1:43–7.

28. Hardy JL, Reeves WC, Rush WA, et al. Experimental infection with western equine encephalomyelitis virus in wild rodents indigenous to Kern County, California. Infect Immun 1974;10:553–64.
29. Ayers JR, Lester TL, Angulo AB. An epizootic attributable to western equine encephalitis virus infection in emus in Texas. J Am Vet Med Assoc 1994;205:600–1.
30. Cilnis MJ, Kang W, Weaver SC. Genetic conservation of highlands J viruses. Virology 1996;218:343–51.
31. Weaver SC, Ferro C, Barrera R, et al. Venezuelan equine encephalitis. Annu Rev Entomol 2004;49:141–74.
32. Aguilar PV, Estrada-Franco JG, Navarro-Lopez R, et al. Endemic Venezuelan equine encephalitis in the Americas: hidden under the dengue umbrella. Future Virol 2011;6:721–40.
33. Forrester NL, Wertheim JO, Dugan VG, et al. Evolution and spread of Venezuelan equine encephalitis complex alphavirus in the Americas. PLoS Negl Trop Dis 2017;11:e0005693.
34. Weaver SC, Salas R, Rico-Hesse R, et al. Re-emergence of epidemic Venezuelan equine encephalomyelitis in South America. VEE Study Group. Lancet 1996; 348:436–40.
35. Crosby B, Crespo ME. In: Venezuelan equine encephalitis. Treasure Island (FL: StatPearls; 2021.
36. Deardorff ER, Estrada-Franco JG, Freier JE, et al. Candidate vectors and rodent hosts of Venezuelan equine encephalitis virus, Chiapas, 2006-2007. Am J Trop Med Hyg 2011;85:1146–53.
37. Beck CE, Wyckoff RW. Venezuelan equine encephalomyelitis. Science 1938; 88:530.
38. Sanmartin-Barberi C, Groot H, Osorno-Mesa E. Human epidemic in Colombia caused by the Venezuelan equine encephalomyelitis virus. Am J Trop Med Hyg 1954;3:283–93.
39. Sudia WD, Newhouse VF, Beadle ID, et al. Epidemic Venezuelan equine encephalitis in North America in 1971: vector studies. Am J Epidemiol 1975;101: 17–35.
40. Weaver SC, Barrett AD. Transmission cycles, host range, evolution and emergence of arboviral disease. Nat Rev Microbiol 2004;2:789–801.
41. Brault AC, Powers AM, Medina G, et al. Potential sources of the 1995 Venezuelan equine encephalitis subtype IC epidemic. J Virol 2001;75:5823–32.
42. Kenney JL, Adams AP, Gorchakov R, et al. Genetic and anatomic determinants of enzootic Venezuelan equine encephalitis virus infection of Culex (Melanoconion) taeniopus. PLoS Negl Trop Dis 2012;6:e1606.
43. Scherer WF, Dickerman RW, Ordonez JV, et al. Ecologic studies of Venezuelan encephalitis virus and isolations of Nepuyo and Patois viruses during 1968-1973 at a marsh habitat near the epicenter of the 1969 outbreak in Guatemala. Am J Trop Med Hyg 1976;25:151–62.
44. Torres R, Samudio R, Carrera JP, et al. Enzootic mosquito vector species at equine encephalitis transmission foci in the Republica de Panama. PLoS One 2017;12:e0185491.
45. Durden LA, Linthicum KJ, Turell MJ. Mechanical transmission of Venezuelan equine encephalomyelitis virus by hematophagous mites (Acari). J Med Entomol 1992;29:118–21.
46. Homan EJ, Zuluaga FN, Yuill TM, et al. Studies on the transmission of Venezuelan equine encephalitis virus by Colombian simuliidae (Diptera). Am J Trop Med Hyg 1985;34:799–804.

47. Sidwell RW, Gebhardt LP, Thorpe BD. Epidemiological aspects of venezuelan equine encephalitis virus infections. Bacteriol Rev 1967;31:65–81.

48. Jose J, Taylor AB, Kuhn RJ. Spatial and temporal analysis of alphavirus replication and assembly in mammalian and mosquito cells. mBio 2017;8. https://doi.org/10.1128/mBio.02294-16.

49. Gardner CL, Burke CW, Tesfay MZ, et al. Eastern and Venezuelan equine encephalitis viruses differ in their ability to infect dendritic cells and macrophages: impact of altered cell tropism on pathogenesis. J Virol 2008;82:10634–46.

50. Del Piero F, Wilkins PA, Dubovi EJ, et al. Clinical, pathologic, immunohistochemical, and virologic findings of eastern equine encephalomyelitis in two horses. Vet Pathol 2001;38:451–6.

51. Bergren NA, Haller S, Rossi SL, et al. "Submergence" of Western equine encephalitis virus: Evidence of positive selection argues against genetic drift and fitness reductions. PLoS Pathog 2020;16:e1008102.

52. Sharma A, Knollmann-Ritschel B. Current understanding of the molecular basis of Venezuelan equine encephalitis virus pathogenesis and vaccine development. Viruses 2019;11. https://doi.org/10.3390/v11020164.

53. Taylor KG, Paessler S. Pathogenesis of Venezuelan equine encephalitis. Vet Microbiol 2013;167:145–50.

54. Trobaugh DW, Klimstra WB. Alphaviruses suppress host immunity by preventing myeloid cell replication and antagonizing innate immune responses. Curr Opin Virol 2017;23:30–4.

55. Nargi-Aizenman JL, Griffin DE. Sindbis virus-induced neuronal death is both necrotic and apoptotic and is ameliorated by N-methyl-D-aspartate receptor antagonists. J Virol 2001;75:7114–21.

56. Azar SR, Campos RK, Bergren NA, et al. Epidemic alphaviruses: ecology, emergence and outbreaks. Microorganisms 2020;8. https://doi.org/10.3390/microorganisms8081167.

57. Castorena KM, Peltier DC, Peng W, et al. Maturation-dependent responses of human neuronal cells to western equine encephalitis virus infection and type I interferons. Virology 2008;372:208–20.

58. Pennick KE, McKnight CA, Patterson JS, et al. Diagnostic sensitivity and specificity of in situ hybridization and immunohistochemistry for Eastern equine encephalitis virus and West Nile virus in formalin-fixed, paraffin-embedded brain tissue of horses. J Vet Diagn Invest 2012;24:333–8.

59. Patterson JS, Maes RK, Mullaney TP, et al. Immunohistochemical diagnosis of eastern equine encephalomyelitis. J Vet Diagn Invest 1996;8:156–60.

60. Saiz JC, Martin-Acebes MA, Blazquez AB, et al. Pathogenicity and virulence of West Nile virus revisited eight decades after its first isolation. Virulence 2021;12:1145–73.

61. Samuel MA, Diamond MS. Pathogenesis of West Nile Virus infection: a balance between virulence, innate and adaptive immunity, and viral evasion. J Virol 2006;80:9349–60.

62. Habarugira G, Suen WW, Hobson-Peters J, et al. West Nile virus: an update on pathobiology, epidemiology, diagnostics, control and "one health" implications. Pathogens 2020;9. https://doi.org/10.3390/pathogens9070589.

63. Moudy RM, Zhang B, Shi PY, et al. West Nile virus envelope protein glycosylation is required for efficient viral transmission by Culex vectors. Virology 2009;387:222–8.

64. Balasuriya UB, Shi PY, Wong SJ, et al. Detection of antibodies to West Nile virus in equine sera using microsphere immunoassay. J Vet Diagn Invest 2006;18: 392–5.

65. International Committee on Taxonomy of Viruses (ICTV). Flaviviridae - flavivirus. ICTV; 2021. Available at. https://talk.ictvonline.org/taxonomy.

66. Mackenzie JS, Gubler DJ, Petersen LR. Emerging flaviviruses: the spread and resurgence of Japanese encephalitis, West Nile and dengue viruses. Nat Med 2004;10:S98–109.

67. Saiz JC. Animal and human vaccines against West Nile Virus. Pathogens 2020; 9. https://doi.org/10.3390/pathogens9121073.

68. Solomon T. Flavivirus encephalitis. N Engl J Med 2004;351:370–8.

69. Sule WF, Oluwayelu DO, Hernandez-Triana LM, et al. Epidemiology and ecology of West Nile virus in sub-Saharan Africa. Parasit Vectors 2018;11:414.

70. Ciccozzi M, Peletto S, Cella E, et al. Epidemiological history and phylogeography of West Nile virus lineage 2. Infect Genet Evol 2013;17:46–50.

71. Fall G, Di Paola N, Faye M, et al. Biological and phylogenetic characteristics of West African lineages of West Nile virus. PLoS Negl Trop Dis 2017;11:e0006078.

72. Hayes CG. West Nile virus: Uganda, 1937, to New York City, 1999. Ann N Y Acad Sci 2001;951:25–37.

73. Ostlund EN, Andresen JE, Andresen M. West Nile encephalitis. Vet Clin North Am Equine Pract 2000;16:427–41.

74. Ostlund EN, Crom RL, Pedersen DD, et al. Equine West Nile encephalitis, United States. Emerg Infect Dis 2001;7:665–9.

75. Trock SC, Meade BJ, Glaser AL, et al. West Nile virus outbreak among horses in New York State, 1999 and 2000. Emerg Infect Dis 2001;7:745–7.

76. Centers for Disease Control and Prevention (CDC). West Nile virus. CDC; 2020. Available at. https://www.cdc.gov/westnile/statsmaps/cumMapsData.html.

77. USDA-APHIS. West Nile virus (WNV). 2020. Available at. https://www.aphis. usda.gov/aphis/ourfocus/animalhealth/animal-disease-information/equine/wnv/ west-nile-virus.

78. European Centre for Disease Prevention and Control. West Nile virus in Europe. 2020. Available at. https://www.ecdc.europa.eu/en.

79. Bertram FM, Thompson PN, Venter M. Epidemiology and clinical presentation of West Nile virus infection in horses in South Africa, 2016-2017. Pathogens 2020;10. https://doi.org/10.3390/pathogens10010020.

80. Venter M, Human S, Zaayman D, et al. Lineage 2 west nile virus as cause of fatal neurologic disease in horses, South Africa. Emerg Infect Dis 2009;15:877–84.

81. Venter M, van Vuren PJ, Mentoor J, et al. Inactivated West Nile Virus (WNV) vaccine, Duvaxyn WNV, protects against a highly neuroinvasive lineage 2 WNV strain in mice. Vaccine 2013;31:3856–62.

82. Salazar P, Traub-Dargatz JL, Morley PS, et al. Outcome of equids with clinical signs of West Nile virus infection and factors associated with death. J Am Vet Med Assoc 2004;225:267–74.

83. Metz MBC, Olufemi OT, Daly JM, et al. Systematic review and meta-analysis of seroprevalence studies of West Nile virus in equids in Europe between 2001 and 2018. Transbound Emerg Dis 2021;68:1814–23.

84. Klenk K, Snow J, Morgan K, et al. Alligators as West Nile virus amplifiers. Emerg Infect Dis 2004;10:2150–5.

85. Goddard LB, Roth AE, Reisen WK, et al. Vector competence of California mosquitoes for West Nile virus. Emerg Infect Dis 2002;8:1385–91.

86. Bunning ML, Bowen RA, Cropp CB, et al. Experimental infection of horses with West Nile virus. Emerg Infect Dis 2002;8:380–6.

87. Fall AG, Diaite A, Seck MT, et al. West Nile virus transmission in sentinel chickens and potential mosquito vectors, Senegal River Delta, 2008-2009. Int J Environ Res Public Health 2013;10:4718–27.

88. Anderson JF, Main AJ, Andreadis TG, et al. Transstadial transfer of West Nile virus by three species of ixodid ticks (Acari: Ixodidae). J Med Entomol 2003;40: 528–33.

89. Bunning ML, Bowen RA, Cropp B, et al. Experimental infection of horses with West Nile virus and their potential to infect mosquitoes and serve as amplifying hosts. Ann N Y Acad Sci 2001;951:338–9.

90. Gardner IA, Wong SJ, Ferraro GL, et al. Incidence and effects of West Nile virus infection in vaccinated and unvaccinated horses in California. Vet Res 2007;38: 109–16.

91. Long MT. West nile virus and equine encephalitis viruses: new perspectives. Vet Clin North Am Equine Pract 2014;30:523–42.

92. Ayala-Nunez NV, Gaudin R. A viral journey to the brain: current considerations and future developments. PLoS Pathog 2020;16:e1008434.

93. Blakely PK, Kleinschmidt-DeMasters BK, Tyler KL, et al. Disrupted glutamate transporter expression in the spinal cord with acute flaccid paralysis caused by West Nile virus infection. J Neuropathol Exp Neurol 2009;68:1061–72.

94. Schuler LA, Khaitsa ML, Dyer NW, et al. Evaluation of an outbreak of West Nile virus infection in horses: 569 cases. J Am Vet Med Assoc 2004;225:1084–9.

95. Ward MP, Levy M, Thacker HL, et al. Investigation of an outbreak of encephalomyelitis caused by West Nile virus in 136 horses. J Am Vet Med Assoc 2004; 225:84–9.

96. Porter MB, Long MT, Getman LM, et al. West Nile virus encephalomyelitis in horses: 46 cases (2001). J Am Vet Med Assoc 2003;222:1241–7.

97. Epp T, Waldner C, West K, et al. Factors associated with West Nile virus disease fatalities in horses. Can Vet J 2007;48:1137–45.

98. American Association of Equine Practitioners. West Nile virus. AAEP; 2021. Available at. https://aaep.org/document/west-nile-virus.

99. Long MT, Gibbs EP, Mellencamp MW, et al. Efficacy, duration, and onset of immunogenicity of a West Nile virus vaccine, live Flavivirus chimera, in horses with a clinical disease challenge model. Equine Vet J 2007;39:491–7.

100. Khatibzadeh SM, Gold CB, Keggan AE, et al. West Nile virus-specific immunoglobulin isotype responses in vaccinated and infected horses. Am J Vet Res 2015;76:92–100.

101. Cantile C, Del Piero F, Di Guardo G, et al. Pathologic and immunohistochemical findings in naturally occurring West Nile virus infection in horses. Vet Pathol 2001;38:414–21.

102. Cantile C, Di Guardo G, Eleni C, et al. Clinical and neuropathological features of West Nile virus equine encephalomyelitis in Italy. Equine Vet J 2000;32:31–5.

103. Sebastian MM, Stewart I, Williams NM, et al. Pathological, entomological, avian and meteorological investigation of a West Nile virus epidemic in a horse farm. Transbound Emerg Dis 2008;55:134–9.

104. Venter M, Steyl J, Human S, et al. Transmission of West Nile virus during horse autopsy. Emerg Infect Dis 2010;16:573–5.

105. American Association of Equine Practitioners (AAEP). Vaccination guidelines. 2020. Available at. https://aaep.org/guidelines/vaccination-guidelines.

106. Berge TO, Banks IS, Tigertt WD. Attenuation of Venezuelan equine encephalomyelitis virus by in vitro cultivation in guinea-pig heart cells. Am J Hyg 1961;73: 209–18.
107. Stromberg ZR, Fischer W, Bradfute SB, et al. Vaccine advances against Venezuelan, Eastern, and Western equine encephalitis viruses. Vaccines (Basel) 2020;8. https://doi.org/10.3390/vaccines8020273.
108. Fine DL, Roberts BA, Teehee ML, et al. Venezuelan equine encephalitis virus vaccine candidate (V3526) safety, immunogenicity and efficacy in horses. Vaccine 2007;25:1868–76.
109. Tauro LB, Rivarola ME, Lucca E, et al. First isolation of Bunyamwera virus (Bunyaviridae family) from horses with neurological disease and an abortion in Argentina. Vet J 2015;206:111–4.
110. Motlou TP, Williams J, Venter M. Epidemiology of shuni virus in horses in South Africa. Viruses 2021;13. https://doi.org/10.3390/v13050937.

Nonarboviral Equine Encephalitides

Ramiro E. Toribio, DVM, MS, PhD

KEYWORDS

- Lyssaviruses • Rhabdoviruses • Rabies • Borna disease • Bornaviruses
- Encephalitis • Encephalomyelitis • Zoonosis

KEY POINTS

- Rabies in equids is rarely diagnosed in the New World, Europe and developed countries but continues to be a problem in the developing world. In developed countries, wildlife is the main source of rabies virus, whereas in the developing world, the main source of rabies virus is the dog.
- Lyssaviruses are emerging pathogens that, similar to rabies, cause inevitably fatal neurologic disease in mammalian species, including horses. Molecular methods have further clarified pathogenic processes shared between the rabies virus and other lyssaviruses.
- Vaccination is the most effective measure to prevent rabies in any species.
- Borna disease is a neurologic condition of horses currently restricted to certain regions of Europe, occasionally reported in other species. It seems to be spreading to other parts of Europe.
- Borna disease remains to be documented in other continents but there is serologic evidence of its presence or a similar virus in Asia, Australia, and North America.

INTRODUCTION

Several viruses transmitted by biological vectors or through direct contact, air, or ingestion cause neurologic disease in equids. Of interest are viruses of the *Togaviridae*, *Flaviviridae*, *Rhabdoviridae*, *Herpesviridae*, *Bornaviridae*, and *Bunyaviridae* families. Many are classified as arboviruses because they use arthropod vectors, whereas others are transmitted directly via ingestion, inhalation, or integument damage. They reach the central nervous system (CNS) through blood, carried by mononuclear cells, or via retrograde axonal transport to the spinal cord or directly to the brain via the olfactory and nasopharyngeal epithelium. Lesions and clinical signs are the result of vascular damage, hemorrhage, thrombosis, edema, inflammation, neuronal and glial cell degeneration and dysfunction, apoptosis, and necrosis. Variable degree of inflammation is

College of Veterinary Medicine, The Ohio State University, 601 Vernon Tharp Street, Columbus, OH 43210, USA
E-mail address: toribio.1@osu.edu

Vet Clin Equine 38 (2022) 323–338
https://doi.org/10.1016/j.cveq.2022.04.007

present with these viruses but lack of an inflammatory response does not rule out their presence. The goal of this article is to provide an overview on pathophysiologic and clinical aspects of nonarboviral equine encephalitides, specifically on lyssaviruses (rabies) and bornaviruses (Borna disease [BD]).

Rabies and Lyssaviruses

Rabies is a severe, progressive, and inevitably fatal neurologic disease (encephalitis) of mammalians. Despite its lethal outcome in people and animals, rabies is perhaps the most neglected zoonotic disease.

Cause

The rabies virus (RABV) belongs to the order *Mononegavirales*, genus *Lyssavirus*, family *Rhabdoviridae* (rhabdos = rod or bullet shape), phylogroup I.[1] In Greek mythology, "Lyssa" was a goddess or spirit of rage, fury, or madness. It is a single-stranded, non-segmented, negative-sense enveloped ribonucleic acid (RNA) virus with a 12 kb genome, measuring 60 × 180 nm (45–100 nm × 100–430 nm).[1] The genome of rhabdoviruses encodes 5 structural proteins: nucleoprotein (N), phosphoprotein (P), matrix protein (M), glycoprotein (G), and RNA-directed RNA polymerase (L) in 3'-N-P-M-G-L-5' order.[1,2] The RNA genome is encapsulated by N to form a tight N-RNA complex known as a ribonucleoprotein (RNP).[1,2] In the lipid bilayer, G forms spikes that wrap the RNP-M complex and binds to surface receptors.[2] RABV is phylogenetically related to other lyssaviruses that cause acute progressive and fatal encephalomyelitis in people and animals.[1–3] To date, at least 17 species of the *Lyssavirus* genus grouped into 3 phylogroups have been described around the world.[1–6] These viruses have antigenic differences but all can cause neurologic disease that is indistinguishable from rabies.[1–5,7]

Bats are hosts for most lyssavirus species, and virus sequence analysis indicates that lyssaviruses coevolved with bats,[3–5,8] mainly in the Palearctic region (Europe, Asia, North Africa, Arabian Peninsula).[8] This is also apparent by the low mortality rate in bats infected with lyssaviruses. There are differences between RABV transmitted from dogs compared with chiropterans and variants circulating foxes and skunks mainly originated from canids. There is evidence that RABV was in the Americas before the arrival of the Europeans.[8]

In addition to *Lyssavirus*, other members of the *Rhabdoviridae* family of veterinary importance include the vesicular stomatitis virus (*Vesiculovirus* genus) and the bovine ephemeral fever virus (*Ephemerovirus* genus).[1] Rhabdoviruses are more stable than other viruses in the environment but are susceptible to commonly used disinfectants.

Epidemiology

Rabies has been documented in all continents with the exception of Australia, New Zealand, Antarctica, and some Pacific islands. However, lyssaviruses in Australia cause signs and outcome comparable to rabies. Canine rabies has been eradicated from many countries. Rabies is rarely diagnosed in developed countries; however, globally there are around 60,000 annual human deaths from rabies of which 95% occur in Africa and Asia, mainly (>99%) from dog bites,[9–13] with the majority being children aged younger than 15 years.[9,10,14] This is shameful and reflects a disconnect between developed and developing countries as most of these deaths could be prevented by implementing canine vaccination programs and public education. In these regions, dog-mediated rabies is linked to poverty, poor health systems, lack of education and expertise, and governmental neglicence.[9,14] Not understanding the implications of dog bites, scarce health centers, inadequate diagnostics, and limited access to biologicals such as vaccines and antiserum are major contributors to mortality. Bringing rabies under control is now a top One Health priority of the World Health Organization (WHO) that has established the ambitious goal of eliminating dog rabies by 2030.[15]

RABV is transmitted to animals and people through bites or scratches from dogs, foxes, raccoons, racoon dogs, skunks, coyotes, mongooses, cats, and bats. In the southern United States, there have been documented human and animal cases from aerosol exposure in caves with high bat density.[16,17]

Of the 17 lyssavirus species described, RABV (carnivore and bat hosts) is the only one in the New World, whereas other species that reside in bats are present in other continents. Based on the type of host, there are 2 epidemiologic cycles: *terrestrial rabies* where RABV is maintained in wild and domestic carnivores and *chiropteran rabies* (or chiropteran lyssavirus infection) where viruses reside in bat colonies (hematophagous, insectivores, frugivores).[5] Clinical signs between these types of rabies are indistinguishable.[5]

Most lyssavirus around the world are maintained in chiropteran hosts[6]; however, in addition to bats, RABV is also maintained in mesocarnivores (dogs, foxes, racoons, racoon dogs, jackals, mongoose, skunks).[6] Infections in people, horses, cattle, and other animals represent dead-end spillover hosts. Canine variants are distributed in mesocarnivores and bat variants are a problem in some regions of Europe and America.[6] Bat lyssaviruses are considered an emerging zoonotic threat.[18] Before 1960, dogs were a common reservoir for RABV in the United States and Europe but currently wildlife (raccoons, skunks, jackals, bats) are the main reservoirs.[19] Most human infections in the United States are from bats.[11]

In the United States, 1 to 3 human cases and in Europe less than 5 human cases are reported annually, with one-third to half related to exposure to rabid dogs in developing countries.[9–11,20–22] These numbers are miniscule compared with the developing world. In the United States and western Europe, canine-transmitted rabies has been eradicated,[9–11,20,23,24] and it is close to eradication in Latin America, with 3 human cases in 2019.[23] Bovine paralytic rabies remains a problem in Latin America.

Even though canine rabies has been eradicated from the United States, surveillance of imported dogs and cats is essential to keep it outside the country.[25] Recent cases of rabies in imported dogs and fraudulent rabies vaccination certificates led the Centers for Disease Control and Prevention (CDC) in 2021 to ban the importation of dogs from 113 countries. Cryptic or cryptogenic rabies refers to infections where there is no history of exposure to vectors.[17] This may be the case for most affected horses.

The prevalence of rabies in animals is very low in developed counties, mainly due to vaccination and reservoir control. In the United States, rabies cases are regional and linked to specific reservoirs. In eastern states (Florida to Massachusetts) is the raccoon, in the Midwest is the skunk, in southern states including Texas are the skunk, fox, and coyote, in western states is the skunk, and in Puerto Rico is the mongoose.[25,26] In Canada, the fox and skunk are the main ones. Cases linked to bats have a wide distribution all over the Americas. In Europe, the red fox accounts for most reported cases. In Latin America, in addition to dogs and small mammals, vampire bats are very important vectors, in particular for cattle and horses.

The dog continues to be the most important vector for rabies in urban areas in Africa and Asia. This is contrary to the New World and Western Europe where most cases are from bats.[11] Human cases associated with the canine variants are extremely rare in the United States and more than 90% are linked to wildlife.[11] Approximately 5000 animal rabies cases are reported annually to the CDC, with the majority (>90%) being in wildlife.[11,25,26] Of these, bats account for 30%, raccoons for 30%, skunks for 20%, and foxes for 7% of the total.[11,25,26] Of the 350 to 400 cases of rabies in domestic animals reported to the CDC annually, most are cats, followed by dogs, cattle, and horses.[25] In Canada, bats account for half of rabid animals, followed by racoons, skunks, and foxes.[25,26] The situation is different in Mexico and the rest of Latin America, where the most diagnosed animals are cattle (chiropteran paralytic rabies).[25,26]

Annually 10 to 30 equine cases are reported in the United States,[25,26] and 20 to 30 in Europe, mainly in eastern Europe.[9] Most are nonvaccinated equids.

Pathogenesis

After viral introduction, rabies incubation is variable, from weeks to months.[2–4,6,10,22] Transmission in almost all cases occurs through bites or scratches from infected animals, exposing tissue to saliva rich in RABV (or lyssavirus). The virus initially replicates in skeletal muscle near the inoculation site. Muscle cells are not as permissive as other cell types for RABV replication, which explains the delay in the development of clinical signs. In addition, unlike other rhabdoviruses, lyssaviruses are not lymphotropic, further delaying initial replication.[4] Viral dose, replication efficiency, and distance to the CNS explains why some animals and people have short or very long incubation times. Glycoprotein G is central to the pathogenesis[27]; it forms spikes (peplomers) on the virus lipid bilayer membrane that are required for receptor binding, internalization, invasion, and immune evasion. The ectodomain of G binds to the nicotinic acetylcholine receptors (nAChRs) on muscle cells to trigger endocytosis.[2,6] From muscle cells, RABV enters the synaptic cleft of the neuromuscular junctions to reach nerve terminals.[6] RABV also binds neuronal cell adhesion molecule (NCAM), p75 neurotrophin receptor and metabotropic glutamate receptor 2 to expedite viral entry, retrograde axonal transport, and neuronal invasion.[2,6]

Once in the axons, via retrograde axoplasmic flow facilitated by NCAM, p75, and dynein, RABV travels centripetally to the spinal cord and brain.[2,6] Initial peripheral neurologic signs develop when the virus reaches the axons, and from that point, the disease progresses rapidly. It has been estimated that the virus travels at 12 to 100 mm per day; therefore, it takes longer for animals with distal bites to develop classic neurologic signs.[28] In the CNS, there is neuron-to-neuron spread via trans-synaptic dissemination.[2,6,28] Simultaneously, the RABV travels in centrifugal (anterograde) direction, mainly via the parasympathetic nervous system, to different organs, including salivary glands and mucosal surfaces innervated by cranial nerves, but also to the skin, cornea, adrenal medulla, and hair follicles.[2,3,6,28] Something unique of RABV compared with other neuroinvasive viruses is that is primarily transported centripetally by motor rather than sensory and autonomic neurons.[2] In the CNS, RABV prefers neurons over glial cells and trans-synaptic spread explains the lack of typical histologic lesions seen with other neurotropic viruses.[2,6,28] RABV virulence depends on its ability to infect neurons and evade the immune system.[2,6,28] However, its effects on neurons are noncytopathic.[2] During the incubation period, the immune response is poor and T cells are ineffective at eliminating the virus, which contributes to the mild inflammatory infiltration noted early on.[2–4,6,28] Type I interferon (IFN) mediates innate antiviral immune responses, which for RABV is insufficient. Neuronal production of IFN-α and IFN-β may slow RABV initial neuroinvasion but in most instances is not effective.[2–4,6,28]

Lyssaviruses cause mitochondrial failure, oxidative injury, degeneration of neuronal process, with dendritic and axonal loss.[2–4,6] Disappearance of intracellular organelles, vesicle and synaptic structures, as well as disruption of cytoskeletal integrity are key mechanisms leading to neuronal failure with minimal structural changes.[2–4,6,29] This ability to avoid immune, inflammatory, and cytolytic host defense mechanisms is regarded as a successful viral adaptation.[2–4,6,28,30,31] Ultimately, RABV causes neuronal death, initially through activation of the apoptotic machinery and later via cell necrosis.[2–4,6,29] These events will also lead to systemic organ failure. Early clinical signs, in particular muscle weakness, are the result of axonal dysfunction. RABV G glycoprotein has neurotoxin-like properties that alter nerve conduction.[32] As the disease progresses, other signs are consequence of altered neuronal activity. Impaired activity of neuronal nAChRs and metabotropic receptors contribute to initial signs, in particular behavioral changes.[2,6,28] Abnormal levels of neurotransmitters such as acetylcholine, dopamine, norepinephrine, serotonin, glutamate, and gamma-aminobutyric acid as well as disruption of ion channels are central disease progression.[28,29]

Rhabdoviruses induce the formation of cytoplasmic inclusions (Negri bodies in lyssavirus) that are minifactories containing all the machinery (N, P, M, G, L) and cellular proteins required for viral replication.[2,3,30,31] Shared mechanisms among lyssaviruses explain similarity in clinical and histologic findings.[5] Viremia is not a feature of lyssaviruses.

Clinical signs

The quote that *"rabies can look like anything"* is valid and valuable for clinicians to keep in mind. Considering the pathogenesis of RABV infection, clinical signs in horses are variable, including lethargy, poor performance, behavioral changes, lameness, colic, urinary incontinence, paralysis, and ataxia. Invariably, once initial signs are evident, the condition progresses rapidly. At terminal stages, horses become recumbent but some may have aggressive behavior. Most horses die or are euthanized within 1 week of initial clinical signs. However, horses can have subtle signs for weeks (R. Toribio, personal communication). Rabies has 3 clinical presentations, in part dictated by the main site for viral replication and neuronal damage. There are *paralytic* (spinal cord), *dumb* (brainstem), and *furious* (cerebral cortex) forms.

In the *paralytic form*, spinal signs are a hallmark and include weakness, lameness, paresis, and ascending paralysis.[33] Other signs include tenesmus, urinary and fecal incontinence, and colon impactions. Some animals may show colic-like signs. It can be difficult to differentiate this presentation from other neurologic diseases, which also has zoonotic implications, because by the time a diagnosis of rabies is made many people have been in contact with the animal. The paralytic form often progresses to other forms. In the *dumb form*, there is lethargy, anorexia, head tilt, nystagmus, circling, ataxia, blindness, cranial nerve paralysis, dysphagia, hypersalivation, tail and anal paralysis, urinary and fecal incontinence as well as extrapyramidal signs including compulsive walking and head pressing.[33,34] In the *furious (encephalitic) form* there is aggression, photophobia, hyperesthesia, ataxia, circling, nystagmus, muscle tremors, pruritus, self-mutilation, opisthotonos, and convulsions.[33] Many of these signs reflect damage to the limbic system. Hydrophobia may be an interpretation of hypersalivation, laryngeal paralysis, dysphagia, and inability to swallow. Around half of diagnosed horses will develop fever that could be result of excessive physical activity or hypothalamic failure. Dysphagia, respiratory failure, and gastrointestinal atony leading to colic could be a consequence of parasympathetic dysfunction.[33] The paralytic and dumb forms are the most common presentations in horses.[34] Self-mutilation is a common sign in donkeys.

Progressive hindlimb ataxia, photophobia, nictitating membrane protrusion, altered behavior, circling, nystagmus, head pressing, cervical ventroflexion, mydriasis, hypersalivation, dysphagia, and convulsions were reported in horses infected with Australian bat lyssavirus.[35] Negri bodies were identified in Purkinje cells from these horses.[35]

Diagnosis

No antemortem diagnostic method is available for equine rabies, and it can only be confirmed at postmortem histologic examination. Clinical signs are nonspecific, and the list of differentials can be extensive. It is important to ask about the core vaccination status. Some animals can present resembling orthopedic problems until they progress to a paralytic form. Others may present with what seems to be abdominal discomfort. Rapid progression and aggressive behavior may raise suspicion. Spinal and cerebral signs can be indistinguishable from alphavirus (Eastern, Western and Venezuelan Equine Encephalomyelitis [EEE/WEE/VEE]), flavivirus (West Nile virus [WNV]), equine herpesvirus-1 (EHV-1), and Bornavirus infections. There could be overlap with parasites (eg, aberrant parasite migration, equine protozoal myeloencephalitis [EPM]), inflammatory or immune-mediate conditions (eg, polyneuritis, meningitis), intoxications (eg, botulism, leukoencephalomalacia, lead poisoning), metabolic disorders (eg, hepatic encephalopathy), space-occupying masses (eg, abscess, neoplasia), orthopedic conditions (eg, trauma, spinal cord compression from cervicovertebral malformation [CVM; wobblers]), and neurodegenerative disorders (equine degenerative myelopathy/neuroaxonal dystrophy [EDM/NAD]).

Laboratory tests are nonspecific. Cerebrospinal fluid (CSF) evaluation can show mononuclear pleocytosis with increased protein; however, a normal CSF does not exclude rabies.[33]

Care must be taken when euthanizing suspect animals. The brain must be processed under biosecurity measures, packaged in a sealed plastic container, cooled (not frozen), placed in a second leakproof container and sent to approved diagnostic entities, frequently a local or state health department. The rest of the animal should not be processed until results are available, which in most instances is less than 48 hours.

The presence of Negri bodies is pathognomonic of lyssavirus infection but their absence does not rule out rabies. The official and gold standard diagnostic method in most countries, including the United States, is the direct fluorescent antibody (DFA) test using monoclonal antibodies on tissue impressions or histologic sections.[3,4,6,11,15,20,28,36] Direct rapid immunohistochemical test (DRIT) is another acceptable method, with 100% sensitivity and specificity compared with DFA, and is recognized by the World Organisation for Animal Health (formerly the Office International des Epizooties [OIE]) as an alternative method for DFA.[3,4,6,28,36] Other methods such as immunohistochemistry, enzyme-linked immunosorbent assay (ELISA), and reverse transcription polymerase chain reaction (RT-PCR) have excellent agreement and can be used for further confirmation.[6] DFA, DRIT, and RT-PCR provide results in less than 4 hours.[6]

At least in people, RT-PCR has shown good antemortem sensitivity using skin biopsies or saliva, and it has been implemented in several countries where rabies is endemic.[6] Molecular methods have been accepted by OIE and WHO; however, for results to be considered valid, the test must be performed by specific laboratories. The mouse intracerebral inoculation is a good diagnostic method but it takes 3 to 4 weeks, restricting its use mainly to virus isolation.[6] New techniques are being evaluated to support the diagnosis of RABV, including flow cytometry.[5,37] Cornea impressions, skin biopsy, and hair follicle have been evaluated in people but not considered reliable in horses.

The rapid fluorescent focus inhibition test (RFFIT) measures RBAV-specific neutralizing antibodies, is used to assess vaccination titers in personnel and is useful to decide on postexposure vaccination (eg, animal workers) but it takes up to 1 week.[6] RFFIT is the WHO gold standard serologic assay for this purpose.[6] Per CDC, titers should not be used to substitute rabies vaccination.

Pathologic condition
Macroscopic changes are minimal compared with other viral encephalitides. There could be hemorrhage and congestion.[33] Histologic lesions are similar between

species, including the presence of Negri bodies, which are centers of viral replication and translation, with viral and cellular proteins.[30,31,38] Negri bodies are sharp round to oval eosinophilic inclusions of variable sizes (0.3–20 μm) in the neuronal perikarya and proximal dendrite, mainly found in cerebellar Purkinje cells, brainstem nuclei neurons, and pyramidal cells in the hippocampus (Ammon's horn) but can also be found in the spinal cord.[2–4,28,35,39] It is estimated that less than 50% of affected animals have Negri bodies, and their absence does not exclude the diagnosis of rabies.[33,34,39] For this reason, DFA is performed in all suspects (100% sensitivity).[39]

Affected horses have nonsuppurative meningoencephalitis, meningomyelitis, ganglioneuritis, perivascular cuffing with lymphocytic infiltration in both gray and white matter. Inflammation is variable but more severe in the brainstem, basal nuclei, thalamus, and hippocampus (encephalitis).[38] RABV effects on neurons are mainly noncytopathic.[2] Chromatolysis, neuronophagia, malacia, gliosis, presence of gitter cells, and satellite glial cell proliferation (Nageotte nodules) are common findings.[28,38] Similar lesions can be observed in the spinal cord (myelitis). One histologic study of 26 cattle and 7 horses found spinal cord lesions in all animals.[38] The study recommended that the spinal cord in all suspect horses must be examined to increase the likelihood of a positive diagnosis.[38] Lesions can be present in the trigeminal ganglion.[35] Immunohistochemistry reveals the presence of RABV in neurons, axons, and dendrites in the cerebral cortex, cerebellum, brainstem, thalamus, hippocampus, and spinal cord horns. RABV can also be found in glial cells, retina, pituitary gland, peripheral ganglia, and adrenal medulla. The cervical spinal cord and brainstem are optimal sites to detect RABV in horses.[40] Histologic lesions similar to rabies, including the presence of Negri bodies, were identified in Purkinje cells of horses naturally infected with Australian bat lyssavirus.[35] Similar to other conditions leading to recumbency, there could be secondary lesions and infections in other body systems.

Treatment

There is no treatment of rabies in animals and people, and postexposure prophylaxis is the most effective method to prevent rabies. Due to lack of antemortem diagnostics, most of these horses receive routine therapy for neurologic disease. Glucocorticoids may delay disease progression and should be avoided when rabies is a top differential.

Prevention

Neglect is perhaps the best term to define the approach of developed countries on rabies in the developing world. Each year hundreds of millions of dollars go to diseases with lower fatality rates and economic impact than rabies, which just receives few million dollars of funding worldwide.[3] Eliminating dog-mediated rabies will save 60,000 lives per year, improve living conditions for millions of people, enhance global health security, and free up billions of dollars in economic resources each year.[41] Surveillance, education, vaccination, and reducing contact with reservoirs have been at the center of successful rabies control strategies in developed and developing countries.

Positive animals should be reported to the local, state, and national authorities based on regulations for each country. Suspect animals should be immediately isolated and proper biosecurity measures implemented, including use of personal protective equipment and thorough disinfection. Biologic fluids, in particular CSF could have RABV, with high zoonotic risk.

A horse bitten by a wild animal should be considered exposed to rabies. Exposed vaccinated horses should be revaccinated and isolated for 45 days.[24] Per the

American Veterinary Medical Association (AVMA), nonvaccinated livestock known to be exposed to a rabid animal should be euthanized immediately.[24] Alternatively, the animal should be isolated for 6 months with no animal or human contact, monitored, and if neurologic signs develop, the animal must be euthanized and the head shipped for testing.[24] It would be unusual for a vaccinated horse to develop rabies. If the animal was vaccinated and develops disease, it should be reported to the manufacturer, local health authorities, and the United States Department of Agriculture (USDA). There is no evidence that rabid horses transmit RABV to other animals but they are a risk, and precautions must be taken. Other animals in the premises should be monitored but the likelihood that other herbivores are infected is extremely low. Human exposure should be reported to local health authorities.

Highly effective inactivated and recombinant rabies vaccines are USDA-approved for horses and other domestic animals. Inactivated vaccines use the same virus as the original Pasteur Merieux human vaccine. The virus is grown in cell culture, inactivated, and prepared with adjuvants. Recombinant vaccines use RABV proteins in vaccinia, adenovirus, canarypox, or other vectors. In the United States, a recombinant vaccine expressing RABV glycoprotein G in a canarypox vector is available for cats (Purevax, Boehringer Ingelheim) but not for horses. Available equine rabies vaccines are monovalent and polyvalent, combining up to 6 antigens (**Table 1**).

Unvaccinated horses require a single dose (pregnant mares 1 month before foaling) with annual revaccination, whereas foals and weanlings should be vaccinated at 3 to 6 months of age and then once a year. Some vaccines in foals require a booster 4 to 6 weeks later. Rabies vaccination is core and most states require the vaccine to be administered by a licensed veterinarian.[42] AVMA defines core vaccinations as those that protect animals from diseases that are endemic, represent a potential public health risk, are required by law, highly infectious, and/or severe to the animal. Vaccination guidelines for horses have been developed by the American Association of Equine Practitioners.[42] There are oral rabies vaccines (ORVs) specific for wild animals and stray dogs that have proven effective in developed and developing countries at reducing human and animal rabies incidence.[5] ORV was credited with controlling fox rabies in parts of Europe.[5] Genetically engineered rabies vaccines have been evaluated in the research setting and proved effective at raising immunity but are not commercially available.

Table 1
USDA-approved rabies vaccines available in the United States for horses

Name	Manufacturer	Dose (mL)	Age of vaccination (mo)	Booster	Route
Rabvac 3[a]	Elanco	2	3	Annually	IM
EquiRab[a]	Merck	1	4	Annually	IM
Potomavac + Imrab[b]	Boehringer-Ingelheim	1	3	Annually	IM
Core Eq Innovator[c]	Zoetis	1	3	Annually	IM
Core Eq Innovator V[d]	Zoetis	1	3	Annually	IM

Abbreviations: EEEV, Eastern equine encephalitis virus; VEEV, Venezuelan equine encephalitis viruses; WEEV, Western equine encephalitis virus; WNV, West Nile virus.
[a] Monovalent.
[b] Bivalent.
[c] Rabies, tetanus, EEEV, WEEV, WNV.
[d] Rabies, tetanus, EEEV, VEEV, WEEV, WNV.

In people exposed to RABV through bites, development of the disease can be prevented by postexposure prophylaxis (wound cleaning, rabies antiserum, vaccination).[5] It consists of thoroughly washing the bite site with soap and viricidal antiseptics (eg, chlorhexidine, povidone iodine, ethanol) for at least 15 minutes followed by administration of immunoglobulins (passive immunity) and vaccination (active immunity).[5] This is rarely done in veterinary medicine, and when animals have been exposed, prophylaxis is restricted to vaccination, isolation, observation, or euthanasia.

In Latin America where bovine and equine rabies is transmitted by vampire bats (eg, *Desmodus rotundus*) ointments based on anticoagulants (eg, brodifacoum) are applied on previous bite sites or on the back of captured bats. Based on their social grooming behavior, a large number of bats are exposed and die.

Public health
Rabies is a fatal zoonosis and despite the lack of evidence that humans can get the virus from infected equids, it is important to take precautions. Ideally, any animal with neurologic disease should be handled by rabies-vaccinated personnel. The use of personal protective equipment is important when working with suspicious animals, dead or alive. It is essential to state in the necropsy request that rabies is a differential. Reducing contact also facilitates contact tracing if the animal tests positive, when a list must be generated to notify exposed people as well as authorities. Depending on the type of contact and rabies vaccination status, additional measures must be coordinated with physicians and local health authorities, which will decide on postexposure treatment, that may or not require rabies vaccination. Measuring titers may be possible but takes time.

Borna Disease

BD is a viral neurologic, typically progressive condition that mainly affects horses and sheep in central Europe, occasionally other domestic and wild animal, and is frequently fatal. The disease has been known to affect horses since the eighteenth century but the term originated from an outbreak at the end of the nineteenth century in Borna, Saxony, Germany.

Cause
BD is caused by bornavirus 1 (mammalian bornavirus-1 [BoV-1]) which is a spherical, enveloped (70–130 nm), negative-sense single-stranded nonsegmented RNA virus with 8.9 kb genome with 6 open reading frames encoding for a nucleoprotein, a phosphoprotein, a glycoprotein (GP-94), protein M, P10 protein, and RNA-polymerase.[43,44] The virus belongs to the *Mononegavirales* order, *Bornaviridae* family, *Orthobornavirus* genus.[43] In addition to mammals, other orthobornaviruses infect passeriform, aquatic, and psittacid birds.[43] BoV-1 isolated in endemic areas are highly conserved (>95% nucleotide homology).[43]

Epidemiology
BD occurs in equids, sheep, goats, dogs, cats, and occasionally in other species.[45–49] Camelids appear to be very susceptible to BoV-1.[46,50] It mainly occurs in Germany, Austria, Switzerland, and Liechtenstein but is sporadically reported in other European countries. This narrow distribution has been attributed to the existence of regional wild reservoirs. It is the main equine neurologic disease in Germany, where is endemic in the central and southern part of the country. Its incidence has decreased in recent decades to 0.02% to 0.04%.[45] However, based on serologic studies in healthy horses (10%–20% seropositivity), most infections in Germany are subclinical or

inapparent.[45,51] In facilities where horses have been diagnosed with BD, up to 50% of horses can be seropositive and are more likely to have additional cases within months.[45] An increase in equine cases occurred recently in Austria, suggesting a novel endemic area.[52] It is important to note that in addition to horses, BD is a major problem in cats in northern Europe (staggering disease), mainly in Sweden.[47]

Equine BD has not been identified clinically in North America or other continents. Perhaps one reason BD has not been diagnosed beyond Europe is because BD is rarely included in the list of differentials for neurologic disorders in horses or ruminants. Of interest, seropositive animals have been identified in North America, Asia, Africa, Middle East, and Australia, although the interpretation of these results has been questioned.[45,53] Equine cases with signs consistent with BD and the presence of high antibody titers are highly suggestive of its presence in Japan.[54] Antibodies against BoV-1 as well as BoV-1 genetic material were found in apparently healthy racehorses in Iran.[55] There is no clear explanation for discrepancies between high seropositivity and low incidence of clinical disease, although similar to other diseases, animal (immunity, genetics, age) and environmental (reservoir, weather) factors are important. The fact that BD in cats has been diagnosed in Asia and Australia further opens the question on whether we are missing the diagnosis of BD in horses in other countries.

BD has a seasonal occurrence with most cases occurring in spring and summer.[45] How animals get infected remains unclear. Infected animals can have viral particles in nasal and lacrimal secretions as well as urine and feces making these important routes of dissemination and transmission.[45,49] Horses with clinical signs can transmit the virus to other horses but are not important for disseminating the virus. The bicolored white-toothed shrew (Crocidura leucodon) is the natural reservoir for BoV-1 in endemic regions of central Europe.[43,56,57] Shrews can shed large amounts of BoV-1 in saliva, urine, lacrimal secretions, and feces and are considered a major source of BoV-1 to infect horses and sheep.[43,56] Squirrels are reservoirs for other orthobornaviruses in Europe including the variegated squirrel bornavirus-1 (VSBV-1).[43,56]

In Europe, Borna disease virus (BDV) has gained attention due to its zoonotic potential, ability to introduce its genetic material into the host genome, and potential association with neuropsychiatric disorders in people.[44,58] Cases of human encephalitis were recently reported in people that received organ transplants but also through natural infection.[43,59] This syndrome is different from the neuropsychiatric presentation.[43,59]

Pathogenesis

In equids, after an incubation that varies from 1 week to 3 months, BoV-1 causes an acute or subacute meningoencephalitis.[45,49,51] Most information on the pathogenesis of BD has been generated in rodents.[43,45,49] It is thought that BoV-1 enters the CNS via retrograde flow from nerve terminals from the olfactory and trigeminal nerves in the nasal and pharyngeal epithelium.[43–45,49] The virus uses GP-94 to enter cells by clathrin-mediated endocytosis in a pH-dependent manner.[43] In infected animals, the virus can be found in nasal and lacrimal secretions making it an important route of dissemination.[48,49] Once in the CNS, BoV-1 replicates in neurons and glial cells (astrocytes, oligodendrocytes) in the brainstem to subsequently disseminate to other areas of the central and peripheral nervous systems.[43,48,49,51]

The role of the type I interferon system in preventing infection seems inconclusive.[43] However, activation of the nuclear factor-κB (NF-κB) pathway suppresses viral replication.[43] Similar to other RNA viruses, its dissemination occurs through axons and nerve fibers. BoV-1 persists for life in nervous tissue of affected animals.[43,48,49,51] Initial clinical signs have been attributed to viral interference with neuronal plasticity, excitability and communication, as well as neurotransmitter release.[43]

In the CNS, BoV-1 causes multifocal lesions (meningoencephalitis, neuronal necrosis, and apoptosis) that are evident in the brainstem and limbic system.[43] Even though BoV-1 is primarily neurotropic, it has been found in other organs (retina, nasal mucosa, parotid gland, heart, lungs, kidneys, liver, bladder) in affected animals.[43,45,48,49,51] Neutralizing antibodies are detected in diseased animals; however, due to the nature of this virus and where it resides, antibodies are not very effective in controlling viral persistence, and animals are carriers for life.[43] Mononuclear cells (CD4+ and CD8+ T lymphocytes) are central to the pathogenesis of this condition.[43,45,49] Excessive mononuclear activity may reactivate or exacerbate clinical signs. Lymphocytes, in particular CD4+, establish a cytotoxic response against infected neurons that results in an inflammatory response. Neuronal death also occurs from the release of cytokines by glial cells and indirect excitotoxicity due to astrocyte failure and increased glutamate levels. At the end, these animals develop a severe mononuclear meningoencephalitis. Virus-induced immunopathologic damage to neurons and glial cells from delayed hypersensitivity is central to the pathogenesis of BD.[43,45] This has been further confirmed in experimental animals where dexamethasone pretreatment ameliorated or prevented clinical disease but did not change viral persistence.[43] Of interest, animals with chronic infection may have minimal inflammatory cell infiltration despite the presence of the virus in neurons and glial cells.[43,45] The fact that the virus has also been found in conjunctival and nasal secretions as well as saliva emphasizes the importance of these fluids as source of dissemination.[43,45]

Clinical signs

The disease has peracute, acute, subacute, and chronic presentations and most affected horses die within 1 month of development of neurologic signs.[45,48] Some horses recover to transition to the chronic form, with minimal, absent, or recurrent clinical signs.[45,48] Lay terms used before it was named BD included hot-headed disease (Hitzige Kopfkrankheit), brain fever, and hypersomnia of horses.[43,45] Neurologic signs are sensory, locomotor, and behavioral. Initial signs are nonspecific and include fever, lethargy, and anorexia. Subsequently, it progresses to changes in behavior and perception, somnolence, stupor, hyporeflexia, hypoesthesia, hypersensitivity, muscle fasciculations, ataxia, conscious and unconscious proprioceptive deficits, dysmetria, vestibular signs, circling, extrapyramidal signs, slow masticatory movements, chewing movements without food, may pause eating with hay in the mouth, tooth grinding, yawning, compulsive and encephalopathic movements, head pressing, hyperexcitability, aggression, recumbency, often leading to death.[45,49,51,52] Nearly all affected horses show abnormal behavior and half develop disturbances of chewing and swallowing.[45] Some animals may develop hyperthermia that is refractory to antipyretics.

Due to lesion localization, cranial nerve deficits are common and include motor and autonomic dysfunction, dysphagia, hypersalivation, headshaking, pharyngeal and laryngeal paralysis, reduced tongue tone, excessive tongue movements, bruxism, trismus, facial nerve paralysis, vestibular dysfunction, strabismus, miosis, anisocoria, poor pupillary light response, blindness, opisthotonos, and death.[45,51] Male horses may extrude the penis without urination. Because many horses have abnormal mastication and swallowing, reduced water and feed intake result in dehydration, colic, weight loss, emaciation, and secondary complications. Many of these signs are not specific to BD, which is important to consider in the differential list.

Diagnosis

Several pathogens can result in similar signs; thus, season, geography, age, and duration of clinical signs should be considered. Differential conditions include rabies, EHV-

1 myeloencephalopathy, botulism, meningitis, parasite migration, EPM, flaviviruses (WNV myeloencephalitis), alphaviruses (Eastern, Western, Venezuelan equine encephalitis—restricted to the Americas), tick-borne diseases (tick paralysis, neuroborreliosis/Lyme disease), toxicities (leukoencephalomalacia), and metabolic disorders (hepatic encephalopathy). Degenerative conditions such as EDM/NAD tend to have different clinical presentation and lesions, with minimal to absent cerebral signs. Metabolic disorders such as hepatic encephalopathy can be easily differentiated with blood chemistry.

Hematology and blood chemistry, similar to most neurologic diseases, are not specific. CSF evaluation may reveal increased protein and mononuclear cells (lymphocytic pleocytosis). There is a poor correlation between serum titers, disease severity, and mortality.[45,49] Healthy animals can be seropositive. Antibodies against BoV-1 in blood and CSF are indicative but not confirmatory of the disease. Indirect immunofluorescence is a reliable method to detect BoV-1 antibodies. Immunohistochemistry and in situ hybridization can be diagnostic and provide information on virus localization. RT-PCR can be useful as antemortem diagnosis using CSF and blood cells, in particular in animals with acute disease. RT-PCR combined with other methods is valuable in the postmortem diagnosis.[49,52] Viral isolation should be considered for further confirmation and for viral genome sequence analysis.

Cause

Gross neurologic lesions are minimal to absent. Histologic changes are present in the brainstem, limbic system (hippocampus, amygdala, thalamus, hypothalamus), spinal cord, and retina. Cerebellar lesions are minimal. Similar to other neurologic viral diseases, there is nonsuppurative meningoencephalitis and lymphocytic perivascular cuffing (CD4+, CD8+), mainly in the gray matter with macrophage and plasma cell infiltration.[43] The effect of BoV-1 on neurons and glial cells is noncytopathic, which may in part explain persistent infections that lead to cell-mediated cytotoxic changes.[43] There is neuronal degeneration, necrosis, neuronophagia, and astrocytosis, mainly in the brainstem and medulla oblongata. Intranuclear eosinophilic inclusion bodies (Joest-Degen bodies) can be present. These inclusions are considered pathognomonic. There could be retinitis. In addition to brain and spinal cord, BDV can be identified in lacrimal and salivary glands.[45] Rabies can be a top differential but unlike BoV-1 that infects neurons and glial cells, RABV only infects neurons. WNV encephalomyelitis has different histologic lesions often involving the spinal cord.

Therapy

Treatment is mainly supportive; most horses do not recover and have to be euthanized.[45,49,51] Antiviral drugs (amantadine) has been used with doubtful results.

Prevention and control

It is recommended to follow biosecurity measures and use personal protection equipment. Affected horses should be isolated and premises disinfected. In endemic areas, BD should be at the top of the differential list. However, it is important to consider other neurologic conditions of horses. BD is likely to be missed due to its similarity to other equine disorders. It has been proposed that New World camelids can be good sentinel animals due to their susceptibility to BoV-1.[50] Experimental vaccines have been evaluated but their efficacy has been questionable.

Implications beyond Europe

Even though seropositive animals to BD have been identified in different continents, the clinical condition remains to be diagnosed outside Europe. It is possible that BD is present in horses in other countries but not diagnosed because it is not included as a differential diagnosis. This is important to consider because horses can be carriers and clinically normal for years, can shed the virus and potentially infect other animals. In addition, horses from endemic areas are imported all over the world.

Public Health

It has been proposed that BoV-1 could be responsible for some neuropsychiatric disorders in people; however, this continues to be a controversial issue. A VSBV-1 has caused fatal neurologic disease in people in Germany.[43,60]

SUMMARY

Rabies and BD are equine viral diseases not transmitted by arthropods with unique pathogenesis. Both induce noncytopathic effect and are incurable. Rabies in equids is rarely diagnosed in the New World, Europe, and developed countries but it continues to be a problem in the developing world. Lyssaviruses are emerging pathogens that, similar to the RABV, cause inevitably fatal neurologic disease in mammalian species, including horses. Vaccination is the most effective measure to prevent rabies in any species. BD is a neurologic condition of horses currently restricted to certain regions of Europe, occasionally reported in other species. There is serologic evidence that BD could be present outside Europe. Therefore, it should be in the list of equine neurologic disorders, in particular in animals that are negative for other conditions.

REFERENCES

1. International Committee on Taxonomy of Viruses (ICTV). Rhabdoviridae - lyssavi rus. ICTV. 2021. Available at: https://talk.ictvonline.org/taxonomy.
2. Davis BM, Rall GF, Schnell MJ. Everything you always wanted to know about rabies virus (but were afraid to ask). Annu Rev Virol 2015;2:451–71.
3. Rupprecht C, Kuzmin I, Meslin F. Lyssaviruses and rabies: current conundrums, concerns, contradictions and controversies. F1000Res 2017;6:184.
4. Rohde RE, Rupprecht CE. Update on lyssaviruses and rabies: will past progress play as prologue in the near term towards future elimination? Fac Rev 2020;9:9.
5. Vega S, Lorenzo-Rebenaque L, Marin C, et al. Tackling the threat of rabies reintroduction in Europe. Front Vet Sci 2020;7:613712.
6. Fooks AR, Cliquet F, Finke S, et al. Rabies. Nat Rev Dis Primers 2017;3:17091.
7. Lecollinet S, Pronost S, Coulpier M, et al. Viral equine encephalitis, a growing threat to the horse population in europe? Viruses 2019;12. https://doi.org/10.3390/v12010023.
8. Hayman DT, Fooks AR, Marston DA, et al. The global phylogeography of lyssaviruses - challenging the 'out of Africa' hypothesis. PLoS Negl Trop Dis 2016;10:e0005266.
9. World Health Organization (WHO). Rabies bulletin. 2021. Available at: https://www.who-rabies-bulletin.org/.
10. Centers for Disease Control and Prevention (CDC). Rabies around the world. 2020. Available at: https://www.cdc.gov/rabies/location/world/index.html.
11. Centers for Disease Control and Prevention (CDC). Rabies in the U.S. 2021. Available at: https://www.cdc.gov/rabies/location/usa/index.html.
12. Minghui R, Stone M, Semedo MH, et al. New global strategic plan to eliminate dog-mediated rabies by 2030. Lancet Glob Health 2018;6:e828–9.
13. Sabeta C, Ngoepe EC. Controlling dog rabies in Africa: successes, failures and prospects for the future. Rev Sci Tech 2018;37:439–49.

14. Dodet B, Tejiokem MC, Aguemon AR, et al. Human rabies deaths in Africa: breaking the cycle of indifference. Int Health 2015;7:4–6.
15. World Health Organization (WHO). New global strategic plan to eliminate dog-mediated rabies by 2030. 2021. Available at: https://www.who.int/news-room/commentaries/detail/new-global-strategic-plan-to-eliminate-dog-mediated-rabies-by-2030.
16. Davis AD, Rudd RJ, Bowen RA. Effects of aerosolized rabies virus exposure on bats and mice. J Infect Dis 2007;195:1144–50.
17. Gibbons RV. Cryptogenic rabies, bats, and the question of aerosol transmission. Ann Emerg Med 2002;39:528–36.
18. Banyard AC, Evans JS, Luo TR, et al. Lyssaviruses and bats: emergence and zoonotic threat. Viruses 2014;6:2974–90.
19. Pieracci EG, Pearson CM, Wallace RM, et al. Vital signs: trends in human rabies deaths and exposures - United States, 1938-2018. MMWR Morb Mortal Wkly Rep 2019;68:524–8.
20. European Centre for Disease Prevention and Control (ECDC). Surveillance and disease data for rabies. 2021. Available at: https://www.ecdc.europa.eu/en/rabies/surveillance-and-disease-data.
21. Gautret P, Diaz-Menendez M, Goorhuis A, et al. Epidemiology of rabies cases among international travellers, 2013-2019: a retrospective analysis of published reports. Trav Med Infect Dis 2020;36:101766.
22. Gossner CM, Mailles A, Aznar I, et al. Prevention of human rabies: a challenge for the European Union and the European Economic Area. Euro Surveill 2020;25. https://doi.org/10.2807/1560-7917.ES.2020.25.38.2000158.
23. Pan American Health Organization (PAHO). PAHO celebrates reduction in new cases of rabies in the Americas 2020. Available at: https://www.paho.org.
24. AVMA. Rabies policy - model rabies control ordinance. 2016. Available at: https://www.avma.org/resources-tools/avma-policies/rabies-policy.
25. Ma X, Monroe BP, Cleaton JM, et al. Rabies surveillance in the United States during 2017. J Am Vet Med Assoc 2018;253:1555–68.
26. Ma X, Monroe BP, Wallace RM, et al. Rabies surveillance in the United States during 2019. J Am Vet Med Assoc 2021;258:1205–20.
27. Dietzschold B, Li J, Faber M, et al. Concepts in the pathogenesis of rabies. Future Virol 2008;3:481–90.
28. Singh R, Singh KP, Cherian S, et al. Rabies - epidemiology, pathogenesis, public health concerns and advances in diagnosis and control: a comprehensive review. Vet Q 2017;37:212–51.
29. Li XQ, Sarmento L, Fu ZF. Degeneration of neuronal processes after infection with pathogenic, but not attenuated, rabies viruses. J Virol 2005;79:10063–8.
30. Nevers Q, Albertini AA, Lagaudriere-Gesbert C, et al. Negri bodies and other virus membrane-less replication compartments. Biochim Biophys Acta Mol Cell Res 2020;1867:118831.
31. Nikolic J, Le Bars R, Lama Z, et al. Negri bodies are viral factories with properties of liquid organelles. Nat Commun 2017;8:58.
32. Hueffer K, Khatri S, Rideout S, et al. Rabies virus modifies host behaviour through a snake-toxin like region of its glycoprotein that inhibits neurotransmitter receptors in the CNS. Sci Rep 2017;7:12818.
33. Green SL, Smith LL, Vernau W, et al. Rabies in horses: 21 cases (1970-1990). J Am Vet Med Assoc 1992;200:1133–7.
34. Green SL. Rabies. Vet Clin North Am Equine Pract 1997;13:1–11.

35. Annand EJ, Reid PA. Clinical review of two fatal equine cases of infection with the insectivorous bat strain of Australian bat lyssavirus. Aust Vet J 2014;92:324–32.
36. Lembo T, Niezgoda M, Velasco-Villa A, et al. Evaluation of a direct, rapid immunohistochemical test for rabies diagnosis. Emerg Infect Dis 2006;12:310–3.
37. Gautret P, Adehossi E, Soula G, et al. Rabies exposure in international travelers: do we miss the target? Int J Infect Dis 2010;14:e243–6.
38. Bassuino DM, Konradt G, Cruz RA, et al. Characterization of spinal cord lesions in cattle and horses with rabies: the importance of correct sampling. J Vet Diagn Invest 2016;28:455–60.
39. Centers for Disease Control and Prevention (CDC). Rabies diagnosis. 2021. Available at: https://www.cdc.gov/rabies/diagnosis/index.html.
40. Stein LT, Rech RR, Harrison L, et al. Immunohistochemical study of rabies virus within the central nervous system of domestic and wildlife species. Vet Pathol 2010;47:630–3.
41. WHO-FAO-OIE-GARC - United Against Rabies. New global strategic plan to eliminate dog-mediated rabies by 2030. 2018. Available at: https://www.who.int/news-room/commentaries/detail/new-global-strategic-plan-to-eliminate-dog-mediated-rabies-by-2030.
42. American Association of Equine Practitioners (AAEP). Vaccination guidelines. 2020. Available at: https://aaep.org/guidelines/vaccination-guidelines.
43. Nobach D, Muller J, Tappe D, et al. Update on immunopathology of bornavirus infections in humans and animals. Adv Virus Res 2020;107:159–222.
44. Lipkin WI, Briese T, Hornig M. Borna disease virus - fact and fantasy. Virus Res 2011;162:162–72.
45. Richt JA, Grabner A, Herzog S. Borna disease in horses. Vet Clin North Am Equine Pract 2000;16:579–95.
46. Schulze V, Grosse R, Furstenau J, et al. Borna disease outbreak with high mortality in an alpaca herd in a previously unreported endemic area in Germany. Transbound Emerg Dis 2020. https://doi.org/10.1111/tbed.13556.
47. Wensman JJ, Jaderlund KH, Holst BS, et al. Borna disease virus infection in cats. Vet J 2014;201:142–9.
48. Richt JA, Pfeuffer I, Christ M, et al. Borna disease virus infection in animals and humans. Emerg Infect Dis 1997;3:343–52.
49. Tizard I, Ball J, Stoica G, et al. The pathogenesis of bornaviral diseases in mammals. Anim Health Res Rev 2016;17:92–109.
50. Malbon AJ, Dürrwald R, Kolodziejek J, et al. New World camelids are sentinels for the presence of Borna disease virus. Transbound Emerg Dis 2022;69:451–64.
51. Ludwig H, Bode L. Borna disease virus: new aspects on infection, disease, diagnosis and epidemiology. Rev Sci Tech 2000;19:259–88.
52. Weissenbock H, Bago Z, Kolodziejek J, et al. Infections of horses and shrews with Bornaviruses in Upper Austria: a novel endemic area of Borna disease. Emerg Microbes Infect 2017;6:e52.
53. Kao M, Hamir AN, Rupprecht CE, et al. Detection of antibodies against Borna disease virus in sera and cerebrospinal fluid of horses in the USA. Vet Rec 1993;132:241–4.
54. Hagiwara K, Okamoto M, Kamitani W, et al. Nosological study of Borna disease virus infection in race horses. Vet Microbiol 2002;84:367–74.
55. Bahmani MK, Nowrouzian I, Nakaya T, et al. Varied prevalence of Borna disease virus infection in Arabic, thoroughbred and their cross-bred horses in Iran. Virus Res 1996;45:1–13.

56. Durrwald R, Kolodziejek J, Weissenbock H, et al. The bicolored white-toothed shrew Crocidura leucodon (HERMANN 1780) is an indigenous host of mammalian Borna disease virus. PLoS One 2014;9:e93659.
57. Nobach D, Bourg M, Herzog S, et al. Shedding of infectious borna disease virus-1 in living bicolored white-toothed shrews. PLoS One 2015;10:e0137018.
58. Kinnunen PM, Palva A, Vaheri A, et al. Epidemiology and host spectrum of Borna disease virus infections. J Gen Virol 2013;94:247–62.
59. Niller HH, Angstwurm K, Rubbenstroth D, et al. Zoonotic spillover infections with Borna disease virus 1 leading to fatal human encephalitis, 1999-2019: an epidemiological investigation. Lancet Infect Dis 2020;20:467–77.
60. Tappe D, Schlottau K, Cadar D, et al. Occupation-associated fatal limbic encephalitis caused by variegated squirrel bornavirus 1, germany, 2013. Emerg Infect Dis 2018;24:978–87.

Equine Herpesvirus-1 Myeloencephalopathy

Nicola Pusterla, DVM, PhD[a],*, Gisela Soboll Hussey, DVM, PhD[b], Lutz S. Goehring, DVM, MS, PhD[c,d]

KEYWORDS

- Equine herpesvirus (EHV)-1 • Equine herpesvirus myeloencephalopathy (EHM)
- Cause • Epidemiology • Pathogenesis • Clinical signs • Diagnosis • Treatment

KEY POINTS

- Equine herpesvirus-1 (EHV-1) is ubiquitous in horses worldwide, and greater than 80% of horses are estimated to be latently infected with the virus.
- Sudden onset of neurologic deficits, including ataxia, paresis, and urinary incontinence; involvement of multiple horses on a premise; and a recent history of fever, abortion, or viral respiratory disease in the affected horse or herd mates, are typical features of EHM outbreaks.
- The mechanism underlying central nervous system (CNS) endothelial infection has yet to be unfolded, as are most of the risk factors that determine its occurrence.
- Antemortem diagnosis of EHM is supported by ruling out other neurologic conditions, demonstrating xanthochromia and an elevated cerebrospinal fluid protein concentration, and identifying or isolating EHV-1 from the respiratory tract, buffy-coat, or cerebrospinal fluid.
- The treatment of EHM is challenging and directed toward supportive nursing and nutritional care, reducing CNS inflammation, minimizing thromboembolic events, and controlling the lymphocyte-associated viremia.
- Early recognition of suspected cases and the close monitoring of high-risk horses represent the most reliable measures at preventing outbreaks of EHM.

[a] Department of Medicine and Epidemiology, School of Veterinary Medicine, University of California, One Shields Avenue, Davis, CA 95616, USA; [b] Department of Pathobiology and Diagnostic Investigation, College of Veterinary Medicine, Michigan State University, 736 Wilson Road, East Lansing, MI 48824, USA; [c] Veterinary Science Department, Institute of Infectious Diseases and Zoonoses, Ludwig-Maximilians University, 13 Veterinärstraße, Munich BY80539, Germany; [d] Department of Veterinary Science, The Maxwell H. Gluck Equine Research Center, College of Agriculture, University of Kentucky, 1400 Nicholasville Road, Lexington, KY 40506, USA
* Corresponding author.
E-mail address: npusterla@ucdavis.edu

Vet Clin Equine 38 (2022) 339–362
https://doi.org/10.1016/j.cveq.2022.05.006
0749-0739/22/© 2022 Elsevier Inc. All rights reserved.

INTRODUCTION

Equine herpesvirus myeloencephalopathy (EHM), although an uncommon manifestation of equine herpesvirus-1 (EHV-1) infection, can cause devastating losses on individual farms, boarding stables, veterinary hospitals, and show and racing venues. Although outbreaks of EHM have been recognized for centuries in domestic horse populations, many aspects of this disease remain poorly characterized. In recent years, an improved understanding of EHM has emerged from experimental studies and from data collected during field outbreaks at riding schools, racetracks, horse shows, and veterinary hospitals throughout North America and Europe. These outbreaks have highlighted the contagious nature of EHV-1 and have prompted a reevaluation of diagnostic procedures, treatment modalities, preventative measures, and biosecurity protocols for this disease. This current review article focuses on recent data related to the cause, epidemiology, pathogenesis, immunity, diagnosis, treatment, and prevention of EHV-1 infection with emphasis on EHM.

CAUSE

EHV-1 is an important, ubiquitous equine viral pathogen that exerts its major impact by inducing respiratory disease in young horses, sporadic abortions or abortion storms in pregnant mares, early neonatal death in foals, and myeloencephalopathy.[1] Although EHM is a relatively uncommon manifestation of EHV-1 infection, it can cause devastating losses and severely impact the equine industry, as exemplified by recent outbreaks at riding schools, racetracks, horse shows, and veterinary hospitals throughout North America, Europe, and New Zealand.[2–6]

EHV-1 is a DNA virus that possesses linear double-stranded genomes composed of a unique long region, joined to a unique short region that is flanked by an identical pair of inverted repeat regions, the terminal repeat, and the internal repeat regions.[7,8] The EHV-1 genome is 150 kilobases in size and encodes for 76 open reading frames or genes. Expression of these genes within infected cells is tightly ordered into a highly controlled cascade.[9] One complete replication cycle takes approximately 20 hours, during which well-ordered sequential events occur, including attachment to the host cell membrane, membrane fusion and penetration, translocation of viral DNA to the nucleus, viral DNA replication and protein synthesis, assembly of the capsid, envelopment, lysis of the cell with release of progeny virions.

Virulence markers distinguishing EHV-1 strains that induce EHM or abortion, or both, have recently been determined. The most important discovery may be the association with a single nucleotide polymorphism at position 2254 in the DNA polymerase gene (ORF 30) and the occurrence of EHM.[10] Analysis of more than 100 EHV-1 outbreaks with various clinical presentations demonstrated that variability of a single amino acid residue at position 752 of the DNA polymerase was found to be strongly associated with the occurrence of EHM, with EHV-1 strains associated with neurologic outbreaks involving a D_{752} genotype, whereas most nonneurologic outbreaks involved an N_{752} genotype.[10,11] The observation that EHV-1 viruses of the D_{752} genotype have a greater potential to induce EHM was recently supported by an experimental study using recombinant viruses with differing polymerase sequences.[12] The N_{752} mutant virus caused no neurologic signs and was associated with reduced levels of viremia, whereas viral shedding was similar between both virus mutants. From an epidemiologic standpoint, it appears that most EHV-1 viruses circulating in the field are of the N_{752} genotype.[13,14] Although EHV-1 D_{752} genotype viruses are more commonly associated with EHM, viruses with an N_{752} genotype are certainly not apathogenic; they have been responsible for approximately 81% to 98% of abortion outbreaks in the United States, United Kingdom, and other countries, and between 15% and 26% of neurologic outbreaks (**Fig. 1**).

EPIDEMIOLOGY

The main epidemiologically relevant features of EHV-1 according to Allen and colleagues[15,16] include the following:

- High incidence of respiratory infection early in life
- Establishment of latency in a high percentage of infected horses
- Possible, frequent reactivation of latent virus with subsequent shedding, resulting in transmission to naïve hosts

Currently, it is estimated that as many as 80% of all horses are latently infected; however, prevalence may vary depending on geographic region.[17] Furthermore, testing technology and tissues sampled for detection of latency affect sensitivity of testing, and actual numbers of latently infected horses may be even higher.[13,14,18] EHV-1 infection is prevalent worldwide and has been reported in several equine breeds and other equids. The only exception to this is Iceland, with its indigenous horse population owing to a century-old import ban for horses onto the island.

EHM is the culmination of several factors acting in concert. These include viral and host characteristics, as well as environmental factors (**Table 1**). EHM has been recognized as a sequel to EHV-1 infection since the mid-1960s. The introduction of rapid and sensitive viral diagnostics at the beginning of this millennium, the launch of ProMED-mail as a system for disease surveillance by the International Society for Infectious Diseases (http://www.isid.org), and rapid communication of equine stakeholders via social media has led to an increase in reported EHM outbreaks.

During the previous century, the peer-reviewed literature has reported on various large-scale EHM outbreaks on stud farms or training facilities (mainly thoroughbred or standardbred) from Western Europe and North America. Recently, reports on

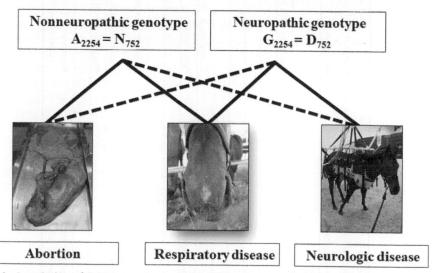

Fig. 1. Association of EHV-1 genotypes of the DNA polymerase (ORF 30) with various disease presentations. Solid lines represent EHV-1 genotypes with greater potential for the development of specific disease forms.

Table 1
Risk factors for disease associated with equine herpesvirus-1

Respiratory Disease	Abortion	EHM
Age <2 y		Age >3 y, further increase in risk in mares over 20 y of age (66%)
	Infection with N752 genotype	Infection with D752 genotype
		Season: Late autumn, winter, spring
		Breed, sex
		Geographic region
		Vaccination against EHV-1 5 wk before event
Crowding & mingling	Crowding & mingling	Crowding & mingling
Past exposure	Past exposure	Past exposure
		Secondary fever several days following primary exposure
		Magnitude and duration of viremia
Stress associated with weaning, transport, introduction of new horses, secondary infection, immune suppression	Stress associated with weaning, transport, introduction of new horses, secondary infection, immune suppression	Stress associated with weaning, transport, introduction of new horses, secondary infection, immune suppression
	Pregnancy in the last trimester	Pregnancy or foal at foot
		Keep in stable
Presence of EHV-1 and/or a shedding horse together with susceptible horses	Presence of EHV-1 and/or a shedding horse together with susceptible horses	Presence of EHV-1 and/or a shedding horse together with susceptible horses

EHM incidence have surfaced from Ethiopia,[19] Croatia after introduction of imported horses from the United States into a local herd,[20] Israel, South Africa, Japan, and the first ever EHM outbreak from New Zealand.[5] Reasons could be differences in distribution of D_{752} versus N_{752} strain variation among horses, or other mechanisms or factors. Interestingly, most outbreaks occur during the cooler months of the year, and most of the reported EHM outbreaks showed D_{752} strain involvement.

The following single-breed (or predominant breed) operations reported EHM outbreaks in the past: (i) thoroughbred,[21] (ii) standardbred,[22] (iii) Lipizzan,[23] (iv) American quarter horse/paint/Appaloosa,[4,24] (v) warmblood,[25] (vi) draft horse (Josie Traub-Dargatz, personal communication, 2016). In contrast, EHM outbreaks have not been described on any sizable Arabian or Icelandic horse operations in endemic areas. Moreover, 2 studies evaluated mixed-breed operations with an EHM outbreak and suggested a lower risk for EHM in small ponies (Shetland or Welsh pony), Arabian horse, and an increased risk for standardbred or Spanish (Baroque) horses, warmblood, and Fjord horses.[26,27]

There is conflicting information about EHM frequencies in donkeys and mules versus horses. A study from the United States found EHM cases exclusively in horses, but not in mules of mixed-breed operations,[28] whereas a study from sub-Saharan Africa described EHM in both donkeys and mules.[19] This information suggests a possible genetic risk factor in the development of EHM.

Age has also been identified as a risk factor. Under experimental settings, EHM is rare in yearling horses upon infection with large doses of neuropathogenic EHV-1 strains. However, the risk for EHM development is increased when adults or old horses are experimentally infected with large doses of neuropathogenic EHV-1 strains.[29] Various outbreak reports describe EHM in horses of any age. However, similar to the observations in experimental settings, foals and yearlings under natural outbreak conditions are only rarely affected by neurologic deficits, whereas adult/older horses are more susceptible and might show more severe clinical signs of EHM during an outbreak.[2] Female sex has been shown to be associated with greater risk to develop EHM.[4]

It is of interest to notice that nowadays many breeding farms frequently vaccinate against EHV-1 in order to prevent abortion. EHM reports from fully vaccinated operations have dwindled, whereas there is a noticeable increase in EHM outbreaks at boarding facilities, housing a mixed breed population that is often completely unvaccinated, or only partially (<15–20%) vaccinated. One risk factor associated with higher EHM risk development during the Ogden outbreak was vaccination in the 5 weeks before the event.[4] It remains to be determined if vaccination against EHV-1 or excessive vaccination outside the recommended guidelines induces an inappropriate immune response that potentially predisposes horses to develop EHM.

EHV-1 herd infection requires horizontal spread of infectious virus and susceptible recipients. EHV-1 can be introduced on a farm via nasal shedding of an acutely infected horse that is (re)introduced into the herd. Alternatively, EHV-1 in a latent-infected horse can reactivate and reappear in the respiratory tract leading to shedding and horizontal spread. EHM outbreaks are more likely confined to a single operation rather than occurring simultaneously at multiple sites following a larger gathering of horses. This suggests that productive reactivation from latency is more likely the source for an outbreak rather than transmission of EHV-1 at an equestrian event.

Long-distance transportation, corticosteroid administration, hospitalization, coinfection, and stress have been incriminated as triggering factors for reactivation. However, even with repetitive sampling of nasal secretions for the detection of EHV-1 from horses under any or a combination of these factors has shown little to no evidence of viral reactivation. Therefore, productive reactivation from latency apparently seems to be a rare event.[30–33]

PATHOGENESIS

The pathogenesis of EHV-1 involves 3 stages of infection in different sites of the body. Primary infection with EHV-1 occurs via the respiratory tract[16] and results in replication and erosion of the respiratory airway epithelium, accompanied by shedding of virus via the nasal secretions. In addition, EHV-1 respiratory epithelial infection induces early innate immune responses that set the stage for induction of downstream adaptive immunity. These responses include induction of type 1 interferons, defensins, regulatory cytokines, and selective chemokine responses that attract immune cells to the site of infection and effect cell-to-cell transfer of virus, orchestration of adaptive immunity, and clinical disease.[34–36] The virus then spreads quickly via the basement membrane to the cells of the lamina propria and the underlying tissues, and by 24 to 48 hours post-infection the virus can be detected in the local lymph nodes of the respiratory tract where further replication and infection of leukocytes occur.[37] Leukocytes harboring infectious virus are released into the bloodstream between days 4 and 10 postinfection and a cell-associated viremia is established. This cell-associated viremia is central in the pathogenesis of EHV-1 because peripheral blood mononuclear cells (PBMCs) are a robust immune and inflammatory cell population in the vasculature, as well as carriers of EHV-1, and transport the virus to sites of secondary infection. Sites of secondary infection include the vasculature of the central nervous system (CNS), pregnant uterus, testis, and the eye,[38] where contact between infected leukocytes and the vascular endothelium leads to endothelial cell infection, inflammation, thrombosis and tissue necrosis, and secondary disease manifestations directly following viremia on days 9 to 13 postinfection. Several recent studies have examined viral and host factors that contribute to the establishment of viremia, virus, and host interaction during viremia, and transfer of virus to vascular endothelial cells at secondary sites of infection. Viral proteins that have thus far been identified to be directly involved in viral spread, and cell-to-cell transfer includes ORF2, ORF17, gB, gD, gp2, ORF30, and UL3.[34,39,40] Cellular mechanisms that contribute to EHM pathogenesis include the induction of interferons, chemokine responses, activation of the MAPK pathway, regulation of adhesion molecules, and cell-to-cell contact.[34,41–43] Furthermore, a dysregulation of hemostasis following EHV-1 infection has been shown in vitro and in vivo and is thought to play an important role in the neuropathogenesis of EHV-1 as well as abortions.[44–46] Finally, there is also evidence that EHV-1-infected lymphocytes are critical for the establishment of EHV-1 latency.[18] Secondary disease manifestations for EHV-1 include EHM, EHV-1 abortions, neonatal foal death, and chorioretinopathies. Although a positive correlation between the duration and magnitude of viremia and incidence of EHM has been identified,[47] EHM is unlikely to occur in the absence of viremia, and only a small percentage (~10%) of viremic horses subsequently develop EHM. Thus, a combination of host and viral factors likely determines whether EHM occurs, and this is of intense interest for the control and prevention of EHM.

In contrast, the incidence of late-term abortions caused by EHV-1 is higher (~50%) than incidence of EHM. This may be related to the hormonal milieu and altered immune system in the last trimester of pregnancy. However, the pathogenesis of EHM and EHV-1 abortion at the vascular endothelium is considered to be similar and likely involves the same host and viral factors. Infection of endothelial cells of the endometrium follows viremia and leads to vasculitis, thrombosis, microcotyledonary infarction, perivascular cuffing, and transplacental spread of virus at the sites of vascular lesions.[48]

The vasculature of the eye is another site of secondary infection for EHV-1. EHV-1-associated chorioretinitis was first described in the late 1980s in llamas and alpacas[49,50] and then in a mare and foal during a natural outbreak of paralytic EHV-1 infection.[51] Interestingly, most ocular infections are subclinical and rarely lead to loss of function or even immediate signs. However, although EHV-1 chorioretinopathies are much less significant economically and clinically, they may offer a unique opportunity to look at EHV-1 infection of the vascular endothelium and serve as a surrogate model to study EHM pathogenesis.[52] The equine ocular fundus is physiologically and anatomically similar to that of the CNS, with similar tight junctions analogous to the blood-brain barrier,[53] but the eye's unique anatomic features permit observation of the chorioretinal vasculature in vivo. Furthermore, incidence of ocular lesions can be greater than 50% following experimental and natural infection.[52] The reason for observation of EHV-1 chorioretinopathies in a much larger percentage of horses than observation of EHM is likely that one can observe subclinical infection in the eye, which is not possible in the spinal cord. Of note is that although postmortem acute inflammation and viral antigen can be detected in the choroidal vasculature at the onset of EHM, ocular lesions are not visible in vivo until the acute disease processes have led to focal disruption of the retinal pigmented epithelium, allowing light to reflect of the tapetum lucidum and appearance of focal or multifocal shotgun lesions (**Fig. 2**). Similarly, EHV-1-associated lesions and viral antigen can be detected in the testicular vasculature of intact males for up to 70 days following experimental infection, but the clinical relevance for breeding and fertility has yet to be determined.[38]

CLINICAL SIGNS

Clinical manifestations of EHV-1 infection include primary respiratory disease, late-term abortions, neonatal foal death, EHM, and chorioretinopathy. EHV-1 has also been shown to infect the male reproductive tract and has been detected in the testicular vasculature and seminal fluid following infection. However, the clinical relevance of these findings has yet to be determined.[38,54–56] Differences in pathogenic potential of viral strains may influence clinical outcome,[10,57] as are several additional host and environmental factors (see **Table 1**).

Equine Herpesvirus Myeloencephalopathy

EHM is a devastating manifestation of EHV-1 infection that affects the CNS. Outbreaks are characterized by a large number of horses affected with mild to moderate respiratory disease and a fever, with 10% to 40% of infected horses developing EHM. In contrast, experimentally, EHM is difficult to induce reproducibly. Clinical signs of EHM appear following the onset of viremia, often following a secondary fever spike and in the absence of respiratory disease. Onset of EHM typically occurs between 6 and 10 days, is often sudden, and reaches peak severity within 2 to 3 days. Experimentally, EHM occurs during or at the end of the cell-associated viremia.[26,58] Clinical signs range from mild, temporary ataxia to paralysis that can lead to recumbency and urinary incontinence, often resulting in euthanasia.[59,60] Commonly, the caudal spinal cord is affected more severely, resulting in weakness of hind limbs, bladder dysfunction, and sensory deficits in the perineal area.[61] Severe cases of EHM can show paresis, paralysis, or even tetraplegia. Less frequently, horses with EHM can develop cortical, brainstem, or vestibular disease characterized by lethargy, recumbency, head tilt, ataxia, and cranial nerve deficits.[62] A recent study determining if the genotype of EHV-1 could impact clinical disease, and outcome in 65 horses with laboratory-confirmed EHM showed that the frequency of lethargy, fever, ataxia, and

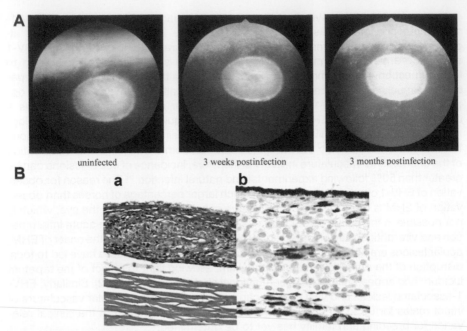

Fig. 2. Development of ocular lesions following experimental infection with EHV-1. (*A*) Fundus photography. (*B*) Eye of a yearling horse, 11 days postequine herpesvirus-1 Ab4 WT infection. (*a*) Dense infiltrates of lymphocytes and histiocytes surround and segmentally ablate the walls of choroidal vessels. Hematoxylin-eosin, original magnification ×200. (*b*) Intracytoplasmic immunoreactivity for EHV-1 antigen within endothelial cells of vessels surrounded by dense inflammatory infiltrates. EHV-1 antigen immunohistochemistry, hematoxylin counterstain, ×400.

outcome was not significantly different between the 2 EHV-1 genotypes.[63] However, urinary incontinence was significantly more frequently reported in horses infected with the D_{752} genotype of EHV-1.[63] Histopathologic changes associated with EHM include vasculitis and thrombosis of small blood vessels in the spinal cord or brain, myelitis with axonal degeneration, perivascular cuffing, and lymphocytic and histiocytic infiltrates. However, histopathologic findings can vary in severity, and often more sensitive diagnostics are needed to confirm a diagnosis. One of the central questions remaining for the pathogenesis of EHM is what other host factors beyond the initial infection of CNS endothelial cells (which is likely common) function as a "2nd hit" and drive EHM pathogenesis. In recent years, a proinflammatory, procoagulant environment as well as modulation of chemoattraction of inflammatory cells and lack of proper activation of interferons and cellular immunity has been identified as a likely contributing host factor.[34,41–43]

Equine Herpesvirus-1 Chorioretinopathy

It has been known for more than 25 years that EHV-1 infection can lead to chorioretinopathy, causing permanent "shotgun" lesions of the retina in a substantial proportion of infected horses.[52] However, the connection between ocular lesions and EHV-1 infection is often not made. Recently, it has been shown that up to 80% of yearling horses can exhibit classical shotgun lesions following experimental infection with EHV-1. Ocular lesions primarily affect the choroidal vasculature and appear between

4 weeks and 3 months after primary infection (see **Fig. 2**).[52] Lesions can be focal, multifocal, or, in rare occasions, diffuse, which affect the entire eye. Clinically, only diffuse lesions have a significant impact and cause loss of vision. Histopathologic changes are also common in the chorioretinal vasculature for at least 3 months following experimental EHV-1 infection and mirror those observed in the CNS and uterus.

DIAGNOSIS

An antemortem diagnosis of EHM is supported by (i) ruling out other neurologic conditions, (ii) demonstrating xanthochromia and an elevated cerebrospinal fluid (CSF) protein concentration, (iii) identifying or isolating EHV-1 from the respiratory tract, buffy-coat, or CSF, and (iii) demonstrating a fourfold increase in antibodies using serum neutralizing, complement fixation, or enzyme-linked immunosorbent assays performed on acute and convalescent serum from affected or in-contact horses 7 to 21 days apart (**Fig. 3**).[64]

Cell Blood Count

Hematological abnormalities in horses with EHM are inconsistent and may include mild anemia and lymphopenia in the early stages, followed a few days later by mild hyperfibrinogenemia.[65] Azotemia and hyperbilirubinemia may occur secondary to dehydration and anorexia, respectively.

Cerebrospinal Fluid Analysis

CSF fluid analysis typically, although not always, reveals xanthochromia, an increased protein concentration (100–500 mg/dL), and an increased albumin quotient (ratio of CSF to serum albumin concentration), which reflects vasculitis with protein leakage

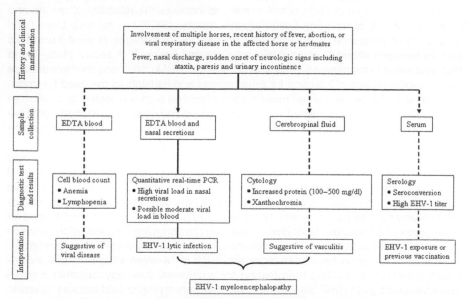

Fig. 3. Flow chart to help support an antemortem diagnosis of EHV-1 infection in a neurologic horse. The dashed arrows represent a presumptive diagnostic pathway, whereas the solid arrows represent a more definitive laboratory pathway.

into the CSF. The nucleated cell count in the CSF is usually normal (0–5 cells/μL) but is occasionally increased.[65] Location of CSF collection may also influence the cytologic results. It is important that the CSF collection matches the neuroanatomical disease location.

Virus Isolation and Detection

Virus isolation, although time-consuming, is generally used in the scientific community to biologically characterize strains. The likelihood of isolating EHV-1 during outbreaks of neurologic disease is increased by monitoring in-contact horses and collecting nasal or nasopharyngeal swab and buffy-coat samples from these animals during the prodromal febrile phase before neurologic signs develop.

Polymerase Chain Reaction Testing

Because of the need for timely laboratory diagnostic, virus isolation has been supplanted by polymerase chain reaction (PCR). PCR detection of EHV-1 is routinely performed on respiratory secretions from the nasal passages or the nasopharynx and from whole blood samples. Because of the risk of carryover contamination, conventional molecular platforms have been replaced by quantitative real-time PCR (qPCR) technology. Advantages of qPCR include quick analytical turn-around time, high sensitivity/specificity, and cost-effectiveness. Furthermore, qPCR represents a major improvement in the detection of infectious pathogens by allowing characterization of disease stage, assessment of risk of exposure to other animals, and monitoring of response to therapy.[66] However, research and diagnostic laboratories should use quantitative methods with the least evidence of variability between samples and extraction protocols. Protocols normalizing results against a preselected volume (ie, eluted DNA or volume of nasal secretions) are more prone to interlaboratory variations than protocols standardizing viral load to the entire swab, a housekeeping gene, or an arbitrarily chosen amount of extracted DNA.[67] It is important that diagnostic laboratories use an internal quality control system to increase the reliability of results and minimize the risk of reporting false-negative results. qPCR has recently been used to document differences in viral loads between disease stages in adult horses as well as between clinically and subclinically infected horses.[68] A recent study found high viral loads in the nasal secretions of horses with EHM confirming their importance as a potential source of infection for other horses and highlighted the need for imposition of strict biosecurity when horses were identified with suspected or confirmed EHM.[68] Follow-up assessment of viral loads in blood and nasal or nasopharyngeal secretions can guide modifications of control measures, including the lifting of quarantine for individual horses that test negative on subsequent sampling.

A recently identified variable region in the EHV-1 genome correlates with neurologic disease.[10] This sequence variation occurs in the DNA polymerase gene (ORF 30) involved in initial viral replication within cells. PCR assays based on ORF 30 have recently been developed and used to differentiate between EHV-1 isolates from neurologically and nonneurologically affected horses. Although the basis for EHV-1 testing for most diagnostic molecular laboratories relies on the genotype discrimination between N_{752} and D_{752}, reports on EHV-1 variants that are not detected via qPCR assays targeting the ORF 30 assays have been reported.[69,70] It is therefore advised to use a diagnostic laboratory that offers both testing for a universal gene (glycoprotein B gene) and a virulence gene (ORF 30). Furthermore, the genotyping of field isolates needs to be interpreted carefully, as between approximately 14% and 24% of EHV-1 isolates from horses with EHM do not have this neuropathogenic marker.[10,11] Strain characterization may be important from a regulatory standpoint but also given that the potential of

EHM development is greater in horses infected with a neuropathogenic genotype (D_{752}). Furthermore, detection of a neurotropic EHV-1 strain may influence therapy, especially in the use of antiviral drugs, such as valacyclovir, used to decrease viremia and prevent the development of neurologic sequelae. Various studies have shown that the EHV-1 genotype impacts the level of viremia with neurotropic strains displaying a higher level of viremia when compared with nonneurotropic strains, while the amount of virus shed is similar between the 2 genotypes (**Fig. 4**).[12,71]

Serologic Analysis

Serology that demonstrates a fourfold or greater increase in serum antibody titer between acute and convalescent samples collected 7 to 21 days apart provides presumptive evidence of infection.[72] However, many horses with EHM do not exhibit a fourfold increase in serum neutralizing titer. This may occur when titers increase rapidly and peak by the time neurologic signs appear. Although serology is limited in confirming EHM in an individual horse, testing of paired serum samples from in-contact animals is recommended given that a significant proportion of these horses will seroconvert, providing indirect evidence of EHV-1 infection. Interpretation of serology is complicated by the fact that the serum neutralization and complement fixation tests used at most diagnostic laboratories do not distinguish between antibodies to EHV-1 and -4.

Histopathologic Examination

Histopathologic examination of the brain and spinal cord is essential in confirming EHV-1 infection in a horse with suspected EHM. Vasculitis and thrombosis of small blood vessels in the spinal cord or brain are consistent histopathologic changes, and virus antigen detection in the CNS is achieved using immunohistochemistry, in situ hybridization, and PCR.[38]

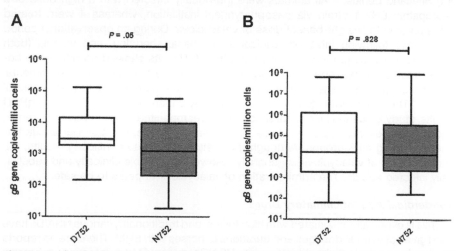

Fig. 4. Viral loads expressed as EHV-1 gB gene copies per million cells in blood (*A*) and nasal secretions (*B*) from horses with EHM infected with neurotropic (N_{752}, n = 24) or nonneurotropic (N_{752}, n = 17) EHV-1. Horizontal bars represent medians.

THERAPEUTIC STRATEGIES

During EHM outbreaks, it is important to differentiate between therapeutic approaches that aim to prevent or minimize the extent of spinal cord damage, and those applicable once myelopathy has developed and the horse is displaying neurologic signs. An important factor for the development of EHM is the magnitude and the duration of viremia. During viremia, there is a constant shower of the neural parenchyma with virus-loaded lymphocytes or monocytes, which are extravasating or interacting with endothelial cell. These interactions allow virus to escape the secure and shielded transport vehicle of cell-associated viremia, granting them access to the vulnerable nervous system. Noteworthy, there is excessive systemic inflammation during EHV-1 viremia with many consequences, one of which is the induction of a procoagulant state.[46]

Therapeutic strategies should focus at (i) lowering viral load in lymphocytes/monocytes during cell-associated viremia; (ii) reducing inflammation; (iii) stopping lymphocyte/monocyte-endothelial cell interactions; (iv) stabilizing vasculature; and (v) supporting healing of damaged tissues.

As inflammation activates coagulation, additional anticoagulation therapy may be warranted. However, and as a word of caution, hemostasis is an intricate interplay between procoagulation, anticoagulation, and fibrinolysis, and it is difficult to intervene without constant monitoring. Furthermore, a main feature of EHM is multiple spinal cord hemorrhage after thrombosis and vasculitis. The following section summarizes available therapeutics, the phase of EHV-1 pathogenesis during which those therapeutics are likely effective, and the evidence for clinical efficacy of therapeutics (**Table 2**).

Antiviral Drugs

Valacyclovir and ganciclovir are analogues to DNA nucleic acid guanine and therefore interfere with viral DNA assembly. However, this requires stages of lytic infection where polymerase activity is upregulated. Pharmacokinetics for both drugs have been established in horses. Valacyclovir efficacy has been evaluated in 2 independent (randomized, placebo-controlled) animal (infection) studies.[73,74] Study 1 used 8 yearling Shetland ponies.[73] All animals were individually infected with a high dose of a neuropathic EHV-1 strain via nasopharyngeal instillation, whereas 4 were treated with appropriate (weight-based) dose of valacyclovir. During an observational period of 21 days following infection, clinical signs, nasal shedding, and viremia (both measured via virus [co-]culture) were monitored. Results showed no difference between treated and placebo-treated group. Study 2 with a more complex experimental design included adult-aged horses, assigned to 2 treatment groups, and one control group.[74] The valacyclovir dose was lower in study 2 than in study 1. Based on qPCR results, study 2 claimed less nasal shedding, lower magnitude and duration of viremia, and a lower severity score for ataxia in the treated groups, yet a similar ataxia frequency among all 3 groups. Although the 2 studies showed conflicting results, the administration of valacyclovir is generally reserved to valuable clinically and subclinically infected equids. The administration of valacyclovir appears to be safe.

Nonsteroidal Anti-Inflammatory Drugs

Viremia is especially associated with high fevers, and traditionally, various NSAIDs have been given at various dosages and durations to horses with EHM. There are no reports of placebo-controlled drug trials using NSAIDs during EHV-1 infection in horses. NSAIDs supposedly lower the proinflammatory state of a horse, which will influence hemostasis as well as adhesion molecule expression on endothelial cells, hence, resulting

Table 2
Drugs commonly used in the treatment of equine herpesvirus-1 myeloencephalopathy

| Drug | Ideal Treatment Time | | | Recommendations |
	Previremia	Viremia	Postviremia	
Valacyclovir (1)	✓	✓	✓	30 mg/kg po tid for 2 d, then 20/kg po bid up to 14 d
Comments: Least likely to have side effects; least likely to interfere with other drugs				
NSAIDs (2)		✓	✓	Cox-2 specific: Full-dose during febrile days, half-dose for 3–5 d beyond fever
Comments: likely to interfere with/potentiate effect of other drugs: 3, 4, 5				
Dexamethasone (3)			✓	0.05–0.07 mg/kg once daily for 5 d; do not combine with NSAIDs
Comments: likely to interfere with/potentiate effect of other drugs				
Heparin (4) (unfractionated/low molecular weight)		✓		50 (unfractionatedr) – 80 (low molecular weight) IU/kg SQ bid for 2–3 d
Comments: likely to interfere with/potentiate effect of other drugs: 2, 3, 5; caution as spinal cord hemorrhage is a hallmark finding during EHM				
Aspirin (5)	✓	✓		5mg/kg po q48h for up to 10 d
Comments: likely to interfere with/potentiate effect of other drugs: 2, 4				
Lidocaine CRI (6)		✓		Bolus followed by CRI maintenance (1.3 mg/kg/min)
Comments: unlikely to interfere with other drugs; unknown effects during periods of blood-brain barrier breeches as occurs during EHM				
Vitamin E (7)	✓	✓	✓	1000–2000 IU po once daily
Comments: unlikely to interfere with other drugs				

in a decreased interaction of leukocytes with endothelial cells. Most of the NSAIDs are also known to decrease activation of platelets reversibly, at the exception of acetylsalicylic acid, which has been shown to irreversibly inhibit cyclooxygenase in platelets. A recent in vitro study determined the effect of EHV-1-infected PBMCs and brain endothelial cells when anti-inflammatories, among which are NSAIDs, corticosteroids, or lidocaine, were added to the model.[75] Anti-inflammatory drugs decreased infection of endothelial cells likely by reducing contact between EHV-1-infected PBMCs and endothelial cells in vitro. NSAIDs should be considered a treatment option during viremia, whereas they may also improve signs of vasculitis.

Corticosteroids

Corticosteroid therapy during EHV-1 infection has not been evaluated in a placebo-controlled experiment. However, corticosteroids are used by some veterinarians based on personal experience at varying concentrations and during different phases of infection. Corticosteroids are potent anti-inflammatories and immunosuppressant drugs. In the previously mentioned in vitro contact model,[75] corticosteroids showed a decrease in endothelial cell infection, suggesting a positive effect when applied during viremia. However, potential side effects of immunosuppression during viremia and viral replication dynamics are still unknown. Corticosteroids are the treatment of choice during vasculitis with their ability to retighten intercellular junctions between endothelial cells. Therefore, there is fair justification to treat horses with early signs of EHM, and the duration of treatment should be based on daily clinical assessment.

Heparin

Coagulation is activated during EHV-1 infection, and apparently more so during the viremic phase. Inflammation is likely the initiator, whereby proinflammatory cytokines activate tissue factor leading to fibrin production.[46] Heparin blocks the activation of factor X of the coagulation cascade, and it activates antithrombin, a capture molecule for thrombin. As thrombin activates the conversion of fibrinogen to fibrin, with thrombin-antithrombin complexes formed, there is a reduction of fibrin production.[76] Furthermore, activated thrombocytes or platelets participate in thrombus formation and growth. Platelets can be activated in vitro by EHV-1, and platelet activation by EHV-1 was decreased, when collected from heparin-treated horses.[44,77] During a naturally occurring EHM outbreak among warmblood horses, empirically determined heparin doses (50 IU/kg subcutaneously twice a day for 3 days) were given to any febrile horse after day 10 of the outbreak.[78] Horses with fever during the first 10 days following the index case served as untreated control. Heparin-treated horses showed a lower EHM incidence than untreated horses, indicating that heparin may be useful for the prevention of EHM during an EHV-1 outbreak. However, these results should be interpreted carefully, as the treated horse group was housed in a different location, where infection dynamics could have been different and/or other undetermined factors could have impacted disease severity. Last but not least and based on the authors' personal experience, EHM numbers typically decrease naturally during the second half of an outbreak. However, based on the pathophysiology of thrombin inhibition and the encouraging field data, the use of heparin may be beneficial in decreasing platelet activation and reducing spinal cord thrombosis and vasculitis. The effect of heparin administered in a procoagulant state during EHV-1 viremia, and the interaction of heparin with other drugs have yet to be investigated. It is the authors' opinion that if heparin administration is considered, it should be limited to the previremic and viremic phase of infection.

Miscellaneous Drugs (Dimethyl Sulfoxide, Lidocaine-Constant Rate Infusion, Aspirin, and Vitamin E)

Dimethyl sulfoxide (DMSO) is an osmotic agent and holds a yet unsubstantiated claim for anti-inflammatory properties. Empirically, DMSO as a 5% to 10% intravenous solution in 0.9% NaCl is used up to twice daily for a period of 3 to 5 days by some veterinarians once EHM clinical signs are noticed. However, DMSO at any concentration has not been tested in a randomized, placebo-controlled experiment.

Lidocaine as a constant rate of infusion (CRI) has been shown to decrease vascular neutrophilic margination through an effect on adhesion molecule upregulation on endothelial cells. A previous report studying the effect of NSAIDs on PBMCs to endothelial cell spread of EHV-1 showed that lidocaine was effective at lowering endothelial cell infection and lysis at a concentration of 1 mg/mL cell culture medium.[75] Outbreak management and personnel availability for monitoring a lidocaine CRI are likely the main limiting factors in applying this medication.

The effect of aspirin has not been critically evaluated during EHM outbreaks. Aspirin has an effect different from other NSAIDs, as it binds irreversibly to platelet cyclooxygenase. In theory, platelets cannot be activated and will not participate in coagulation and thrombus formation. The use of aspirin should be limited to the previremic and viremic periods. Because of the risk of spinal cord hemorrhage, aspirin should be used with caution.

Vitamin E is routinely used for the treatment of various traumatic, degenerative, and infectious neurologic disorders.[79] To the authors' knowledge, there is no harm of supplementing with vitamin E, although there is no evidence to support its benefit.

In summary, there are too few placebo-controlled studies to evaluate the efficacy of most drugs currently used in the treatment of EHM.

IMMUNITY AND IMMUNE EVASION
Immunity to Equine Herpesvirus-1

Over the past decades, much effort has been placed on trying to understand what parts of the immunity correlate with protection to aid with vaccine development and to predict which horses might be most at risk for developing EHM. Although some progress has been made toward an understanding of what aspects of immunity are relevant for protecting horses from EHV-1, there are many questions remaining. For one, we need to define better what protection entails. An ideal vaccine would protect from respiratory disease, abortions, and EHM, prevent shedding and viremia as well as establishment of latency. However, prevention of latency seems unrealistic at this point, and although current vaccines can limit viral nasal shedding and respiratory disease, reduction of viremia is more limited, as is prevention of abortion. Finally, there are no vaccines that have been shown to be effective in preventing EHM. To complicate things further, it is challenging to compare immune responses at different sites of the body (respiratory tract, blood, and CNS/reproductive organs) and some EHV-1 target sites, including the CNS, are difficult to access. In recent years, several exciting in vitro models have been developed that are starting to shed light on different aspects of EHV-1 pathogenesis, but many studies do not differentiate well between responses at the respiratory tract versus responses during viremia and responses in immune privileged vascular endothelia. In addition, many models remain artificial because simulating in vivo infection conditions via cell-to-cell contact is complicated, as is creating immune privilege in a dish.

What is known is that following natural infection there is a short period of immunity that protects against reinfection, and horses are likely protected from all clinical disease manifestations as well as shedding and viremia.[58] It is also known that this immunity includes a combination of virus-neutralizing antibodies, which play a role in reduction of nasal viral shedding,[58] cytotoxic T-lymphocytes (CTLs), which are most critical for protection from secondary clinical disease and viremia,[47,80] as well as multiple components of mucosal and systemic innate immunity.[81,82] At this point, the only identified reliable correlate of immunity for protection from EHM is the precursor frequencies of CTLs (pCTL),[80] but good laboratory assay systems for regularly evaluating pCTL are lacking. Some studies have identified high preinfection EHV-1-specific immunoglobulin G (IgG) and IgG3/7 (IgGb) titers in serum as well as a rapid induction of IgG3/7 in the absence of interferon-α (IFN-α), IFN-γ, and CC chemokine motif ligand (CCL2), CCL3, CD14, and CCL11 in nasal secretions following infection as an indicator of protection from respiratory disease, shedding, and viremia,[83] but notably, these studies did not include horses that showed clinical EHM or abortions, and thus, predictions may not apply the same way to secondary EHV-1 manifestations. An earlier study compared a modified live vaccine and an inactivated vaccine and found that protection from EHM was associated with increased IgG3/7 and decreased IgG3/5 levels and lower IgG3/5 to IgG3/7 or IgG1 ratios in serum prechallenge.[84] These are interesting observations; however, it is not clear whether the identified immunologic parameters actually "protect" from the virus or merely correlate with an induction of cellular immunity, including pCTLs, which were not measured in either study. A third study that used the neuropathic strain Ab4 and induced clinical EHM in 3 out of 8 yearling horses identified decreased induction of IFN-alpha and increased induction of interleukin-10 (IL-10) in nasal secretions collected from horses that went on to develop clinical EHM. These results suggest that a shift from a TH1-type cellular immunity to a TH2-type immunity may correlate with an increased risk for developing EHM.[57] However, studies that include more horses that are affected by clinical EHM would be needed to confirm host risk factors for EHM and correlates for protection from EHM. Several additional recent studies using in vitro models of respiratory epithelial cell, blood, and vascular endothelial infection have identified induction and modulation of several key host factors that are likely involved in the pathogenesis of EHM.[85] These include selective modulation of chemokine responses and modulation of interferon responses, controlling production and transfer of new virions in PBMCs, and regulating cell adhesion between PBMCs and endothelial cells.[34,40,43,86] These more recent findings may offer new opportunities for controlling EHV-1 secondary disease and extend existing in vivo findings.

Immune Evasion by Equine Herpesvirus-1

On the flip side, difficulties in developing successful strategies to induce long-lasting immunity to EHV-1 are likely due to the immunomodulatory properties of EHV-1, similar to what has been described for other herpesviruses.[87–89]

Immune evasion strategies used by EHV-1 include interference and modulation of NK-cell lysis, alteration of cytokines regulating B- and T-cell responses, alteration of the chemokine network resulting in loss of efficient antigen presentation and selective chemo-attraction of immune cells, inhibition of antibody-dependent cytotoxicity, induction of T-regulatory cells, and alteration of CTL responses.[89] All of these mechanisms likely contribute to and explain the short-lived immunity following infection, and many viral genes have been identified over the past decade and are potential targets for successful preventative or therapeutic approaches. Earlier research focused on induction of CTL responses and identified the UL49.5 and ORF1 proteins to interfere with MHC-I antigen presentation and induction of CTL responses.[88,90,91] Another viral modulatory gene that has been described a while ago is glycoprotein G. This gene has been found to function as a viral chemokine-binding protein that selectively inhibits IL-8 and CCL-3-mediated chemotaxis of phagocytes (neutrophils and macrophages).[92,93] Furthermore, in recent years, glycoprotein B, glycoprotein D, US3, ORF2, and ORF17 have been identified to play a role in cell-to-cell transfer of EHV-1,[39,40] and gP2 and neuropathic strains of EHV-1 have been shown to selectively stimulate CXCR3 ligands CXCL9 and CXCL10 production by the respiratory epithelium to facilitate attraction and infection of CD4, CD8, and monocytic CD172[+] cells.[34] Interestingly, infected monocytic CD172[+] have subsequently been shown to upregulate α4β1, αLβ2, and αVβ3 integrin-mediated adhesion to endothelial cells and activation of ERK/MAPK signaling pathways, which are important mechanisms stimulated during viremia in EHV-1-infected horses.[40,42] Finally, there is evidence that EHV-1 targets the induction of the type I interferon response in equine endothelial cells[43] and that there might be differences in sensitivity to interferons between neuropathic and abortigenic strains of EHV-1.[35] Other viral modulatory genes are likely present and may be identified in the future.

CONTROL STRATEGIES

Currently available vaccines do not reliably block infection, the development of viremia, or the establishment of latency, and EHM has been observed in horses regularly vaccinated against EHV-1.[2,4] Furthermore, vaccination has been cited as a potential risk factor for the development of EHM, although the supporting evidence is far from conclusive. The significant reduction in viral shedding observed in vaccinated horses provides reasonable justification for booster vaccination of nonexposed horses at risk for infection in order to reduce viral shedding in the event of exposure to EHV-1. By enhancing herd immunity, it is hoped that the level of infectious virus circulating in the at-risk population and, in turn, that the risk of individual horses in the population developing disease will be reduced. This approach also relies on the assumption that the immune system of most mature horses has been primed by prior exposure to EHV-1 antigens through "field" infection or vaccination and can therefore be boosted within 7 to 10 days of administration of a single dose of vaccine. Although the validity of this approach has not been critically evaluated for the prevention of EHM, its implementation seems rational when faced with one or more horses with confirmed clinical EHV-1 infection of any form. Whereas booster vaccination of horses that are likely to have been exposed is not recommended, it is rational to booster vaccinate nonexposed horses, as well as those that must enter a premise with a recent outbreak history, if they have not already been vaccinated against EHV-1 during the previous 90 days. Horse owners must develop an understanding of the concept of boosting herd immunity to help protect individual horses rather than having, an as yet unattainable, expectation that the attending veterinarian can reliably protect an individual horse from developing potentially fatal EHM by administering one of the currently available vaccines.

Although there is no reliable method of preventing EHM, implementation of routine management practices aimed at reducing the likelihood of introducing and disseminating EHV-1 infection is justified. To prevent EHM within veterinary clinics and hospitals, all horses presenting with significant fevers and nonspecific clinical signs that may or may not include neurologic deficits should be strictly isolated until a diagnosis is secured. Such an approach can prevent the later quarantine of an entire hospital should EHV-1 infection be diagnosed subsequently. Blood and nasal secretions of suspect horses should be tested by qPCR for EHV-1, and other infectious agents, until these tests and accompanying clinical signs confirm or rule out active EHV-1 infection. Once EHV-1 infection is confirmed, strict isolation procedures and secondary quarantine of both the clinic and the source stable of the particular horse should be used. At stables and farms, all newly arrived horses should be isolated for at least 3 weeks. Footbaths, boot covers, and coveralls should be provided and adequately maintained for sanitary purposes. Separate equipment, tack, bedding, and feedstuffs should be used in the care of these animals. Grooms and other personnel should be instructed to work with these animals last in the course of their daily routine. Exercise periods should be confined to a time when other horses are not present in the training areas, and riders should wear protective clothing and clean and thoroughly disinfect their boots, tack, and hands after contact with such animals. Horses returning from shows or extended traveling events should be isolated according to their particular circumstances. Minimum isolation precautions include the prevention of fomite transmission through "nose-to-nose" contact or the indirect transmission of infective nasal secretions by mechanical transmission through stable employees or horse owners. All horse vans and trailers should be thoroughly cleaned and disinfected after use. Prevention of EHM following horse shows, races, or other athletic events is problematic. Although the requirement of an "active vaccination status" before admittance and during extended stays at such events may lessen the probability of outbreaks of the respiratory form of EHV-1 infection, no vaccine currently offers protection against the development of EHM. Consequently, the effectiveness of any such strategy in this context is questionable. The examination of at-risk horses for clinical signs of disease, including twice daily assessment of rectal temperature, remains the most effective tool in determining possible sources of virus introduction.

Following the identification of a horse with clinical signs consistent EHM, such as fever, nasal discharge, and the acute onset of neurologic deficits, measures must be instituted immediately to confirm the diagnosis and control disease spread. It is known that nasal secretions of horses with EHM contain extremely large amounts of replicating virus, and these secretions contribute to the spread of disease to other susceptible individuals. Therefore, horses suspected of having EHM must be removed from the stable environment as quickly as possible and placed in strict isolation. Failure to remove such animals facilitates the continued viral contamination of the environment and contributes to disease spread. A recent study tested the viability of EHV-1 in the environment and showed that the virus could be recovered up to 48 hours from various materials (leather, polyester-cotton fabric, wood shavings, straw, plastic) and environmental conditions (4°C, indoors and outdoors) with persistence decreasing over time.[94] These results highlight the need for barrier precautions to prevent the spread of EHV-1 via contaminated material and environment. Clinically affected horses should remain in strict quarantine until such time as they are proven either not to have EHV-1 infection or to have fully recovered and have remained asymptomatic for 21 days. Horses known to have had direct contact with a suspected EHM case should be maintained in their existing barns and segregated from other horses during exercise periods until a diagnosis is made. Once confirmed, appropriate quarantine restricting the movement of all potentially exposed horses is necessary to prevent the spread of disease to other locations. Aerosol transmission is considered less important than direct contact or spread of secretions on fomites between horses by handlers. These procedures may begin with the focal quarantine of individuals in the immediate area of exposure, such as a single barn or other unit of housing within a facility. Horses in the immediate focal contact area of the clinically affected (index) individual should be monitored twice daily for fever, and if found to be febrile should be tested for EHV-1 infection by qPCR. If after focal quarantine measures, additional clinically ill or EHV-1 positive horse or horses are identified at other locations within the facility, additional quarantine of exposed horses should be instituted and the area under quarantine may be expanded to include other affected barns or the entire stable area. An optimum strategy is the imposition of a series of focal quarantine procedures in an expanding series of "concentric rings" of disease control. Individual animals that have tested positive for EHV-1 infection within the designated quarantine area, whether subclinical or not, should be periodically retested until disease is confirmed or eliminated based on lack of clinical signs and a negative EHV-1 qPCR test result. Quarantine should be maintained until absence of further clinical cases and positive tests from exposed horses suggest no new cases are occurring. At this point, areas of the facility under focal quarantine may have their restrictions rescinded in a reverse concentric ring approach.

The effectiveness of medical intervention to reduce the likelihood of EHM development in horses with early signs (fever) is unproven and the justification is theoretic. The goal of such medical strategy is aimed at decreasing viremia with the use of antiviral drugs, at preventing interactions between infected PBMCs and endothelial cells of the CNS by using NSAIDs and at minimizing sequelae resulting from infected endothelial cells by using antithrombotic or rheological drugs. The random treatment of exposed but subclinical horses with any of the above listed drugs should be discouraged.

SUMMARY

Although EHM is a relatively uncommon manifestation of EHV-1 infection, it can cause devastating losses during outbreaks. Antemortem diagnosis of EHM relies mainly on the molecular detection of EHV-1 in nasal secretions and blood. Management of horses affected by EHM is aimed at supportive nursing and nutritional care, at reducing CNS inflammation, and preventing thromboembolic sequelae. Horses exhibiting sudden and severe neurologic signs consistent with a diagnosis of EHM pose a definite risk to the surrounding horse population. Consequently, early intervention to prevent the spread of infection is required. Disease control measures, such as isolation of affected horses, segregation and monitoring of exposed horses, and quarantine measures, should be established in order to prevent the spread of the virus. Although there are several vaccines available against both the respiratory and the abortigenic form of EHV-1 infection, currently no vaccine has a claim for the prevention of EHM.

CLINICS CARE POINTS

- EHM is a rare complication of EHV-1 infection All different EHV-1 genotypes have been associated with EHM Clinical diagnosis of EHM is supported through qPCR detection of EHV-1 in nasal secretions and/or blood Because EHM cases shed high levels of EHV-1, it is imperative to quickly isolate suspected or confirmed cases Early medical intervention improves the outcome of EHM cases No vaccine has a claim for the protection against EHM Biosecurty is the most effective strategy to reduce the risk of EHV-1 spread and therefore, reduce the risk of EHM outbreak.

REFERENCES

1. Ostlund EN. The equine herpesviruses. Vet Clin North Am Equine Pract 1993;9: 283–94.
2. Henninger RW, Reed SM, Saville WJ, et al. Outbreak of neurologic disease caused by equine herpesvirus-1 at a university equestrian center. J Vet Intern Med 2007;21:157–65.

3. Burgess BA, Tokateloff N, Manning S, et al. Nasal shedding of equine herpesvirus-1 from horses in an outbreak of equine herpes myeloencephalopathy in Western Canada. J Vet Intern Med 2012;26:384–92.

4. Traub-Dargatz JL, Pelzel-McCluskey AM, Creekmore LH, et al. Case-control study of a multistate equine herpesvirus myeloencephalopathy outbreak. J Vet Intern Med 2013;27:339–46.

5. McFadden AM, Hanlon D, McKenzie RK, et al. The first reported outbreak of equine herpesvirus myeloencephalopathy in New Zealand. N Z Vet J 2016;64: 125–34.

6. Pronost S, Legrand L, Pitel PH, et al. Outbreak of equine herpesvirus myeloence-phalopathy in France: a clinical and molecular investigation. Transbound Emerg Dis 2012;59:256–63.

7. Crabb BS, Studdert MJ. Expression of small regions of equine herpesvirus 1 glycoprotein C in Escherichia coli. Vet Microbiol 1995;46:181–91.

8. Telford EA, Watson MS, McBride K, et al. The DNA sequence of equine herpes-virus-1. Virology 1992;189:304–16.

9. Gray WL, Baumann RP, Robertson AT, et al. Regulation of equine herpesvirus type 1 gene expression: characterization of immediate early, early, and late tran-scription. Virology 1987;158:79–87.

10. Nugent J, Birch-Machin I, Smith KC, et al. Analysis of equid herpesvirus 1 strain variation reveals a point mutation of the DNA polymerase strongly associated with neuropathogenic versus nonneuropathogenic disease outbreaks. J Virol 2006;80: 4047–60.

11. Perkins GA, Goodman LB, Tsujimura K, et al. Investigation of the prevalence of neurologic equine herpes virus type 1 (EHV-1) in a 23-year retrospective analysis (1984-2007). Vet Microbiol 2009;139:375–8.

12. Goodman LB, Loregian A, Perkins GA, et al. A point mutation in a herpesvirus po-lymerase determines neuropathogenicity. PLoS Pathog 2007;3:e160.

13. Allen GP, Bolin DC, Bryant U, et al. Prevalence of latent, neuropathogenic equine herpesvirus-1 in the Thoroughbred broodmare population of central Kentucky. Equine Vet J 2008;40:105–10.

14. Pusterla N, Mapes S, Wilson WD. Prevalence of equine herpesvirus type 1 in tri-geminal ganglia and submandibular lymph nodes of equids examined postmor-tem. Vet Rec 2010;167:376–8.

15. Allen GP, Bryans JT. Molecular epizootiology, pathogenesis, and prophylaxis of equine herpesvirus-1 infections. Prog Vet Microbiol Immunol 1986;2:78–144.

16. Allen GP. Equid herpesvirus 1 and equid herpesvirus 4 infections. In: Coetzer JAWT, RC, editors. Infectious diseases of livestock. Newmarket (Can-ada): Oxford University Press; 2004. p. 829–59.

17. Dunowska M. A review of equid herpesvirus 1 for the veterinary practitioner. Part B: Pathogenesis and epidemiology. N Z Vet J 2014;62:179–88.

18. Giessler KS, Samoilowa S, Soboll Hussey G, et al. Viral load and cell tropism dur-ing early latent equid herpesvirus 1 infection differ over time in lymphoid and neu-ral tissue samples from experimentally infected horses. Front Vet Sci 2020;7:621.

19. Negussie H, Gizaw D, Tessema TS, et al. Equine herpesvirus-1 myeloencephal-opathy, an emerging threat of working equids in Ethiopia. Transbound Emerg Dis 2017;64:389–97.

20. Barbić L, Lojkić I, Stevanović V, et al. Two outbreaks of neuropathogenic equine herpesvirus type 1 with breed-dependent clinical signs. Vet Rec 2012;170:227.

21. Greenwood RE. Simson AR Clinical report of a paralytic syndrome affecting stal-lions, mares and foals on a thoroughbred studfarm. Equine Vet J 1980;12:113–7.

22. Thomson GW, McCready R, Sanford E, et al. Case report: An outbreak of herpesvirus myeloencephalitis in vaccinated horses. Can Vet J 1979;20:22–5.
23. Chowdhury SI, Kubin G, Ludwig H. Equine herpesvirus type 1 (EHV-1) induced abortions and paralysis in a Lipizzaner stud: a contribution to the classification of equine herpesviruses. Arch Virol 1986;90:273–88.
24. Friday PA, Scarratt WK, Elvinger F, et al. Ataxia and paresis with equine herpesvirus type 1 infection in a herd of riding school horses. Vet Intern Med 2000;14: 197–201.
25. van Maanen C, Sloet van Oldruitenborgh-Oosterbaan MM, Damen EA, et al. Neurological disease associated with EHV-1-infection in a riding school: clinical and virological characteristics. Equine Vet J 2001;33:191–6.
26. Goehring LS, van Winden SC, van Maanen C, et al. Equine herpesvirus type 1-associated myeloencephalopathy in The Netherlands: a four-year retrospective study (1999-2003). J Vet Intern Med 2006;20:601–7.
27. Goehring LS, Klouth E, Reese S. Clinical evidence of breed predilection for equine herpesvirus-1 associated myeloencephalopathy (EHM). Proceedings of the 100th Conference of Research Workers in Animal Diseases, Chicago, IL, November 2–5, 2019, pp. 78.
28. Pusterla N, Mapes S, Wademan C, et al. Investigation of the role of mules as silent shedders of EHV-1 during an outbreak of EHV-1 myeloencephalopathy in California. Vet Rec 2012;170:465.
29. Giessler KS, Goehring LS, Jacobs S, et al. Use of the old horse model to identify host factors contributing to EHM pathogenesis. Proceedings of the 101st Conference of Research Workers in Animal Diseases, Chicago, IL, December 5 8, 2020, pp. 269.
30. Pusterla N, Mapes S, Madigan JE, et al. Prevalence of EHV-1 in adult horses transported over long distances. Vet Rec 2009;165:473–5.
31. Pusterla N, Hussey SB, Mapes S, et al. Molecular investigation of the viral kinetics of equine herpesvirus-1 in blood and nasal secretions of horses after corticosteroid-induced recrudescence of latent infection. J Vet Intern Med 2010;24:1153–7.
32. Carr E, Schott H, Pusterla N. Absence of equid herpesvirus-1 reactivation and viremia in hospitalized critically ill horses. J Vet Intern Med 2011;25:1190–3.
33. Sonis JM, Goehring LS. Nasal shedding of equid herpesvirus type 1 and type 4 in hospitalized febrile horses. J Equine Vet Sci 2013;33:756–9.
34. Poelaert KCK, Van Cleemput J, Laval K, et al. Equine herpesvirus 1 infection orchestrates the expression of chemokines in equine respiratory epithelial cells. J Gen Virol 2019;100:1567–79.
35. Poelaert KCK, Van Cleemput J, Laval K, et al. Abortigenic but not neurotropic equine herpes virus 1 modulates the interferon antiviral defense. Front Cell Infect Microbiol 2018;8:312.
36. Van Cleemput J, Poelaert KCK, Laval K, et al. An alphaherpesvirus exploits antimicrobial β-defensins to initiate respiratory tract infection. J Virol 2020;94. e01676-19.
37. Kydd JH, Smith KC, Hannant D, et al. Distribution of equid herpesvirus-1 in the respiratory tract–associated lymphoid tissue: implications for cellular immunity. Equine Vet J 1994;26:470–3.
38. Holz CL, Sledge D, Kiupel M, et al. Histopathological findings following experimental equine herpesvirus 1 infection of horses. Front Vet Sci 2019;6:59.

39. Spiesschaert B, Goldenbogen B, Taferner S, et al. Role of gB and pUS3 in equine herpesvirus 1 transfer between peripheral blood mononuclear cells and endothelial cells: a dynamic in vitro model. J Virol 2015;89:11899–908.

40. Pavulraj S, Kamel M, Stephanowitz H, et al. Equine herpesvirus type 1 modulates cytokine and chemokine profiles of mononuclear cells for efficient dissemination to target organs. Viruses 2020;12:999.

41. Laval K, Favoreel HW, Poelaert KC, et al. Equine herpesvirus type 1 enhances viral replication in CD172a+ monocytic cells upon adhesion to endothelial cells. J Virol 2015;89:10912–23.

42. Zarski LM, Weber PSD, Lee Y, et al. Transcriptomic profiling of equine and viral genes in peripheral blood mononuclear cells in horses during equine herpesvirus 1 infection. Pathogens 2021;10:E43.

43. Oladunni FS, Sarkar S, Reedy S, et al. Equid herpesvirus 1 targets the sensitization and induction steps to inhibit the type I interferon response in equine endothelial cells. J Virol 2019;93. e01342-19.

44. Stokol T, Yeo WM, Burnett D, et al. Equid herpesvirus type 1 activates platelets. PLoS One 2015;10:e0122640.

45. Wilson ME, Holz CL, Kopec AK, et al. Coagulation parameters following equine herpesvirus type 1 infection in horses. Equine Vet J 2019;51:102–7.

46. Goehring LS, Soboll Hussey G, Gomez Diez M, et al. Plasma D-dimer concentrations during experimental EHV-1 infection of horses. J Vet Intern Med 2013;27: 1535–42.

47. Allen GP. Risk factors for development of neurologic disease after experimental exposure to equine herpesvirus-1 in horses. Am J Vet Res 2008;69:1595–600.

48. Gardiner DW, Lunn DP, Goehring LS, et al. Strain impact on equine herpesvirus type 1 (EHV-1) abortion models: Viral loads in fetal and placental tissues and foals. Vaccine 2012;30:6564–72.

49. House JA, Gregg DA, Lubroth J, et al. Experimental equine herpesvirus-1 infection in llamas (*Lama glama*). J Vet Diagn Invest 1991;3:137–43.

50. Rebhun WC, Jenkins DH, Riis RC, et al. An epizootic of blindness and encephalitis associated with a herpesvirus indistinguishable from equine herpesvirus I in a herd of alpacas and llamas. J Am Vet Med Assoc 1988;192:953–6.

51. Whitwell KE, Blunden AS. Pathological findings in horses dying during an outbreak of the paralytic form of Equid herpesvirus type 1 (EHV-1) infection. Equine Vet J 1992;24:13–9.

52. Hussey GS, Goehring LS, Lunn DP, et al. Experimental infection with equine herpesvirus type 1 (EHV-1) induces chorioretinal lesions. Vet Res 2013;44:118.

53. Matthews A. Fundus. Equine ophthalmology. An atlas and text. In: Barnett K, editor. London: Elsevier Health Sciences; 2004. p. 235–8.

54. Walter J, Balzer HJ, Seeh C, et al. Venereal shedding of equid herpesvirus-1 (EHV-1) in naturally infected stallions. J Vet Intern Med 2012;26:1500–4.

55. Hebia-Fellah I, Léauté A, Fiéni F, et al. Evaluation of the presence of equine viral herpesvirus 1 (EHV-1) and equine viral herpesvirus 4 (EHV-4) DNA in stallion semen using polymerase chain reaction (PCR). Theriogenology 2009;71:1381–9.

56. Tearle JP, Smith KC, Boyle MS, et al. Replication of equid herpesvirus-1 (EHV-1) in the testes and epididymides of ponies and venereal shedding of infectious virus. J Comp Pathol 1996;115:385–97.

57. Holz CL, Nelli RK, Wilson ME, et al. Viral genes and cellular markers associated with neurological complications during herpesvirus infections. J Gen Virol 2017; 98:1439–54.

58. Slater J. Equine Herpesviruses. In: Debra DS, Long MT, editors. Equine infectious diseases. St. Louis: Saunders Elsevier; 2007. p. 151–68.
59. Goehring LS, van Maanen C, Sloet van Oldruitenborgh-Oosterbaan MM. Neurological syndromes among horses in The Netherlands. A 5 year retrospective survey (1999-2004). Vet Q 2005;27:11–20.
60. Lunn DP, Mayhew I. Neurological examination of the horse. Equine Vet Educ 1989;1:94–101.
61. Dunowska M. A review of equid herpesvirus 1 for the veterinary practitioner. Part A: Clinical presentation, diagnosis and treatment. N Z Vet J 2014;62:171–8.
62. Estell KE, Dawson DR, Magdesian KG, et al. Quantitative molecular viral loads in 7 horses with naturally occurring equine herpesvirus-1 infection. Equine Vet J 2015;47:689–93.
63. Pusterla N, Hatch K, Crossley B, et al. Equine herpesvirus-1 genotype did not significantly affect clinical signs and disease outcome in 65 horses diagnosed with equine herpesvirus-1 myeloencephalopathy. Vet J 2020;255:105407.
64. Lunn DP, Davis-Poynter N, Flaminio MJ, et al. Equine herpesvirus-1 consensus statement. J Vet Intern Med 2009;23:450–61.
65. Wilson WD. Equine herpesvirus 1 myeloencephalopathy. Vet Clin North Am Equine Pract 1997;13:53–72.
66. Pusterla N, Wilson WD, Mapes S, et al. Characterization of viral loads, strain and state of equine herpesvirus-1 using real-time PCR in horses following natural exposure at a racetrack in California. Vet J 2009;179:230–9.
67. Pusterla N, Hussey SB, Mapes S, et al. Comparison of four methods to quantify equid herpesvirus 1 load by real-time polymerase chain reaction in nasal secretions of experimentally and naturally infected horses. J Vet Diagn Invest 2009;21: 836–40.
68. Pusterla N, Mapes S, Wilson WD. Use of viral loads in blood and nasopharyngeal secretions for the diagnosis of EHV-1 infection in field cases. Vet Rec 2008;162: 728–9.
69. Paillot R, Sutton G, Thieulent C, et al. New EHV-1 variant identified. Vet Rec 2020; 186:573.
70. Sutton G, Thieulent C, Fortier C, et al. Identification of a new equid herpesvirus 1 DNA polymerase (ORF30) genotype with the isolation of a C_{2254}/H_{752} strain in French horses showing no major impact on the strain behaviour. Viruses 2020; 12:1160.
71. Allen GP, Breathnach CC. Quantification by real-time PCR of the magnitude and duration of leucocyte-associated viraemia in horses infected with neuropathogenic vs. non-neuropathogenic strains of EHV-1. Equine Vet J 2006;38:252–7.
72. McCartan CG, Russell MM, Wood JL, et al. Clinical, serological and virological characteristics of an outbreak of paresis and neonatal foal disease due to equine herpesvirus-1 on a stud farm. Vet Rec 1995;136(1):7–12.
73. Garré B, van der Meulen K, Nugent J, et al. In vitro susceptibility of six isolates of equine herpesvirus 1 to acyclovir, ganciclovir, cidofovir, adefovir, PMEDAP and foscarnet. Vet Microbiol 2007;122:43–51.
74. Maxwell LK, Bentz BG, Bourne DW, et al. Pharmacokinetics of valacyclovir in the adult horse. J Vet Pharmacol Ther 2008;31:312–20.
75. Goehring LS, Brandes K, Ashton LV, et al. Anti-inflammatory drugs decrease infection of brain endothelial cells with EHV-1 in vitro. Equine Vet J 2017;49: 629–36.
76. DeNotta SL, Brooks MB. Coagulation assessment in the equine patient. Vet Clin North Am Equine Pract 2020;36:53–71.

77. Stokol T. Veterinary Pathology - A path forward with directions and opportunities. Front Vet Sci 2016;3:76.
78. Walter J, Seeh C, Fey K, et al. Prevention of equine herpesvirus myeloencephalopathy - Is heparin a novel option? A case report. Tierarztl Prax Ausg G Grosstiere Nutztiere 2016;44:313–7.
79. Finno CJ, Valberg SJ. A comparative review of vitamin E and associated equine disorders. J Vet Intern Med 2012;26:1251–66.
80. Kydd JH, Wattrang E, Hannant D. Pre-infection frequencies of equine herpesvirus-1 specific, cytotoxic T lymphocytes correlate with protection against abortion following experimental infection of pregnant mares. Vet Immunol Immunopathol 2003;96:207–17.
81. Soboll Hussey G, Ashton LV, Quintana AM, et al. Innate immune responses of airway epithelial cells to infection with equine herpesvirus-1. Vet Microbiol 2014;170:28–38.
82. Soboll Hussey G, Hussey SB, Wagner B, et al. Evaluation of immune responses following infection of ponies with an EHV-1 ORF1/2 deletion mutant. Vet Res 2011; 42:23.
83. Schnabel CL, Babasyan S, Rollins A, et al. An equine herpesvirus type 1 (EHV-1) Ab4 open reading frame 2 deletion mutant provides immunity and protection from EHV-1 infection and disease. J Virol 2019;93:e01011–9.
84. Goodman LB, Wagner B, Flaminio MJ, et al. Comparison of the efficacy of inactivated combination and modified-live virus vaccines against challenge infection with neuropathogenic equine herpesvirus type 1 (EHV-1). Vaccine 2006;24: 3636–45.
85. Kamel M, Pavulraj S, Osterrieder K, et al. EHV-1 pathogenesis: current in vitro models and future perspectives. Front Vet Sci 2019;6:251.
86. Oladunni FS, Reedy S, Balasuriya UBR, et al. The effect of equine herpesvirus type 4 on type-I interferon signaling molecules. Vet Immunol Immunopathol 2020;219:109971.
87. Van de Walle GR, Jarosinski KW, Osterrieder N. Alphaherpesviruses and chemokines: pas de deux not yet brought to perfection. J Virol 2008;82:6090–7.
88. Koppers-Lalic D, Reits EA, Ressing ME, et al. Varicelloviruses avoid T cell recognition by UL49.5-mediated inactivation of the transporter associated with antigen processing. Proc Natl Acad Sci U S A 2005;102:5144–9.
89. Van der Meulen KM, Favorell HW, Pensaert MB, et al. Immune escape of equine herpesvirus 1 and other herpesviruses of veterinary importance. Vet Immunol Immunopathol 2006;111:31–40.
90. Soboll Hussey G, Ashton LV, Quintana AM, et al. Equine herpesvirus type 1 pUL56 modulates innate responses of airway epithelial cells. Virology 2014; 464-465:76–86.
91. Ma GG, Osterrieder N, Van de Valle GR. Identification and characterization of equine herpesvirus type 1 pUL56 and its role in virus-induced downregulation of major histocompatibility complex class I. J Virol 2012;86:3554–63.
92. Van de Walle GR, May ML, Sukhumavasi W, et al. Herpesvirus chemokine-binding glycoprotein G (gG) efficiently inhibits neutrophil chemotaxis in vitro and in vivo. J Immunol 2007;179:4161–9.
93. Van de Walle GR, Sakamoto K, Osterrieder N. CCL3 and viral chemokine-binding protein gg modulate pulmonary inflammation and virus replication during equine herpesvirus 1 infection. J Virol 2008;82:1714–22.
94. Saklou NT, Burgess BA, Ashton LV, et al. Environmental persistence of equid herpesvirus type-1. Equine Vet J 2021;53:349–55.

Traumatic Nervous System Injury

Yvette S. Nout-Lomas, DVM, PhD

KEYWORDS

- Traumatic brain injury • Spinal cord injury • Peripheral nerve injury • Head trauma
- Pathophysiology • Plasticity • Diagnostic imaging • Rehabilitation

KEY POINTS

- Evaluation for fractures of skull and vertebrae is important for diagnosis, therapy, and prognosis.
- Ongoing secondary injury can lead to worsening of clinical signs over the initial few days; however, improvement thereafter is possible.
- Treatment in the acute stage is focused on reducing edema and inflammation, whereas treatment thereafter is focused on the reestablishment of neural pathways through exercise and rehabilitation.
- Advancements in the fields of equine diagnostic imaging, medicine, surgery, and rehabilitation will lead to improved prospects for horses that suffer neurotrauma.

Trauma to the nervous system in horses occurs through accidents that usually cause blunt force trauma and occasionally penetrating injuries. For nervous tissue damage to occur, skull or vertebral body fractures are not always necessary; however, careful evaluation for fractures of the skull and vertebrae is recommended as type and location of fracture can affect treatment and prognosis. Injury to the temporohyoid apparatus can lead to the fracture of portions of this apparatus, including petrous temporal bone fracture, and result in vestibular disease, cranial nerve disease, and occasional brain stem or hindbrain disease. Although this condition can have an acute onset of neurologic deficit, the underlying disease is more long-standing.

Central nervous system (CNS) trauma accounts for 22% to 24% of neurologic disorders seen in equine hospitals, with spinal cord injury (SCI) being the most common (56%–77% vs 23%–44% brain and cranial nerves).[1,2] Studies investigating fatalities associated with high-speed equestrian sports found skull and axial spine fractures in 5% to 10% of fatalities.[3–6] It must be noted that distal limb injuries are the most common cause of racing fatalities[3–6] and in some cases more than one site of injury

The author has no disclosures to declare.
Department of Clinical Sciences, Johnson Family Equine Hospital, Colorado State University, 2230 Gillette Drive, Fort Collins, CO 80523-1678, USA
E-mail address: Yvette.Nout-Lomas@colostate.edu

is found. For example, a recent case was described in which a preexisting sesamoid bone lesion resulted in fracture and the subsequent fall resulted in acute SCI and death.[7]

CLASSIFICATION AND MECHANISMS OF INJURY

The most common mechanisms of trauma in the horse are rearing and falling over backwards, struggling from entrapment in fences or after being cast, collision and kick injuries, and recovery from anesthesia. Although head trauma often results in skull fractures, traumatic brain injury (TBI) is an uncommon sequela. Feary and colleagues[8] reported that 65% of horses with TBI had skull fractures. Injuries to the brain can be mild with temporary loss of function and occur without structural damage to the brain (concussion) or they can be associated with vascular and brain tissue damage of various degrees of severity. The classification of TBI is shown in **Table 1**.[9]

Most of the horses that sustain a poll injury and TBI through rearing and falling backward are less than 1 year of age.[8] This is likely due to a combination of behavioral responses, because the suture between the basilar bones remains open until 2 to 5 years of age. Basilar (basisphenoid and basioccipital) and temporal bone fractures (**Fig. 1**) are the most common skull fractures seen after this type of trauma and were seen in 44% of TBI cases.[8] Fracture of the basilar bones is a result of the strong traction forces of the longus and rectus capitis ventralis muscles, and in most cases, the fracture site is stable with minimal displacement. Despite this, serious damage of associated soft tissue such as subdural or subarachnoid bleeding around the brain

Table 1			
Classification of traumatic brain injury			
Mechanism	Blunt	High or low velocity	Most common in the horse
	Penetrating	Gunshot wound	
	Blast	Shock wave	
Severity	Mild		Neurologic examination
	Moderate		
	Severe		
Morphology	Skull fracture	Vault	
		Basilar	Most common in the horse
	Intracranial lesions	Focal	
		Diffuse	
Tissue Injury	Concussion	Temporary loss of function	
		No structural damage	
	Contusion	Bruise	Swelling and hemorrhage
	Laceration	Tears	
	Diffuse axonal injury	Microscopic	Common in high-velocity injuries
		Eventual axonal loss	
	Brain swelling and ischemia	Continued swelling results in reduced CPP	Hours to days following injury
	Vascular injuries	Epidural hematoma	
		Subdural hematoma	
		Intracerebral hematoma	
		Subarachnoid hemorrhage	

Abbreviation: CPP, cerebral perfusion pressure.

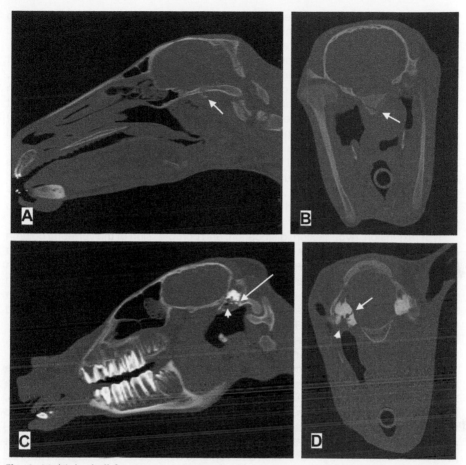

Fig. 1. Multiple skull fractures in a 3-month-old Quarter Horse foal with TBI. This foal was being haltered and abruptly turned its head, crashed into a wall, fell down, and was unable to get up and developed persistent nystagmus. Pre-contrast computed tomography images taken with a bone algorithm show multiple basisphenoid fractures (*white arrow*): one with an avulsion into the right longus capitis muscle (*A*: sagittal; *B*: transverse) and a fracture of the left petrous temporal bone through the internal acoustic meatus (*white arrow*) with intracranial gas and fluid in the left tympanic membrane (*white arrowhead*; *C*: sagittal; *D*: transverse). The foal also had a fractured transverse process of C7. No structural abnormalities were noted in the foal's brain and spinal cord. This foal recovered over a period of 7 days following management that included hyperosmolar (mannitol) and antiinflammatory [dimethylsulfoxide (DMSO), nonsteroidal antiinflammatory drugs (NSAIDs), vitamin E] treatments.

stem and cranial nerve damage may occur. The cerebellum is seldom severely damaged after poll impact, whereas the cerebral parenchyma is more commonly injured after being subjected to the rapid acceleration—deceleration forces. Also, optic nerves and other attachments may be torn from the cerebral hemispheres.[10] Impact to the dorsal surface of the head may result in damage to the frontal or parietal bones with subsequent cerebral cortical injury or, more commonly, damage to the cervical vertebrae with subsequent SCI. Also, cranial nerve XII may be injured as it exits the hypoglossal foramen. Furthermore, occipital cortical injury may occur and with frontal injuries the optic nerves may be stretched as described for poll impact injuries.

Recently, a case of coup contrecoup TBI was reported in a horse.[11] In these injuries, there are two primary locations of TBI: the coup injury adjacent to the point of impact and the contrecoup injury in a location greater than 90° from the site of coup impact, often directly opposite the site of the coup impact. Another phenomenon that can occur is gas accumulation secondary to trauma or infection which can be present around the cranial vault (pneumocranium), within the cranial vault (pneumocephalus) and the spinal canal (pneumorrhachis).[12] Any extensive trauma involving the frontal bones, the sinuses, ethmoids, and cribiform plate can result in a pneumocephalus, and the leakage of cerebrospinal fluid (CSF) from the nares, ears, or wounds indicates a communication between the outside and the CSF space. Although, in most reported equine cases, pneumocephalus was an incidental finding, it can result in fatal complications through the spread of infection and development of tension pneumocephalus.[12,13]

Hyperextension, hyperflexion, dislocation, and compression of the vertebral column can result in varying severities of osseous and soft tissue damage and SCI. When a horse nosedives with the head under the body, neck hyperflexion can lead to damage in the occipital–atlanto-axial and caudal cervical regions. Although neck injuries with subsequent SCI are seen most commonly in horses,[1,2] lumbar fractures have been identified as the most common of vertebral fractures seen in racing injuries,[6,14] and recent evidence suggests that in racehorses preexisting pathology at the L5–L6 vertebral junction likely predisposes horses to catastrophic lumbar fractures.[15] In foals, fractures have also been reported secondary to osteomyelitis.

In both TBI and SCI, primary and secondary injury mechanisms after trauma contribute to the damage to the nervous system. Primary injury mechanisms are those that occur at the time of insult and include mechanical disruption of tissue damage. Secondary injury mechanisms, on the other hand, occur after the initial trauma and take place up to months after the initial trauma. A plethora of secondary injury mechanisms involving molecular, cellular, and biochemical events that lead to delayed but progressive tissue damage have been and continue to be discovered (**Fig. 2**, **Table 2**). Secondary injury mechanisms are considered the reason for expansion and exacerbation of initial damage. These secondary changes partially explain the reasons many patients have only limited endogenous recovery, and identifying and understanding provide novel targets for treatment discovery.[9,16–19]

Traumatic peripheral nerve injury occurs through stretch, compression, or laceration and is classified according to the degree of damage (**Fig. 3**).[20] In the horse, peripheral nerve injuries are most commonly caused by crashes and accidents whereby limbs get stuck resulting in stretch or compression injuries. They can also be caused by lacerations and iatrogenically during intramuscular injections. Peripheral nerve injuries tend to occur in areas where the nerve runs close to the skin over a bony protuberance and is less protected by soft tissues; thus, injuries are often associated with wounds and fractures.

CLINICAL SIGNS AND DIAGNOSTICS

Clinical signs of TBI include mentation changes such as dullness, obtundation, coma, and death. TBI can also result in ataxia, recumbency, and seizures as well as clinical signs related to specific sites of damage, such as nystagmus, head tilt, leaning, ocular changes (blindness, strabismus, abnormal pupil size, pupillary asymmetry, and loss of pupillary light reflex), dysphagia, cranial nerve dysfunction, epistaxis, and otorrhea.

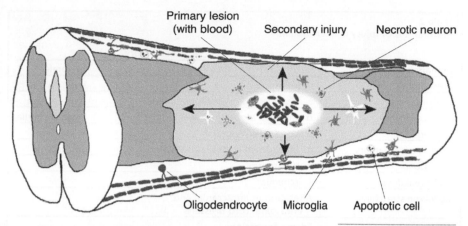

Primary lesion
(with blood)   Secondary injury   Necrotic neuron

Oligodendrocyte   Microglia   Apoptotic cell

TRENDS in Molecular Medicine

Fig. 2. Secondary SCI. Initial trauma to the cord is directed to the central gray matter, where frank destruction occurs. The initial injury is followed by a cascade of biochemical events (secondary injury) that is thought to enlarge the area of cell death through necrosis and apoptosis. Neurons and glial cells at the margins of the expanding lesion represent a target for neuroprotection. When axons in the white matter are damaged, Wallerian degeneration can induce microglial activation and apoptotic cell death of oligodendrocytes long after the initial injury. This later microglial activation represents another potential target for treatments that reduce microglial activation and/or oligodendrocyte apoptosis. (*From*: Beattie MS. Inflammation and apoptosis: linked therapeutic targets in spinal cord injury. Trends Mol Med 2004;10:580-583[16]; with permission.)

Clinical signs of SCI are depend on the localization and severity of the impact, Although most horses with SCI have normal brain function, it is possible for animals to incur both TBI and SCI. Polytrauma could affect treatment and prognosis. Depending on the site of SCI or peripheral nerve injury, clinical signs can be quite variable, ranging from perineal hypalgesia and tail weakness to incontinence, gait abnormalities, and recumbency.[9] The evaluation of recumbent horses is difficult, but the utilization of reflex pathways is often possible and can be helpful. In horses, the motor nucleus of the phrenic nerve is located in the ventral horn of the spinal cord, and the nerve variably arises between C4 and C7. Input to the phrenic nerve is from the respiratory center located in the brainstem. Injuries along this tract can lead to respiratory compromise and, when severe, death. Clinical signs of peripheral nerve injuries are shown in **Table 3**[21] and include an abnormal stance or gait, reduced cutaneous sensation, and muscle atrophy. Muscle atrophy develops rapidly and continues until the nerve heals. Affected muscles lose approximately half their mass by 2 weeks after injury.

The diagnosis of traumatic nervous system injury is based on history and clinical signs. Ancillary diagnostics are useful to obtain a specific diagnosis and evaluate the extent of injuries and dysfunction. The goals of neuroimaging are to determine the extent and type of primary injury, plan therapeutic and possible surgical approaches to reduce secondary injury, and ascertain prognosis. In horses, computed tomography (CT) or MRI may be performed but availability is limited, cost may be prohibitive, and there is a risk of additional injury during recovery from general anesthesia. However, the benefits of improved patient management generally outweigh these limitations. For spinal imaging in adult horses, MRI is not yet available. CT (see **Fig. 1**) is

Table 2
Mechanisms of injury in neurotrauma

Primary Injury	Secondary Injury	
	CNS	Systemic
Mechanical	Vascular	Hypoxia
a. Contusion	a. Blood pressure dysregulation	Hypotension
b. Laceration	b. Impaired blood flow autoregulation	Hyperglycemia
Hemorrhage	c. Blood flow mismatch	Fever
Diffuse axonal injury	d. Breakdown of BBB and BSCB	Seizures
Hematoma	e. Vasospasm	
BBB breakdown	f. Ischemia	
Cell/Axon stretching	Alteration in intracranial and intraspinal cord pressure	
Synapse loss	Edema formation Inflammatory/Immunologic tissue response a. Astrogliosis b. Lymphocyte infiltration c. Activated and phagocytic monocytes d. Glial/Fibrous scar e. Extracellular matrix proteins—CSPGs f. Myelin-associated proteins—NOGO, ROCK Oxidative stress a. Reactive oxygen species b. Lipid peroxidation Cell death a. Necrosis b. Apoptosis Excitotoxicity and neurotransmitter accumulation Serum proteins, calpain proteinases, and metalloproteinases Altered homeostasis a. Impaired energy metabolism b. Mitochondrial dysfunction c. Ionic concentration alterations (calcium, sodium) Changes in gene expression Infection	

Abbreviations: BBB, blood brain barrier; BSCB, blood spinal cord barrier; CNS, central nervous system; CSPGs, chondroitin sulfate proteoglycans; NOGO, neurite outgrowth inhibitor; ROCK, Rho-associated protein kinase.

optimal for evaluating TBI 3 to 24 hours after injury, whereas MRI is superior after 49 to 72 hours or when results of the CT do not explain severity of clinical signs.[22] Primary brain injuries often are classified as intra-axial (within brain parenchyma; eg, axonal injury, cortical contusion, and intracerebral hematoma) and extra-axial (outside of the brain; for example, epidural and subdural hematoma, subarachnoid and intraventricular hemorrhage). Secondary brain injuries that can be detected include those that produce a mass effect such as hemorrhage and edema and more specific details of those finding such as type of edema and age of hemorrhage.[22] Other diagnostic

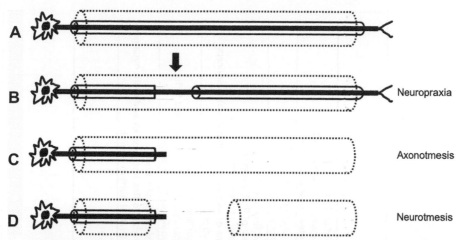

Fig. 3. Classification of peripheral nerve injury. An intact peripheral nerve (*A*) contains of multiple fascicles that consist of many Schwann cell-myelinated axons surrounded by endoneurium. Fascicles are surrounded by perineurium and vessels. The entire peripheral nerve is covered by epineurium. Neuropraxia (*B*) results in bruising and inflammation of the nerve; axonal integrity is maintained. Axonotmesis (*C*) is a more severe injury, resulting from a crushing of the nerve; the axon is severed but various portions of the endoneurium, perineurium, fascicular arrangement, and epineurium are preserved. Neurotmesis (*D*) is the most severe; there is complete disruption of nervous and perineural tissues.

imaging techniques that can be useful in the horse are radiography, myelography, and CT myelography. If CT is not available, radiographs of skull or vertebral column are recommended that should include dorsoventral, lateral, and oblique views. Myelography and CT myelography are useful in cases of cervical SCI.[23]

Electrodiagnostic testing can be useful for the diagnosis and determination of extent and prognosis of peripheral nerve injuries. For example, electromyography can be used to determine which nerves are involved in peripheral nerve injuries. It takes days to weeks before a muscle will develop abnormalities such as fibrillation potentials, positive sharp waves, and complex repetitive discharges after losing nerve input.[24]

The identification of biofluid-based biomarkers to detect ongoing injury, to stratify the need for monitoring and interventions, and to provide prognostic information in TBI and SCI is underway. For example, a serum biomarker test for ubiquitin carboxy-terminal hydrolase L1 and glial fibrillary acidic protein (GFAP) is now used in human TBI and can distinguish mild TBI from no injury controls but can also distinguish those mild TBI subjects with CT-detectable pathoanatomical lesions from those that are CT normal.[25] In human SCI, the combination of inflammatory (interleukin 6 and 8 and monocyte chemoattractant protein-1) and structural (tau, S100β, and GFAP) biomarkers in CSF was used to correctly predict the failure to see functional improvement with an accuracy of over 90%.[26] In dogs with SCI, serum or plasma GFAP predicts both recovery of ambulation and development of progressive myelomalacia with an accuracy of greater than 80%.[27]

MANAGEMENT AND PROGNOSIS

Treatment of neurotrauma is aimed at reducing effects of secondary damage (neuroprotection) and encouraging neural repair (neuroregeneration; **Fig. 4**).[17,28–33] First and

Table 3
Clinical signs of peripheral nerve injuries

		Pectoral Limb			Pelvic Limb
Suprascapular	C6–C7	Lateral rotation and subluxation of shoulder Atrophy of supraspinatus and infraspinatus	Gluteal	L5–S2	Mild abduction Outward rotation of stifle Gluteal muscle atrophy
Axillary	C7–C8	Atrophy of deltoid	Obturator	L4–L6	Abduction of rear limbs Lateral slipping
Musculocutaneous	C7–C8	Overextension of elbow Hypalgesia medial forearm Atrophy of brachialis and biceps brachii	Femoral	L4–L5	Inability to bear weight Lack of limb extension Absent patella reflex Loss of sensation (medial thigh) quadriceps atrophy
Radial	C8–T1	Non-weight-bearing Inability to extend/lock elbow Dorsum of pastern on ground	Sciatic	L6–S1	Poor limb flexion Extended stifle and hock/flexed fetlock Hypalgesia (stifle down)
Median and Ulnar	C8–T2	Goose-stepping gait Dragging of toe Hyperextension of carpus, fetlock, and pastern	Peroneal	L5–S1	Knuckling of fetlock Unable to flex hock and extend digits hypalgesia (cranial portion of limb)
Brachial plexus	C6–T2	Signs of radial and suprascapular nerve injury Atrophy of supra and infraspinatus, triceps, and extensor carpi radialis			

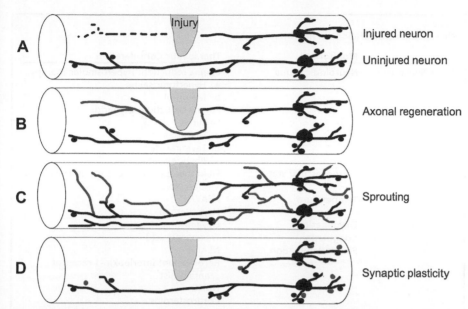

Fig. 4. Cellular mechanisms of neural repair. Injuries to the CNS typically damage certain axonal pathways but spare parallel pathways (*A*). Three main mechanisms for cellular events that support recovery and repair. An injured axon can grow back over long distances by regeneration (*B*), or uninjured and injured fibers that are rostral and caudal to the injury can sprout to form new connections (*C*), or plastic changes of presynaptic and postsynaptic connections throughout the nervous system can occur (*D*).

foremost, this involves management of any acute systemic comorbidities that can negatively impact prognosis including hypoxia, hypotension, hyperglycemia, fever, and seizures. Mean arterial pressure should be maintained within the normal range and seizures treated and prevented. Intravenous hyperosmolar treatments and surgical decompression aim to relieve pressures caused by ongoing edema and hemorrhage, thereby reducing secondary hypoxia and ischemia.[29,34] When hypertonic saline and mannitol are compared, there is not a large difference in efficacy and mortality; however hypertonic saline seems preferred over mannitol for refractory increased intracranial pressure.[35] In some cases, the surgical decompression of the nervous tissue or stabilization of unstable fractures is warranted. Early decompression after SCI is associated with improved sensorimotor recovery, and in humans, the first 24 to 36 hours after SCI seems to represent a crucial time window to achieve optimal neurologic recovery with decompressive surgery.[36] Similarly, in TBI cases, the rapid surgical correction of displaced and compressive fractures is needed. However, current evidence from multicenter clinical trials suggests that decompressive craniectomy for mild-to-moderate intracranial hypertension is not superior to medical management for patients with diffuse TBI.

Neuroprotection using antiapoptotic, anti-inflammatory, and excitatory neurotransmitter antagonists remains a promising strategy to treat SCI (**Table 4**). The role of methylprednisolone (MP) in the management of SCI has been investigated in depth; however, its use remains contentious. Although MP initially showed promise, more recent studies have questioned its use citing numerous systemic adverse effects. Despite this and because of the lack of alternative treatment options, MP and other corticosteroids are still widely used by veterinarians and physicians. At present,

Table 4
Therapeutic considerations in neurotrauma

	Monitoring	Therapeutic Consideration
Acute/Subacute	Neurologic status	Edema reduction: Hyperosmolar therapy:
		a. Hypertonic saline
		b. Mannitol
		Edema reduction: Glyburide
		Seizures:
		a. Diazepam
		b. Levetiracetam
		c. Phenobarbital
	Cardiovascular status	Fluid therapy—Judicious use of crystalloids
		Vasopressors
	Temperature	NSAIDs
		Hypothermia
	Oxygenation	Oxygen
	Coagulation	Tranexamic acid
	Pain/Inflammation	NSAIDs
		Recombinant interleukin-1 receptor antagonist
		DMSO
		Corticosteroids
		Gabapentin
		Minocycline
		Granulocyte colony-stimulating factor
		Vitamin E
	Neuroimaging	Immobilization/protective padding
		Exercise restriction
		Surgical stabilization or decompression
	Reducing excitotoxicity	Riluzole
	Infection	Antibiotics
Long-term	Neurologic status	Vitamin E
		Cellular therapies:
		a. Mesenchymal stem cells
		b. Olfactory ensheathing cells
		c. Schwann cells
		d. Neural stem cells
		e. Activated autologous macrophages
		f. Embryonic stem cells
		g. Pluripotent stem cells
		Biomaterials
		Rehabilitation
		Electrostimulation

Abbreviations: DMSO, dimethylsulfoxide; NSAIDs, nonsteroidal anti-inflammatory drugs.

evidence regarding use of corticosteroids remains contentious, and ultimately, further investigation into the use of steroids is required to determine its utility in treating patients with SCI.[37] Other drugs currently being explored in clinical trials include riluzole, a glutamate blocker, cytokine granulocyte colony stimulating factor which promotes cell survival and inhibits tumor necrosis factor-α and interleukin-1β, and glyburide.[28,32] Glyburide has been shown to reduce cytotoxic edema and cell lysis after acute SCI and has been shown to be safe in dogs that are undergoing anesthesia, imaging, and surgery for treatment of their acute SCI.[38] Tranexamic acid is an antifibrinolytic agent and its use has been associated with decreased mortality in humans TBI.[29]

There is evidence for a neuroprotective role of vitamin E in conditions that produce neuronal excitotoxicity and during brain development.[39] A better knowledge of systemic and local mechanisms of neuroprotection by the different forms of vitamin E is necessary to better understand what its role could be in neurotrauma. When there are open wounds, open fractures, or gas is identified within the cranial vault, antimicrobial treatment should be initiated to prevent establishment of a CNS infection.[12] Trimethoprim–sulfamethoxazole is an excellent candidate for broad-spectrum long-term antibiotic treatment of CNS infections in the horse. Minocycline is another antibiotic with anti-inflammatory properties including inhibition of tumor necrosis factor-α, interleukin-1β, cyclooxygenase-2, and nitric oxide synthase. Studies have shown decreased lesions sizes, decreased neuron loss, and improved motor scores in patients treated with minocycline.[28,32]

Cell-based therapies are promising modalities of regeneration and mechanisms of action include cellular replacement, neurotrophic support, immunomodulation, and induction of plasticity at existing synapses. A wide number of cell types have been studied or are being evaluated in ongoing studies (see **Table 4**). Transplantable biomaterials, such as hydrogels and collagen, are attractive candidates to improve and promote cell survival and differentiation, respectively, by serving as structural frameworks and delivery vehicles. Advanced fabrication and tissue engineering techniques including use of implantable bridges (nerve conduits and scaffolds) manufactured using 3D printing, electrospinning, and cell sheet technologies seem very promising methodologies that allow for the combination of structural repair through

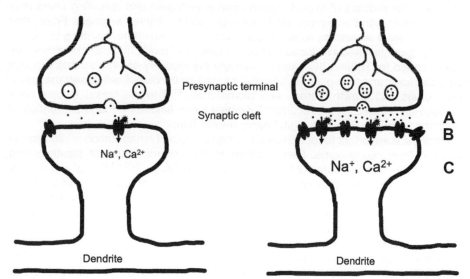

Fig. 5. Mechanisms of synaptic plasticity. Following an action potential, synaptic transmission occurs through neurotransmitter release, binding of neurotransmitter to postsynaptic receptors, and opening of ion channels in the postsynaptic neuron. This allows electrical current to flow in or out of the cell to propagate transmission of an impulse. The strength of synapses can be increased or decreased. Very active synapses are likely to become stronger (long-term potentiation), and those that are less active, or less effective at causing an action potential, tend to become weaker (long-term depression). Synaptic plasticity occurs through changes in either the amount of neurotransmitter released (A) or the number of postsynaptic receptors available (B). Both have the effect of altering how much electrical current flows through the ion channels (C).

Table 5
Examples of systems circuitry level and cellular–molecular approaches to repairing the central nervous system

Systems Circuitry Level Approaches Macroscopic	Cellular–Molecular Interventions Microscopic
1. Increase excitability of intact neural elements 2. Induce circuit plasticity across lesions	1. Replacement of lost tissue 2. Create permissive milieu for neuroregeneration 3. Induction of plasticity 4. Requires surgical administration
Rehabilitation paradigms: 1. Without neural interfaces 2. With neural interfaces	Cellular replacement therapy Induction of axonal growth via molecular mechanisms optogenetic modulation
Electrical stimulation strategies	Immunotherapy
	Enhancement of neurotrophic guidance

incorporation of cells, with sustained release of therapeutic drugs, growth factors, or genes after SCI.[17,30,33]

Injured peripheral nerves have the capacity to regenerate and reinnervate their target organs. Axons can grow at a rate of 1 mm/d.[21] Nerve fibers distal to the injury site undergo Wallerian degeneration, and the denervated Schwann cells proliferate, elongate, and line the endoneurial tubes to guide and support regenerating axons. However, the process of axonal regeneration is inefficient and sprouting fibers may not reconnect with the appropriate fascicle beyond the injured segment. Fibers that reach the target muscle do so in substantially reduced numbers, resulting in incomplete reinnervation and a reduced number of functional motor units. Similar strategies as described for TBI and SCI exist to promote the recovery of function that includes surgical repair and transplant techniques, as well as the use of cell-based therapies, local drugs and growth factors, and biomaterials.[40,41] In the horse, studies have focused on recovery of left recurrent laryngeal nerve function[42,43] and prevention of neuroma formation following digital nerve transection.

Finally, it is important to recognize the important role of rehabilitation in recovery of function from neurotrauma. Rehabilitation techniques make use of plasticity and learning that occurs throughout the nervous system (**Fig. 5**).[30,31,44] Spinal and cortical plasticity mechanisms play an important role in recovery of function, and the techniques that include exercise and electrical stimulation of pathways can enhance recovery of function (**Table 5**). Combinatorial therapies that include use of biomaterials, stem cells, growth factors, and drugs may achieve axonal regeneration but not necessarily functional recovery. Formation and remodeling of functional circuits also depend on rehabilitation exercises that include exercise training, electrical stimulation, and brain–computer interfaces.[30,31] The author stresses return to exercise and rehabilitative techniques to optimize functional recovery in horses with neurotrauma.

CLINICS CARE POINTS

- Horses with central nervous system trauma should undergo thorough neurologic and neuroimaging evaluation.

- Horses can respond well to neuroprotective (fluids, hyperosmolar, anti-inflammatory, surgery) and neuroregenerative (exercise, rehabilitation) therapies.
- Prognosis depends on severity of primary damage and ability to mitigate secondary damage within the first few days.

REFERENCES

1. Feige K, Fürst A, Kaser-Hotz B, et al. Traumatic injury to the central nervous system in horses: occurrence, diagnosis and outcome. Equine Vet Educ 2000;12: 220–4.
2. Tyler CMDR, Begg AP, Hutchins DR, et al. A survey of neurological diseases in horses. Aust Vet J 1993;70:445–9.
3. DeLay J. Postmortem findings in Ontario racehorses, 2003-2015. J Vet Diagn Invest 2017;29:457–64.
4. Rosanowski SM, Chang YM, Stirk AJ, et al. Descriptive epidemiology of veterinary events in flat racing Thoroughbreds in Great Britain (2000 to 2013). Equine Vet J 2017;49:275–81.
5. Wylie CE, McManus P, McDonald C, et al. Thoroughbred fatality and associated jockey falls and injuries in races in New South Wales and the Australian Capital Territory, Australia: 2009-2014. Vet J 2017;227:1–7.
6. Sarrafian TL, Case JT, Kinde H, et al. Fatal musculoskeletal injuries of Quarter Horse racehorses: 314 cases (1990-2007). J Am Vet Med Assoc 2012;241: 935–42.
7. Samol MA, Uzal FA, Blanchard PC, et al. Sudden death caused by spinal cord injury associated with vertebral fractures and fetlock failure in a Thoroughbred racehorse. J Vet Diagn Invest 2021;33:788–91.
8. Feary DJ, Magdesian KG, Aleman MA, et al. Traumatic brain injury in horses: 34 cases (1994-2004). J Am Vet Med Assoc 2007;231:259–66.
9. Nout-Lomas YS. Central Nervous System Trauma. In: Furr MO, Reed SM, editors. Equine neurology. Second edition. Ames, Iowa, USA: Blackwell Publishing; 2015. p. 406–28.
10. Martin L, Kaswan R, Chapman W. Four cases of traumatic optic nerve blindness in the horse. Equine Vet J 1986;18:133–7.
11. Morgan RE, Dunkel B, Spiro S, et al. Computed tomographic and magnetic resonance imaging of a coup contrecoup traumatic brain injury in a horse. Equine Vet Educ 2022;34(4):e151–6.
12. Dunkel B, Corley KT, Johnson AL, et al. Pneumocephalus in five horses. Equine Vet J 2013;45:367–71.
13. Hirsch JE, Huber MJ, Hedstorm OR. Intraventricular tension pneumocephalus secondary to head trauma in a horse. Equine Vet Educ 2006;18:145–7.
14. Stover SM, Murray A. The California Postmortem Program: leading the way. Vet Clin North Am Equine Pract 2008;24:21–36.
15. Collar EM, Zavodovskaya R, Spriet M, et al. Caudal lumbar vertebral fractures in California Quarter Horse and Thoroughbred racehorses. Equine Vet J 2015;47: 573–9.
16. Beattie MS. Inflammation and apoptosis: linked therapeutic targets in spinal cord injury. Trends Mol Med 2004;10:580–3.
17. Ashammakhi N, Kim HJ, Ehsanipour A, et al. Regenerative therapies for spinal cord injury. Tissue Eng B Rev 2019;25:471–91.

18. Orr MB, Gensel JC. Interactions of primary insult biomechanics and secondary cascades in spinal cord injury: implications for therapy. Neural Regen Res 2017;12:1618–9.
19. Orr MB, Gensel JC. Spinal cord injury scarring and inflammation: therapies targeting glial and inflammatory responses. Neurotherapeutics 2018;15:541–53.
20. Seddon HJ. A classification of nerve injuries. Br Med J 1942;2:237–9.
21. Furr MO. Disorders of the peripheral nervous system. In: Furr MO, Reed SM, editors. Equine neurology. Second edition. Ames, Iowa: Blackwell Publishing; 2015. p. 429–36.
22. Scrivani PV. Neuroimaging in horses with traumatic brain injury. Equine Vet Educ 2013;25:499–502.
23. Gough SL, Anderson JDC, Dixon JJ. Computed tomographic cervical myelography in horses: Technique and findings in 51 clinical cases. J Vet Intern Med 2020; 34:2142–51.
24. Williams DC. Electrodiagnostics: EMG. Proceedings; ACVIM Brain Camp - On Line 2020.
25. Bazarian JJ, Biberthaler P, Welch RD, et al. Serum GFAP and UCH-L1 for prediction of absence of intracranial injuries on head CT (ALERT-TBI): a multicentre observational study. Lancet Neurol 2018;17:782–9.
26. Kwon BK, Streijger F, Fallah N, et al. Cerebrospinal fluid biomarkers to stratify injury severity and predict outcome in human traumatic spinal cord injury. J Neurotrauma 2017;34:567–80.
27. Zidan N, Fenn J, Griffith E, et al. The Effect of electromagnetic fields on postoperative pain and locomotor recovery in dogs with acute, severe thoracolumbar intervertebral disc extrusion: a randomized placebo-controlled, prospective clinical trial. J Neurotrauma 2018;35:1726–36.
28. Rouanet C, Reges D, Rocha E, et al. Traumatic spinal cord injury: current concepts and treatment update. Arq Neuropsiquiat 2017;75:387–93.
29. Khellaf A, Khan DZ, Helmy A. Recent advances in traumatic brain injury. J Neurol 2019;266:2878–89.
30. Yang B, Zhang F, Cheng F, et al. Strategies and prospects of effective neural circuits reconstruction after spinal cord injury. Cell Death Dis 2020;11:439.
31. Krucoff MO, Miller JP, Saxena T, et al. Toward functional restoration of the central nervous system: a review of translational neuroscience Principles. Neurosurgery 2019;84:30–40.
32. Torregrossa F, Salli M, Grasso G. Emerging therapeutic strategies for traumatic spinal cord injury. World Neurosurg 2020;140:591–601.
33. Jeong HJ, Yun Y, Lee SJ, et al. Biomaterials and strategies for repairing spinal cord lesions. Neurochem Int 2021;144:104973.
34. Nout YS, Mihai G, Tovar CA, et al. Hypertonic saline attenuates cord swelling and edema in experimental spinal cord injury: a study utilizing magnetic resonance imaging. Crit Care Med 2009;37:2160–6.
35. Gu J, Huang H, Huang Y, et al. Hypertonic saline or mannitol for treating elevated intracranial pressure in traumatic brain injury: a meta-analysis of randomized controlled trials. Neurosurg Rev 2019;42:499–509.
36. Badhiwala JH, Wilson JR, Witiw CD, et al. The influence of timing of surgical decompression for acute spinal cord injury: a pooled analysis of individual patient data. Lancet Neurol 2021;20:117–26.
37. Canseco JA, Karamian BA, Bowles DR, et al. Updated review: the steroid controversy for management of spinal cord injury. World Neurosurg 2021;150:1–8.

38. Jeffery N, Boudreau CE, Konarik M, et al. Pharmacokinetics and safety of oral glyburide in dogs with acute spinal cord injury. PeerJ 2018;6:e4387.
39. Galli F, Azzi A, Birringer M, et al. Vitamin E: emerging aspects and new directions. Free Radic Biol Med 2017;102:16–36.
40. Simon NG, Franz CK, Gupta N, et al. Central adaptation following brachial plexus injury. World Neurosurg 2016;85:325–32.
41. Gordon T. Peripheral nerve regeneration and muscle reinnervation. Int J Mol Sci 2020;21:8652.
42. Rossignol F, Brandenberger O, Perkins JD, et al. Modified first or second cervical nerve transplantation technique for the treatment of recurrent laryngeal neuropathy in horses. Equine Vet J 2018;50:457–64.
43. Gutierrez-Nibeyro SD, Werpy NM, White NA 2nd, et al. Outcome of palmar/plantar digital neurectomy in horses with foot pain evaluated with magnetic resonance imaging: 50 cases (2005-2011). Equine Vet J 2015;47:160–4.
44. Grau JW, Baine RE, Bean PA, et al. Learning to promote recovery after spinal cord injury. Exp Neurol 2020;330:113334.

Rehabilitation Strategies for the Neurologic Horse

Sherry A. Johnson, DVM, MS

KEYWORDS

• Neurologic • Rehabilitation • Physiotherapy • Balance • Stability

KEY POINTS

• Manual physical therapy exercises aimed at improving core stability, balance, flexibility, and neuromotor control are some of the most effective strategies for equine neurologic rehabilitation.

• The most efficient neurologic rehabilitation programs use regular, longitudinal patient assessments followed by appropriate adaptation of protocols with both injury-specific and whole-body considerations.

• Specific rehabilitation protocols for the neurologic horse must consider owner, trainer, and associated personnel safety in the handling of ataxic horses.

• Appropriate incorporation of any modality or therapeutic exercise into a successful rehabilitation program relies on an accurate diagnosis and consideration of any orthopedic comorbidities.

INTRODUCTION

Sports medicine and rehabilitation is quickly becoming one of the most progressive and exciting sectors within the equine practice. While the human athletes have embraced the vital role physical therapy and rehabilitation play in the longevity of successful careers, the equine sports medicine community has been slower to identify and incorporate rehabilitative approaches maximally beneficial for specific diagnoses. Barriers to this progress include the lack of universal recommendations regarding the timing, frequency, and specific indications of modalities in conjunction with widely varied therapeutic approaches. Whether human or equine, specific neurologic rehabilitation goals to decrease pain, improve flexibility, increase strength and restore maximal neuromotor control are believed to result in recoveries with less convalescence, less morbidity, and ultimately improved function. The most effective rehabilitation programs use regular, longitudinal patient assessments followed by appropriate adaptation of protocols with both injury-specific and whole-body considerations. Specific

Department of Clinical Sciences, Orthopaedic Research Center at the C. Wayne McIlwraith Translational Medicine Institute, College of Veterinary Medicine and Biomedical Sciences, Colorado State University, Fort Collins, CO 80523, USA
E-mail address: sherryjdvm@gmail.com

Vet Clin Equine 38 (2022) 379–396
https://doi.org/10.1016/j.cveq.2022.05.007
0749-0739/22/Published by Elsevier Inc.
vetequine.theclinics.com

rehabilitation protocols for the neurologic horse must also consider owner, trainer, and associated personnel safety in the handling of ataxic horses, for which subsequent risks and precautions must be thoroughly assessed.

This article will discuss various physical modalities, therapeutic exercises, and strategies being currently used to rehabilitate the neurologic horse. Appropriate incorporation of any modality or therapeutic exercise into a successful rehabilitation program relies on an accurate diagnosis. Unfortunately, universal recommendations regarding the timing, frequency, and specific indications of many of the below-described modalities are still lacking. As further research is able to define specific parameters, significant advancements within the neurologic rehabilitation field can be expected. Example rehabilitation program elements and dynamic progression considerations for the neurologic horse are included at the end of this article for clinician consideration (**Table 1**).

EVALUATION OF THE NEUROLOGIC HORSE FOR REHABILITATION PROTOCOL CONSTRUCTION

Similar to the evaluation of horses with appendicular orthopedic injury, the neurologic horse must be thoroughly examined before rehabilitation protocol construction for which a sample evaluation checklist is provided (Supplementary Item 1). In the evaluation of the neurologic horse, specific attention should be paid to the grade of ataxia, proprioceptive deficits, cervical range of motion, ability to maintain both static and dynamic postural control and any secondary muscle weakness and/or atrophy in addition to previously described neurologic clinical impressions.[1] This information should be collected during both passive (palpation) and dynamic (active) examination, and oftentimes will require experimentation with various physical therapy tools to gauge suitability (ground poles, theraband, balance pads, and so forth) before formal adoption into the rehabilitation program. As specific diagnosis as possible must be achieved in each neurologic case, acknowledging that economic constraints may limit the diagnostic information able to be obtained. With the incorporation of advanced imaging techniques such as cervical computed tomography (CT) in conjunction with myelographic evaluation, the spectrum of pathologic change within the cervical region has been greatly expanded to further characterize specific disease processes contributing to clinical signs (**Fig. 1**), and therefore targeted with multi-modal rehabilitation. In absence of postmortem evaluation, however, specific neurologic diagnoses may not be achieved even in cases with unlimited diagnostic imaging and ante-mortem testing, highlighting a significant source of vulnerability for accurate prognosis and rehabilitative management. Despite these diagnostic limitations, the clinician can use physical examination findings and functional weaknesses to construct a useful rehabilitative program that targets balance, neuromotor control, and global strength using a variety of therapeutic strategies and commercially available physical therapy equipment.

PHYSIOTHERAPEUTIC STRATEGIES TO IMPROVE POSTURAL STABILITY AND BALANCE ACQUITY

Physiotherapeutic exercises aimed at stimulating motor control, flexibility, and stability are regularly used in human physical therapy programs to improve neurologic function. The use of such exercises has been shown to reduce pain, improve neuromotor control and circumvent orthopedic reinjury.[2–4] Human athletes that incorporate specific core balance exercises into their rehabilitation programs are significantly less likely to suffer reinjury during a 12-month period following injury, compared with those individuals with similar injuries that did not emphasize core strength (7% reinjury rate

Table 1
Table outlining components of a generalized rehabilitation program for a horse with mild to moderate neurologic deficits

		First 30 d	60 d	90 d	120 d	180 d
Controlled Exercise	Controlled Walk/Trotting	10 min, 2x/day, walk pace only	15 min, 2x/day, walk pace only	20 min, 2x/day ± weighted surcingle for one session, walk pace only	20 min, 2x/day ± weighted surcingle for one session with 5 min interval trot	25 min, 2x/day, +/− weighted surcingle for one session with 10 min interval trot
	Resistance Band	1st 5 min of each walk session (hind end band only)	1st 10 min of each walk session (hind end band only)	Hind end band for one full exercise session; belly band for 1st 5 min of the opposite session	Hind end band for one full exercise session; belly band for 1st 10 min of the opposite session	Hind end & belly band for one full exercise session; nothing on for the opposite session
	Ground Poles	1–2 passes over 3 poles, 0" & spaced evenly	2–3 passes over 3 poles, (poles 1 & 3 at 0" and middle pole raised 4–6") & spaced evenly	3–5 passes over 4 poles, (poles 1 & 3 raised 4–6", poles 2 & 4 at 0"); spaced evenly	5–7 passes over 5 poles, (poles 1, 3 & 5 raised 4–6" and at opposite slants and poles 2 & 4 at 0") & spaced unevenly Serpentine through 3 poles in figure-8 configuration x 2, alternate directions	7–9 passes over 6 poles, (poles 1, 3 & 5 raised 7–9" and at opposite slants and poles 2 & 4 raised 4–6" and at opposite slants) & spaced unevenly; alternate direction of approach Serpentine through 3 poles in figure-8 configuration x 3 alternate directions
	Backing	/	Back 10 strides straight on flat, firm footing	Back through ground poles arranged in an L-shape x3	Back up a small incline 3x	Back up and down a small incline x3
	Tactile Stimulators	/	/	Bell boots worn on both hindlimbs 1st 5 min of exercise session	Bell boots worn on both hindlimbs 1st 10 min of exercise session	700g pastern weights on both hindlimbs 1st 5 min of exercise session

(continued on next page)

Table 1
(continued)

		First 30 d	60 d	90 d	120 d	180 d
Physiotherapeutic Exercises	Core Exercises	Caudal tail pulls x5 reps Lateral cervical bending to the level of the stifle x5 reps each direction Ventral cervical flexion to the level of the chest x5 reps	Caudal tail pulls x5 reps Lateral cervical bending to the level of the hock x5 reps each direction Ventral cervical flexion to the level of the carpi x5 reps	Caudal tail pulls x5 reps Lateral cervical bending to the level of the hind fetlock x5 reps each direction Ventral cervical flexion to the level of the front fetlock x5 reps	Caudal tail pulls x5 reps, lateral tail pulls x5 reps on each side, sternal lifts x5 reps	Caudal tail pulls x5 reps, lateral tail pulls x5 reps on each side, wither pulls x5 reps on each side, sternal lifts x5 reps
	Balance Pad Work	Green (firm) pads both forelimbs 5 min	Blue (soft) pads both forelimbs 5 min Green (firm) pads both hindlimbs for 5 min	Blue (soft) pads both forelimbs with simultaneous green (firm) pads both hindlimbs for 5 min	Blue (soft) pads both forelimbs with simultaneous green (firm) pads both hindlimbs for 5 min while performing ventral cervical flexions x5 reps	Pads on all four limbs, alternate color for each limb at each session for 5 min while performing: caudal tail pulls x5, ventral cervical flexions x5, lateral cervical bending x5 each direction
	Perturbations	LF & RF perturbations x3 reps, holding pressure for each repetition for 1–3 s	LF & RF perturbations x5 reps, holding pressure for each repetition for 3–5 s	LF & RF perturbations x5 reps, holding pressure for each repetition for 3–5 s with opposite forelimb on green (firm) pad	LF & RF perturbations x5 reps, holding pressure for each repetition for 3–5 s with opposite forelimb on blue (soft) pad	LF & RF perturbations x5 reps, holding pressure for each repetition for 3–5 s with opposite forelimb on blue (soft) pad & LH/RH limbs on green (firm) pads

Whole-Body Vibration	Theraplate	/	15 min, 2x/day	20 min, 2x/day	20 min, 2x/day while performing lateral cervical bending x5 reps each direction	20 min, 2x/day while performing sternal lifts, caudal tail pulls & lateral cervical bending x5 reps each direction
Aquatic Exercise	Underwater Treadmill	/	/	Increase by 1 minute/session from 5 min; gradually increase water depth to the level of the shoulder	20 min, 1x/day with water at the level of the shoulder	30 min, 1x/day with alternating water depths

Specific diagnosis, presence of orthopedic comorbidities, behavioral considerations, and equipment availability ultimately dictate this framework's suitability for each patient. This table is not meant to be blanketly applied to all neurologic cases, but rather provided to give the clinician a framework of gradual, titrated use of a variety of physical therapy components. All neurologic rehabilitation programs should be overseen by the primary care veterinarian with regular, longitudinal monitoring to ensure each protocol is productive for the horse and safe for associated personnel.

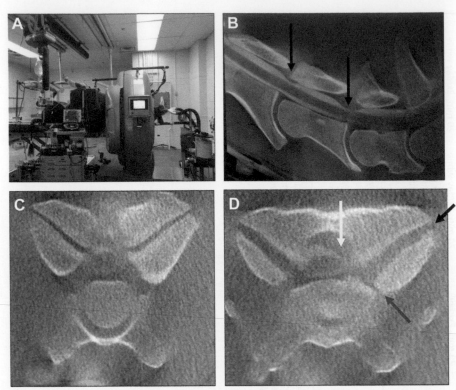

Fig. 1. Horse placed under general anesthesia for cone-beam computed tomographic (CT) guided myelographic evaluation at Colorado State University (*A*). This case was subsequently diagnosed with dynamic spinal cord compression at C5/6 and C6/7 on sagittal plane CT images (*black arrows, B*) in addition to left-sided extradural compression at C6/7 (*yellow arrow D*), left facet widening with marked osteoarthritis (*black arrow, D*) and left spinal nerve root compression on transverse plane CT images (*red arrow, D*). This patient's more normal C4/5 articular facet in the transverse CT plane is presented for comparison (*C*).

in the balance training group vs 29% reinjury rate in the control group).[3] Strengthening, improving proprioception and balance control following injury remains a central focus of human physical therapy programs, and while standardized investigations have yet to focus on equine applications, there are several mechanisms through which neuro-motor control can be recruited to aid the clinician in neurologic rehabilitation outcome. Improving postural stability and balance control through improving strength, size, and symmetry of the spinal stabilizer muscle multifidus remain one of the most promising targets for the equine clinician.[5,6] This muscle can be targeted through the use of physiotherapeutic exercises,[5] various forms of perturbation [6] and even whole-body vibration.[7]

Therapeutic Exercises

Pursuant to the neurologic equine patient, several core strengthening exercises and their role in activating deep, stabilizing epaxial musculature to subsequently improve postural motor control and alter kinematics have been investigated.[5,6,8,9] Both baited and passive exercises offer opportunities to facilitate stretching during dynamic phases and strengthening during static phases of the exercise. Institution of dynamic

Ventral Cervical Flexion to Chest

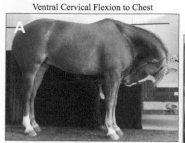

Biomechanical Target Regions:
Cranial cervical spine
Cranial thoracic spine
Rectus abdominus

Ventral Cervical Flexion to Carpi

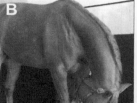

Biomechanical Target Regions:
Middle cervical spine
Cranial to central thoracic spine
Rectus abdominus

Ventral Cervical Flexion to Front
Fetlocks

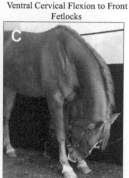

Biomechanical Target Regions:
Entire cervical spine
Entire T/L spine & LS
Rectus abdominus

Fig. 2. Ventral cervical flexion exercises performed at 3 different levels: chest (*A*), carpi (*B*) and front fetlocks (*C*). Corresponding anatomic regions targeted with each exercise listed, respectively, for each level based on research performed by[8,9] that found the largest angular changes to occur within the cranial and caudal cervical regions (<10° change within the middle cervical spine). Incorporation of these exercises must align with the rehabilitative goal of improving cervical range of motion, augmenting core stability, and stretching the thoracolumbar region. (Photos courtesy of Equine Sports Medicine & Rehabilitation, Whitesboro, TX.)

mobilization exercises over a 3-month time period has been shown to increase both size and symmetry of the multifidus muscle as assessed through longitudinal ultrasonographic evaluation.[5] A recent investigation demonstrated a positive association between postural stability and multifidus muscle hypertrophy in lame horses undergoing individualized rehabilitation programs.[6] While blanket recommendations regarding the prescription of the below listed exercises is not advised, the stretches listed below offer means through which various regions of the cervical and thoracolumbar spine may be targeted (**Figs. 2** and **3**).

In the author's experience, these dynamic exercises are most effectively instituted as part of an individualized program, then progressively modified to increase in difficulty. Depending on the neuroanatomic localization of the lesion, targeting various regions of the cervical spine is possible based on the level of dynamic bending.[8,9] As the patient improves in flexibility and ability to complete various physiotherapeutic exercises the clinician can then begin to increase the level of difficulty by altering static postural (stance) position (limb protracted vs retracted, for example), or combining these exercises with other physical therapy aides (resistance bands and/or balance pads, for example). Suitability for these exercises must be assessed carefully in terms of a patient's ability to safely and comfortably perform them in light of the specific neurologic diagnosis. More physiologic benefit will be achieved when fewer repetition of these types of stretches can be correctly performed in contrast to agitation with increased repetitions using an incorrect form, so care must be taken to ensure the exercises are performed in as pain-free state as possible.

Significant muscle hypertonicity and spasming contributing to the avoidance of these exercises may be alleviated by first applying heat therapy to the cervical or

Lateral Cervical Bending to Stifle Level

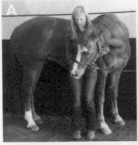

Lateral Cervical Bending to Hock Level

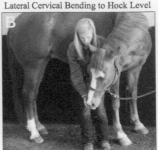

Lateral Cervical Bending to Hind Fetlock Level

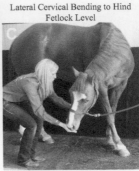

<u>Biomechanical Target Regions</u>:
Lower cervical spine
Cranial thoracic spine
Abdominal musculature

<u>Biomechanical Target Regions</u>:
Middle cervical spine
Central thoracic spine
Abdominal musculature

<u>Biomechanical Target Regions</u>:
Entire cervical spine
Entire T/L spine
Abdominal musculature

Fig. 3. Lateral cervical bending exercises performed at 3 different levels: stifle (*A*), hock (*B*) and hind fetlocks (*C*). Corresponding anatomic regions targeted with each exercise listed, respectively, for each level based on research performed by[10] that evaluated lateral cervical bending at the levels of girth, hip or tarsus for which they noted activation through the multifidus and longus colli muscles. They also noted that the further caudally horses were bending, the more the caudal cervical and thoracolumbar regions were activated. Incorporation of these exercises must align with the rehabilitative goal of improving cervical range of motion, augmenting core stability, and increasing lateral spinal motion. (Photos courtesy of Equine Sports Medicine & Rehabilitation, Whitesboro, TX.)

thoracolumbar regions for 15 to 30 minutes. Heat therapy may also be combined with massage using a variety of commercially available human self-massage tools that in the author's experience are suitable for equine use due to various pressure and intensity settings that can be adjusted as needed. This warm-up period can help increase soft tissue extensibility, improve pain and increase flexibility which may ultimately result in improved function.

Forms of Balance Perturbation

Neuromotor control retraining is a fundamental aspect of human physical therapy programs in both elderly and individuals with neurologic conditions.[11] Perturbation-based balance training involves repeated postural perturbations to improve control of rapid balance reactions.[11] This form of training, combined with physical exercise has been shown to dramatically improve functional outcomes and reduce falls.[11,12]

Perturbation training specifically has not yet been studied in horses, but it is well accepted that postural stability is integral in maintaining equine balance, protecting the spinal column, and allowing more accurate reactions to destabilizing forces.[6] Improving postural stability in neurologic horses, therefore, represents a key rehabilitative target to improve both static and dynamic function. A variety of physical therapy aides can be used by the practitioner in veterinary-guided rehabilitative management of the neurologic horse, including recently developed foam pad systems (**Fig. 4**).[a] The

---

[a] Sure Foot Equine, Washington, VA.

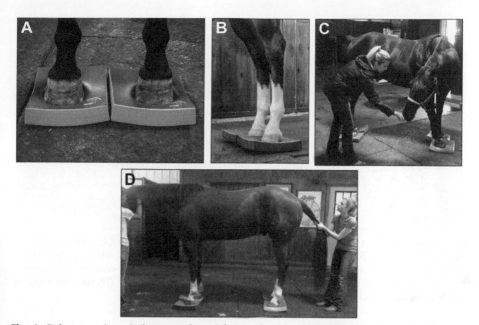

Fig. 4. Balance pad use in horses referred for professional rehabilitation: (*A*) Bilateral fore-limb application while standing on medium density (*purple*) Sure Foot balance pads; (*B*) Bilateral hindlimb application while standing on firm density (*green*) Sure Foot balance pads. (*C*) Bilateral forelimb application with blue pads (soft) and bilateral hindlimb green (firm) pad application while performing lateral cervical bending to the level of the hock for increasing balance acquity challenge. (*D*) Multi-limb green (firm) and blue (soft) application while performing a caudal tail pull for additional balance perturbation. (Photos courtesy of Equine Sports Medicine & Rehabilitation, Whitesboro, TX.)

pads are commercially available in a variety of firmness, and can be used for forelimb, hindlimb or multi-limb use. The goal of the use of these pads is to challenge and/or exacerbate postural weakness to stimulate and ultimately improve neuromuscular function. Depending on the severity of neurologic dysfunction, the author typically begins with forelimb, firm-pad application on a smooth, nonslick surface to ensure safety for both horse and handler. Once the horse acclimates both physically and behaviorally to forelimb, firm-pad application, the author typically then gradually incorporates more soft pads, and eventual hindlimb and/or all four-limb application. Once the balance pad is mastered in a standard application fashion (on a flat, nonslick surface), the clinician can then begin to incorporate further challenges to the neurologic system by introducing manual perturbation or combining pad application with core exercises (see **Fig. 4**).

The author also finds the pads to be a worthwhile diagnostic tool due to the fact that subtle neurologic deficits may go undetected during the normal, dynamic examination, but be exacerbated with a balance challenge. It often times is unclear whether subtle body swaying while on the pads indicates true neurologic dysfunction, core weakness, or a combination of both, but the author believes global function can be improved through titrated retraining exercises. The clinician must be fully mindful of concurrent orthopedic injuries for strategic pad use so as not to exacerbate existing injuries through soft-pad use.

Manual perturbation exercises also represent an avenue through which the clinician can stimulate neuromuscular feedback in the neurologic horse. Obvious safety

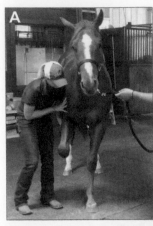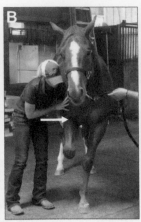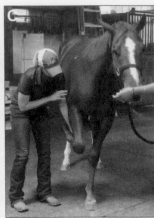

Fig. 5. Manual right forelimb perturbation prepressure application (*A*), during pressure application for 3 to 5 seconds (*white arrow, B*) and on gradual release during balance recuperation (*C*). Such exercises represent an avenue through which the clinician can dynamically stimulate neuromuscular feedback in the neurologic horse. (Photos courtesy of Equine Sports Medicine & Rehabilitation, Whitesboro, TX.)

considerations must be thoroughly evaluated, but if deemed physically stable enough, perturbation challenges can be introduced by lifting a forelimb or hindlimb and gently applying steady pressure for 3 to 5 seconds toward the weight-bearing limb, followed by gradual pressure release (**Fig. 5**) and subsequent balance recuperation. Surface changes and/or incline/decline work can also be introduced as horses progress through a rehabilitative program, and can eventually incorporate a variety of proprioceptive stimulation tools such as ground poles, tactile stimulators, or resistance bands.

Proprioceptive Stimulation and Strengthening Tools

Because declines in muscular strength can be quite dramatic in human neurologic conditions and often exacerbate concurrent weakness, human neuromotor physical therapy programs focus heavily on maintaining as much muscular strength as possible in the rehabilitative setting. Resistance band training is successfully used in human physical therapy programs to improve core strength and stability.[13–15] The use of various strength training aids within the equine rehabilitation setting has been of recent interest, including the use of a system of elastic resistance bands, full-body wraps, and Pessoa lines.[16–18] Commonly referred to as a Theraband,[19–21] the two-piece equine elastic band system is thought to stimulate core abdominal muscles with the abdominal band and engage hindlimb musculature with the hindquarter band (**Fig. 6**). Its use in horses at a trot was recently investigated and found to reduce mediolateral and rotational movement throughout the thoracolumbar region.[17] Further studies investigating more long-term use and potential mechanistic pathways will help refine its use in the neurologic rehabilitation setting. Also pertinent to the rehabilitation of the axial skeleton is the use of training lines. Pessoa training aids were demonstrated to increase both lumbosacral angles and thoracolumbar dorsoventral excursion when used in horses being lunged at a jog,[18] but care must be used when prescribing their use in neurologic horses with concurrent cervical pain. Also recently

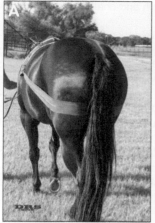
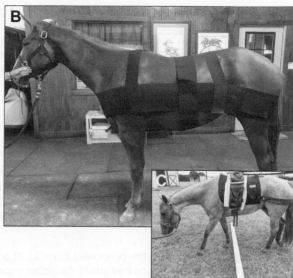

Fig. 6. Incorporation of various forms of resistance band systems that are commercially available including hind end Theraband system (EquiCore Concepts, LLC [*A*]) and Eagle Pro-SIx's full-body wrap (*B*). Multi-modal incorporation of resistance band work can be accomplished by combining its use with ground pole and weighted surcingle use (*C*). (Photos courtesy of Equine Sports Medicine & Rehabilitation (Whitesboro, TX) and DRS Photography.)

available to the clinician is a commercially available full-body resistance band wrap[b] that the author has used in select neurologic cases (see **Fig. 6**). Formal studies are lacking on this tool specifically, but it is the author's impression that the full-body wrap provides tactile stimulation in a stabilizing manner that can be used during controlled exercise sessions, self-exercise (turnout), or as part of a multi-modal, cross-training rehabilitative program (in combination with ground poles, tactile stimulators, core stretches, and so forth). With its continued use and protocol refinement, further recommendations can be expected.

Specific to equine neurologic dysfunction, other physical therapy aides such as ground poles and tactile stimulators offer clinicians passive means of engaging neuromotor control during activities in daily rehabilitation or training. Ground poles when arranged at various distances, heights and configurations can encourage increases in thoracolumbar excursion, active range of joint motion, and limb suspension.[22] Swing and stance phase kinematics while going over ground poles have been previously investigated,[22,22] with several interesting findings related to their incorporation into neurologic rehabilitation. Ground pole exposure was noted specifically to increase forelimb braking, increase the activity of forelimb adductors, and activate flexor muscles.[22,22] Their gradual integration into neurologic rehabilitation programs can aid the clinician in augmenting controlled proprioceptive challenges, activating specific muscle groups, and increasing the activity of muscles responsible for downward speed transitions (braking). Hill work and incorporating backing exercises into hill work can

[b] Eagle ProSix Bark River, MI 49807.

also be used to simultaneously improve muscular strength and challenge proprioceptive acuity.

The effects of tactile stimulators on biomechanical stimulation have also been previously investigated.[22,23] When 9 sound horses were evaluated with or without 55g
weighted tactile stimulators on the hind pasterns, higher foot flight arcs, reduced
hind stance duration, and increased concentric activity of tarsal musculature were
appreciated.[23] In subsequent investigation, this same research group evaluated 4
types of tactile stimulators including a strap, tactile stimulators only, a 700g limb
weight only, and a 700g limb weight with tactile stimulators.[22] Authors noted that
the highest foot flight arc was appreciated with the 700g weight with tactile stimulator.
Lowest hoof flight arcs were observed with no stimulation or loose straps only.[22]
Incorporation of various forms of tactile stimulators can be used for forelimb or hindlimb use within the neurologic rehabilitative setting including bell boots, homemade
tactile stimulators, or custom-made 700g pastern weights (**Fig. 7**).

AQUATIC THERAPY

In the rehabilitation setting, the proposed benefits of aquatic exercise include buoyancy, viscosity, and resistance that promote global improvements in muscular timing,
strength, and neuromotor control.[24] Several options to use aquatic therapy for the
equine athlete are currently available including above-ground underwater treadmills,
in-ground underwater treadmills, and swimming pools (circular or straight).[19] Investigations into the benefits of aquatic therapy for the equine patient have thus far reported subsequent physiologic responses,[25–27] biomechanical effects [28] its role in
mitigating carpal osteoarthritis [29] and improvements in postural sway.[24] Alterations
in limb kinematics secondary to varying water depths provide the clinician a means
of targeting or sparing flexion/extension joint angles depending on the rehabilitation
goals of the specific patient.[30] It was also recently demonstrated that walking slowly
(0.8 m/s) on a water treadmill reduced forelimb protraction-retraction range of motion

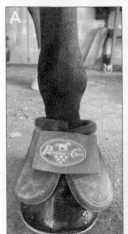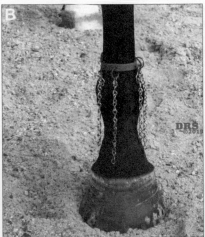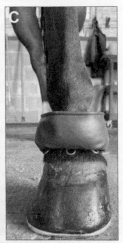

Fig. 7. Incorporation of various forms of tactile stimulators can be used for forelimb or hindlimb use within the neurologic rehabilitative setting including bell boots (*A*), homemade
tactile stimulators (*B*) or custom-made 700g pastern weights with the option to attach
tactile stimulators (*C*, Mark Williams/Scott McClure). (Photos courtesy of Equine Sports Medicine & Rehabilitation (Whitesboro, TX) and DRS Photography.)

and increased hindlimb protraction-retraction range of motion compared with walking on a dry treadmill at normal speed (1.6 m/s).[31,32] Based on these findings, the authors concluded that forelimb protraction was decreased while hindlimb retraction was increased during water treadmill exercise, which could be used to design rehabilitation programs.[31] When axial rotation, lateral bending and pelvic flexion were evaluated in a population of riding horses, significant increases in rotation and flexion of the back were noted at higher water depths.[33] Additionally, pelvic flexion was significantly increased at higher water levels.[33] Similarly, increases in cranial thoracic extension and thoracolumbar flexion were appreciated in 14 horses walking in high water compared with water at lower depths.[33]

The safety and suitability of exposing neurologic horses to aquatic work must be carefully considered in light of equipment available, rehabilitative goal, and severity of neurologic dysfunction secondary to a specific diagnosis. The benefits of improving postural sway as a means of increasing global strength and stability through underwater treadmill exercise are well documented,[24] but severe neurologic dysfunction may prohibit the clinician from safely exposing select cases to this rehabilitative therapy. In the author's experience, the decision to incorporate aquatic work can be aided through the use of safety benchmark assessments such as: (1) grade of ataxia at a walk on firm, flat footing; (2) grade of ataxia while performing incline/decline exercise; and (3) exacerbation of ataxia while lightly sedated. Should the assigned ataxic grade be > 2 according to the modified ataxia-grading scale of 0 to 4 [34-38] for any condition, it is the author's experience that aquatic exercise should be avoided until neurologic improvement can be achieved. In cases whereby a ramp must be navigated in and/ or out of the underwater treadmill the neurologic horse's ability to safely perform incline and decline work on a dry, flat surface should be assessed before the commencement of aquatic exercise involving ramp entry and/or exit. Additionally, clinicians should be mindful that the lower cervical region is put into significant (temporary) extension during decline ramp entry into a high water depth in-ground linear underwater treadmill unit, so if neurologic signs or cervical pain seem to be significantly worsened on dry, flat ground with elevated head and/or neck carriage, this clinical exacerbation may prohibit this specific form of aquatic exercise and require the use of an underwater treadmill unit capable of adjusting water depth appropriately. Should underwater treadmill work be able to be safely incorporated, gradual increases in exposure time and water depth can be considered to achieve rehabilitative goals of improving neuromotor strength, timing, control, and overall stability in the neurologic horse. Concurrent orthopedic morbidities must also be considered in terms of water depth, time, and frequency of exposure to aquatic exercise.

WHOLE-BODY VIBRATION

Of recent interest within the equine community has been the use of low-amplitude, low-frequency mechanical vibration therapy. Although empirically prescribed, perceived benefits reported by owners and horsemen include general relaxation and overall well-being. Acute hematologic and clinical effects of horses undergoing vibration therapy have been recently described, noting no adverse effects following vibration sessions [Carstanjen]. Within the neurologic rehabilitative setting, there has been recent interest in the effects of prolonged vibration therapy on the cross-sectional area and symmetry of the multifidus muscle.[7] A significant increase in multifidus muscle cross-sectional size and symmetry was found following 60 days of twice daily, 30-minute whole-body vibration sessions.[7] Known for its role in spinal stabilization and postural muscle acuity as previously discussed, the development of the multifidus muscle is thought to have potential as an osteoarthritis deterrent [Hides x3] and axial skeleton stabilizer,[6] making it a potential therapeutic target for neurologic rehabilitation programs. With further experimentation expected, insight into more specific protocol applications and incorporation can be expected.

SUMMARY

Rehabilitation of the neurologic horse represents a unique challenge for the equine practitioner, but can often be rewarding due to dramatic clinical improvements in balance, neuromotor control, flexibility, and global strength. Safety of the horse and personnel interacting with the horse during rehabilitative activities must be considered first and foremost. In the author's experience, manual physical therapy exercises aimed at improving core stability, balance, flexibility, and neuromotor control are integral for the most effective rehabilitation outcomes rather than machines alone. Neuroanatomic localization and diagnosis specificity enable the practitioner to determine suitability for such rehabilitative tasks, and with the advent of evolving strategies and commercially available equipment, the bandwidth for professionally guided programs under direct veterinary supervision and for at-home use are continuously being developed and expected to improve traditional outcomes.

CLINICS CARE POINTS

- The multifidus muscle remains one of the most promising rehabilitative targets for improving spinal stabilization. It can be targeted specifically through the use of physiotherapeutic exercises, various forms of perturbation and even whole body vibration.

- For the evaluation of the neurologic horse, specific attention should be paid to grade of ataxia, proprioceptive deficits, cervical range of motion, ability to maintain both static and dynamic postural control and any secondary muscle weakness and/or atrophy.

- The clinician can utilize physical examination findings and functional weaknesses to construct a useful rehabilitative program that targets balance, neuromotor control and global strength using a variety of therapeutic strategies and commercially available physical therapy equipment.

DISCLOSURE

S.A. Johnson is a cofounder and partner of Equine Core, Inc (Fort Collins, CO), and a partner in Equine Sports Medicine & Rehabilitation (Whitesboro, TX).

REFERENCES

1. Alcott CJ. Evaluation of ataxia in the horse. Equine Vet Educ 2015. https://doi.org/10.1111/eve.12461.
2. Kavcic N, Grenier S, McGill SM. Determining the Stabilizing Role of Individual Torso Muscles During Rehabilitation Exercises. Spine 2004;29(11):1254–65.
3. Holme E, Magnusson SP, Becher K, et al. The effect of supervised rehabilitation on strength, postural sway, position sense and re-injury risk after acute ankle sprain. Scan J Med Sci Sports 1999;9:104–9.
4. Salavati M, Akhbari B. Effect of spinal stabilization exercise on dynamic postural control and visual dependency in subjects with chronic non-specific low back pain. J Bodyw Mov Ther 2016;20:441e8.

5. Stubbs NC, Kaiser LJ, Hauptman J, et al. Dynamic mobilisation exercises increase cross sectional area of musculus multifidus. Equine Vet J 2011;43(5): 522–9.

6. Ellis KL, King MR. Relationship between postural stability and paraspinal muscle adaptation in lame horses undergoing rehabilitation. J Eq Vet Sci 2020;91:1–8.

7. Halsberghe BT, Gordon-Ross P, Peterson R. Whole body vibration affects the cross-sectional area and symmetry of the m. multifidus of the thoracolumbar spine in the horse. Eq Vet E 2017;29(9):494–9.

8. Clayton HM, Kaiser LJ, Lavagnin M, et al. Dynamic mobilisations in cervical flexion: effects on intervertebral angulations. Equine Vet J 2010;42:688–94.

9. Clayton HM, White AD, Kaiser LJ, et al. Hindlimb response to tactile stimulation of the pastern and coronet. Equine Vet J 2010;42(3):227–33.

10. Clayton HM, Kaiser LJ, Lavagnino M, Stubbs NC. Evaluation of intersegmental vertebral motion during performance of dynamic mobilization exercises in cervical lateral bending in horses. Am J Vet Res 2012;73(8):1153–9.

11. Mansfield A, Wong JS, Bryce J, et al. Does perturbation-based balance training prevent falls? Systematic review and meta-analysis of preliminary randomized controlled trials. Phys Ther 2015;95(5):700–9.

12. Gerards MHG, McCrum C, Mansfield A, et al. Perturbation-based balance training for falls reduction among older adults: Current evidence and implications for clinical practice. Geriatr Gerontol Int 2017;17:2294–303.

13. Kell RT, Asmundson GJG. A comparison of two forms of periodized exercise rehabilitation programs in the management of chronic nonspecific low-back pain. J Strength Cond Res 2009;23:513–23.

14. Macedo LG, Maher CG, Latimer J, et al. Motor control exercise for persistent, nonspecific low back pain: a systematic review. Phys Ther 2009;89:9 25.

15. Sundstrup E, Jakobsen MD, Andersen CH, et al. Evaluation of elastic bands for lower extremity resistance training in adults with and without musculo- skeletal pain. Scand J Med Sci Sports 2014;24:e353–9.

16. Goff LS. Equine therapy and rehabilitation. In: McGowan CM, editor. Animal physiotherapy; assessment, treatment and rehabilitation of animals. Oxford (England): Blackwell Publishing Ltd; 2007. p. 239–50.

17. Pfau T, Simons V, Rombach N, et al. Effect of a 4-week elastic resistance band training regimen on back kinematics in horses trotting in-hand and on the lunge. Equive Vet J 2017;49:829–35.

18. Walker VA, Dyson SJ, Murray RC. Effect of a Pessoa training aid on temporal, linear and angular variables of the working trot. Vet J 2013;198:404–11.

19. Haussler KK, King MR. Physical rehabilitation. In: McIlwraith CW, Frisbie DD, Kawcak CE, et al, editors. Joint disease in the horse. 2nd edition. St Louis (MO): Elsevier; 2016. p. 243–65.

20. Brown S, Stubbs NC, Kaiser LJ, et al. Swing phase kinematics of horses trotting over poles. Equine Vet J 2015;47:107–12.

21. Clayton HM, Stubbs NC, Lavagnino L. Stance phase kinematics and kinetics of horses trotting over poles. Equine Vet J 2015;47:113–8.

22. Clayton HM, Kaiser LJ, Stubbs NC. Hind limb flexion response to different types of tactile devices. Am J Vet Res 2011;72:1489–95.

23. Clayton HM, White AD, Kaiser LJ, et al. Hindlimb response to tactile stimulation of the pastern and coronet. Equine Vet J 2010;42(3):227–33.

24. King M, Haussler K, Kawcak C, et al. Effect of under-water treadmill exercise on postural sway in horses with experimentally induced carpal osteoarthritis. Am J Vet Res 2013;74:971–82.

25. Hobo S, Yosjida K, Yoshihara T. Characteristics of respiratory function during swimming exercise in Thoroughbreds. J Vet Med Sci 1998;60(6):687–9.

26. Voss B, Mohr E, Krzywanek H. Effects of aqua-treadmill exercise on selected blood parameters and on heart-rate variability of horses. J Vet Med A Physiol Pathol Clin Med 2002;49(3):137–43.

27. Nankervis KJ, Williams RJ. Heart rate responses during acclimation of horses to water treadmill exercise. Equine Vet J 2006;36(Suppl):110–2.

28. Scott R, Nankervis K, Stringer C, et al. The effect of water height on stride frequency, stride length and heart rate during water treadmill exercise. Equine Vet J 2010;38(Suppl):662–4.

29. King MR, Haussler KK, Kawcak CE, et al. Biomechanical and histologic evaluation of the effects of underwater treadmill exercise on horses with experimentally induced osteoarthritis of the middle carpal joint. Am J Vet Res 2017;78(5):558–69.

30. Mendez-Angulo JL, Firshman AM, Groschen DM, et al. Effect of water depth on amount of flexion and extension of joints of the distal aspects of the limbs in healthy horses walking on an underwater treadmill. Am J Vet Res 2013;74(4): 557–66.

31. Nankervis KJ, Lefrancois K. A comparison of protraction-retraction of the distal limb during treadmill and water treadmill walking in horses. J Eq Vet Sci 2018; 70:57–62.

32. Mooij MJW, Jans W, den Heijer GJL, et al. Biomechanical responses of the back of riding horses to water treadmill exercise. Vet J 2013;198:120–3.

33. Nankervis KJ, Finney P, Launder L. Water depth modifies back kinematics of horses during water treadmill exercise. Equine Vet J 2016;48:732–6.

34. Reed SM. Neurologic exam. J Equine Vet Sci 2003;23:484–92.

35. Carstanjen B, Balali M, Gajewski Z, et al. Short-term whole body vibration exercise in adult healthy horses. Pol J Vet Sci 2013;16(2):403–5.

36. Hides J, Richardson C, Jull G. Multifidus muscle recovery is not automatic after resolution of acute, first-episode low back pain. Spine 1996;21:2763–9.

37. Hides JA, Jull GA, Richardson CA. Long-term effects of specific stabilizing exercises for first-episode low back pain. Spine 2001;26:E243–8.

38. Hides J, Gilmore C, Stanton W, et al. Multifidus size and symmetry among chronic LBP and healthy asymptomatic subjects. Man Ther 2008;13:43–9.

SUPPLEMENTARY ITEM 1: A SAMPLE EVALUATION CHECKLIST THAT CAN BE INCORPORATED FOR THE THOROUGH EXAMINATION OF THE NEUROLOGIC HORSE FOR REHABILITATION PROTOCOL CONSTRUCTION.

100-POINT REHABILITATION EVALUATION

Equine Sports Medicine and Rehabilitation

eCORE

Horse: _____ Date: _____ Evaluator: _____

Conformation Notes: _____ Stance/Posture At Rest: _____ Feet: _____

	WNL	Mildly Abnormal	Moderately Abnormal	Markedly Abnormal	Notes
LF Brachiocephalicus Sensitivity					
LF Retraction					
LF Protraction					
LF Scapular Glide					
LF Shoulder Circumductions					
LF Perturbations					
LF Wither Pulls Standing Square					
RF Brachiocephalicus Sensitivity					
RF Retraction					
RF Protraction					
RF Scapular Glide					
RF Shoulder Circumductions					
RF Perturbations					
RF Wither Pulls Standing Square					
Sternal Lifts					
LS Tucks					
Left TMJ Palpation					
Poll Palpation/Manip					
Left Lateral Cervical Bending					
Left Cervical Facet Palpation (C2-C7)					
Right TMJ Palpation					
Right Lateral Cervical Bending					
Right Cervical Facet Palpation (C2-C7)					
Ventral Cervical Flexion					
Left Lateral Tail Pulls					
Right Lateral Tail Pulls					
Caudal Tail Pulls					
Direct DSP Palpation					
Direct Tuber Sacrale Compression					
Myofascial Restriction Left Side					
Myofascial Restriction Left Side					
T/L Left Lateral Bending					
T/L Right Lateral Bending					
Lumbar Left Lateral Bending					
Lumbar Right Lateral Bending					
Sensitivity off cranial aspect tuber coxae LH					
Sensitivity off cranial aspect tuber coxae RH					
LH tuber coxae DV excursion					
RH tuber coxae DV excursion					
LF RC/MC Joints					
LF Fetlock Joint					
LF DIP Joint					
LF Medial/Lateral Splint Bones					
LF PSL Palpation					
LF LSB Palpation					
LF MSB Palpation					
LF Tendon Sheath Palpation/Sensitivity					
LF Hoof Integrity					
RF RC/MC Joints					
RF Fetlock Joint					
RF DIP Joint					
RF Medial/Lateral Splint Bones					
RF PSL Palpation					
RF LSB Palpation					
RF MSB Palpation					
RF Tendon Sheath Palpation/Sensitivity					
RF Hoof Integrity					

	WNL	Mildly Abnormal	Moderately Abnormal	Markedly Abnormal	Notes
Pelvic Symmetry – tuber sacrale, tuber coxae and tuber ischia					
LH Middle Gluteal Development/Trigger Points					
LH Biceps Femoris Development					
LH Circumductions Square					
LH Circumductions Retracted					
LH Circumductions Protracted					
LH Protraction					
LH Retraction					
LH Perturbations					
LH Stifle – MFT/FP/LFT effusion					
LH Stifle ROM – flexion and extension					
LH Tarsal Palpation – TCJ, TMT, DIT					
LH Tarsal ROM					
LH PSL Palpation					
LH Medial/Lateral Splint Bones					
LH LSB Palpation					
LH MSB Palpation					
LH Fetlock Joint (effusion and ROM)					
LH Tendon Sheath Palpation/Sensitivity					
LH PIP Joint					
LH DIP Joint					
LH Hoof Integrity					
RH Middle Gluteal Development/Trigger Points					
RH Biceps Femoris Development					
RH Circumductions Square					
RH Circumductions Retracted					
RH Circumductions Protracted					
RH Protraction					
RH Retraction					
RH Perturbations					
RH Stifle – MFT/FP/LFT effusion					
RH Stifle ROM – flexion and extension					
RH Tarsal Palpation – TCJ, TMT, DIT					
RH Tarsal ROM					
RH PSL Palpation					
RH Medial/Lateral Splint Bones					
RH LSB Palpation					
RH MSB Palpation					
RH Fetlock Joint (effusion and ROM)					
RH Tendon Sheath Palpation/Sensitivity					
RH PIP Joint					
RH DIP Joint					
RH Hoof Integrity					
Ground Poles					
hind end Theraband					
Abd Theraband					
Surfaces					
Backing					
MISC NOTES					

Vestibular Disease

Monica Aleman, MVZ Cert, PhD

KEYWORDS

- Balance • Brainstem • Hair cells • Nystagmus • Semicircular

KEY POINTS

- The vestibular system is the primary specialized proprioception system responsible for maintaining balance (equilibrium) relative to gravity and orientation of the eyes, neck, trunk, and limbs during rest and movement.
- The vestibular system has peripheral and central components.
- Most of the clinical signs of vestibular disease are ipsilateral to the side of the lesion.
- Common clinical signs of disease include head tilt, pathologic nystagmus, ventrolateral strabismus, body leaning, moving in tight circles, and ataxia.
- Acute profound vestibular signs should not always prompt euthanasia since complete resolution might be possible depending on cause.

INTRODUCTION

The vestibular system is a specialized sensory system responsible for maintaining the position of the eyes, neck, trunk, and limbs relative to the position or movement of the head at any time.[1,2] Two vestibular reflexes are important in the stabilization of eyes, neck, trunk, and limbs position in space.[1] These reflexes are the vestibulo-ocular and vestibulospinal reflexes.[1,3] Therefore, dysfunction of the vestibular system will result in multiple clinical signs involving the position of the areas previously mentioned. To understand disease processes, it is important to review functional neuroanatomy (anatomy and pathways associated with the vestibular system).[2]

The vestibular system is a special proprioception system that receptor develops in conjunction with the special somatic afferent system (auditory system), derived from the ectoderm and contained in a mesoderm-derived structure with fluid-filled lumen.[2] These receptors are located in the inner ear.[2] The reader is referred elsewhere for a detailed description of the embryologic development of this system.[2] The inner ear is composed of the cochlea, vestibule, and 3 semicircular canals, which form the bony labyrinth of the petrous temporal bone.[1,2] All 3 areas contain perilymph similar to cerebrospinal fluid (CSF).[2] The vestibule and semicircular canals serve vestibular function, whereas the cochlea is involved in auditory function.[1] The bony labyrinth

SVM: Department of Medicine and Epidemiology, University of California, Tupper Hall 2108, One Shields Avenue, Davis, CA 95616, USA
E-mail address: mraleman@ucdavis.edu

Vet Clin Equine 38 (2022) 397–407
https://doi.org/10.1016/j.cveq.2022.05.008
0749-0739/22/© 2022 Elsevier Inc. All rights reserved.

Abbreviations	
BAER	Brainstem auditory evoked responses
CN	Cranial nerve
MLF	Medial longitudinal fasciculus
THO	Temporohyoid osteoarthropathy
VS	Vestibular system

has 2 openings: vestibular and cochlear window.[2] Within the bony labyrinth is the membranous labyrinth, which comprises the cochlear duct, utricle, saccule, and the 3 semicircular canals (**Fig. 1**).[2,4] These areas contain endolymph derived from blood vessels and absorb back into blood vessels.[2] The semicircular canals consist of 3 tubular structures projecting from the vestibule and oriented at 90° from each other.[2] These structures are the anterior (vertical), posterior (vertical), and lateral (horizontal) semicircular canals.[2] The end of each canal is dilated into an ampulla, which is connected to the vestibule.[4] Within the ampulla, sensory receptors and cristae ampullaris in the membranous labyrinth are responsible for the detection of angular movements of the head.[1] On the surface of the crista, a gelatinous structure composed of a protein-polysaccharide material called the cupula extends across the ampulla.[2] This neuroepithelium is composed of 2 cell types: hair cells and supporting cells.[2] The dendritic areas of the vestibular nerve form synapsis with the hair cells.[2] The hair cells serve as transducers with high sensitivity to mechanical stimulation (mechanoreceptors) and direction.[2] The hair cells have 40 to 80 hairs or modified microvilli (stereocilia) and a single modified cilium (kinocilium).[2] The hairs project into the cupula, and

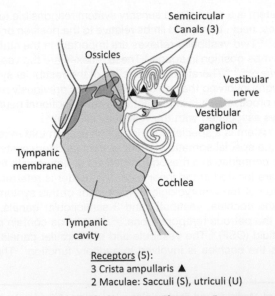

Fig. 1. Sensory receptors of the vestibular system. There are 5 sensory receptors on each side of the peripheral component of the vestibular system. These sensory receptors include the crista ampullaris within the ampulla at the end of each semicircular canal and the maculae (2): sacculi and utriculi. These receptors contain specialized hair cells that deflect transforming movement into electrical signals transmitted to the terminal axons of the vestibular nerve.

movement of fluid in the semicircular ducts causes deflection of the cupula.[2] The activity of vestibular neurons is going to be excited or inhibited depending on the direction of the deflection of the cupula to maintain dynamic equilibrium while the head moves in any plane or angular rotation.[2] For in-depth description of the effects of deflection of the cupula and movement of endolymph in the semicircular ducts, the reader is referred elsewhere.[2]

There are 2 additional sensory receptors within the vestibule: the macula of the utricle and macula of the saccule, which contain specialized hair cells (see **Fig. 1**).[2] The maculae has a mucopolysaccharide otolithic membrane that embeds calcium carbonate crystals known as otoliths.[2] The maculae sense static position (static equilibrium) of the head and respond to linear acceleration, deceleration, and gravitational forces.[2] The hair cells of the maculae alter their resting membrane potential when the hairs are bent by the action of the surrounding endolymph due to linear movement or from effects of gravity.[1]

Anatomically, the VS consists of central and peripheral components (**Figs. 2 and 3**).[1] The dendritic zone of the vestibular nerve (CN VIII) forms a synapsis with the hair cells of each crista ampullaris and the macula utriculi and macula sacculi. The vestibular axons along the axons of the cochlear division course through the internal acoustic meatus at the level of the cerebellomedullary angle.[2] In the vestibular ganglion, the cell bodies of these bipolar sensory neurons (neuron 1 in the pathway, see **Figs. 2 and 3**) form the vestibular ganglion.[2] Most of the vestibular axons from these neurons project to the 4 ipsilateral vestibular nuclei neurons (neuron 2).[1] Axons from the vestibular nuclei project to the brainstem, cerebellum, and spinal cord.[2] However, some axons of the vestibular nerve bypass the vestibular nuclei in the brainstem and project directly to the cerebellum.[1] Projections to and from the cerebellum are through the caudal cerebellar peduncle.[2]

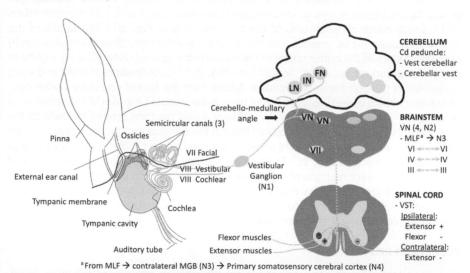

Fig. 2. The vestibular system. This figure depicts the peripheral and central components of the vestibular system. Cerebellum: Cd, caudal; FN, fastigial nucleus; IN, interpositus nucleus; LN, lateral nucleus; Vest, vestibular. Brainstem: VII, facial motor nuclei; motor nuclei of VI, abducens; IV, trochlear; III, oculomotor; MLF, medial longitudinal fasciculus; VN, vestibular nucleus (4 = 4 ipsilateral VN); double discontinued arrow, ipsilateral and contralateral projections. Spinal cord: MGB, medial geniculate body in the thalamus; N1, neuron 1 in the pathway; N2, neuron 2; N3, neuron 3; N4, neuron 4; VST, vestibulospinal tract.

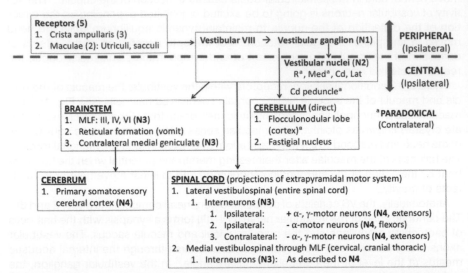

Fig. 3. Vestibular system pathways to brainstem, cerebellum, and spinal cord. [a]Paradoxical, vestibular disease if lesions occur in the rostral or medial vestibular nuclei, flocculonodular cerebellar cortex, and caudal cerebellar peduncle. α, alpha motor neuron; γ, gamma motor neuron; motor nuclei of III, oculomotor; IV, trochlear; VI, abducens; Cd, caudal; Lat, lateral; Med, medial; MLF, medial longitudinal fasciculus; N1, neuron 1; N2, neuron 2; N3, neuron 3; N4, neuron 4 within the vestibular pathway; R, rostral.

The central VS is composed of 4 vestibular nuclei (rostral, caudal, medial, and lateral) located at each side of the medulla oblongata, and the flocculonodular lobes and fastigial nuclei on each side of the cerebellum (see **Fig. 2**)[1,2] The axons of the rostral vestibular nuclei project rostrally in the medial longitudinal fasciculus (MLF) of the brainstem to the motor nuclei of the oculomotor (cranial nerve [CN] III), trochlear (CN IV), and abducens (CN VI) nerves (see **Fig. 2**).[1,3] Coordination of head and eyes movement is through these projections. Axons from the lateral vestibular nuclei neurons project in the lateral vestibulospinal tract in the ventral funiculus of the spinal cord (see **Fig. 3**).[2] Axons from the medial vestibular nuclei neurons project medially to the MLF through the medial vestibulospinal tract in the cervical and thoracic spinal cord.[2] Axons of the vestibulospinal tracts synapse on interneurons in the ventral gray matter of the spinal cord (see **Fig. 2**).[1] These interneurons are facilitatory to the ipsilateral α-motor and γ-motor neurons of the extensors of the limb and inhibitory to the ipsilateral flexors of the limbs (see **Fig. 2**). Concurrently, the interneurons project to the contralateral side and are inhibitory of the extensor of the limbs. Therefore, the VS confers increased ipsilateral extensor tone and decreased contralateral extensor tone.[1]

VESTIBULAR DISEASE

Two important reflexes are responsible for maintaining balance of the eyes, head, neck, trunk, and limbs during rest and movement: vestibulo-ocular (physiologic nystagmus) and vestibulospinal (extensor tone) reflexes.

Nystagmus

Physiologic nystagmus, also known as the vestibulo-ocular reflex, is a normal rapid involuntary rhythmic oscillation of the eyes usually horizontal in the direction of the head movement.[1,3] This eye movement is almost always equal for both eyes.[3] As the head turns, the eyes move slowly in the direction opposite to the head movement followed by a faster movement toward a more central position.[1] Eye movements involve coordination of the extraocular muscles of the eye through input to the oculomotor (main), trochlear, and abducens motor nuclei.[1,3] Because the oculomotor nuclei provides input to most of the extraocular muscles, disorders in this nuclei or with vestibular disease will result in ipsilateral ventrolateral strabismus. This strabismus will be present at all times with lesions in the oculomotor nuclei or nerve but might vary or be inducible with vestibular disease.

Nystagmus can be induced in normal individuals after rotation, for example (postrotational nystagmus).[3] This is challenging to induce and evaluate in equine. If nystagmus is observed when there is no movement or rotation of the head, this is called *spontaneous nystagmus* and is usually pathologic.[3] The slow phase of the nystagmus tends to indicate the side of the lesion, whereas the fast phase indicates the side away from the lesion and represents a quick recovery to a more central axis of vision.[3] If nystagmus only occurs when the head is placed in an unusual position (eg, lateral, facing up), this is called *positional nystagmus*.[3] Nystagmus affects vision due to inability to focus a visual field; this gets exacerbated at night or in dark areas because visual compensation is important in vestibular disease. Therefore, vestibular deficits are exacerbated under dark conditions.

The types of nystagmus described in the aforementioned paragraph are called jerk nystagmus on which a slow and fast phase occur whether physiologic or pathologic.[5,6] Pathologic nystagmus can be congenital or acquired.[5] Another type of nystagmus is called *pendular nystagmus*[5]; this is a sinusoidal oscillation in which there are no slow or fast phases and the eye moves slow in a pendular fashion.[5] The direction of the pendular nystagmus can be horizontal, vertical, or a combination and involving both eyes, different in both eyes, or even monocular.[5] This type of nystagmus can be congenital or acquired and is rare in equine species. The author has seen this type of pendular nystagmus in neonatal foals born blind. Acquired pendular nystagmus has been observed rarely in adult horses.

Pathologic forms of nystagmus in equine occur more commonly with peripheral disease such as trauma, otitis media/interna, temporohyoid osteoarthropathy (THO), and idiopathic vestibular disease, and with brainstem disease as with trauma, bacterial meningoencephalitis, neoplasia, and equine protozoal myeloencephalopathy.[7] Less common in equine, vestibular disease can occur with caudal cerebellar disease (mass-occupying lesions, vascular accidents),[8,9] and rarely with rostral visual pathway, thalamic, and cerebral hemispheres disease.

Pathologic nystagmus is usually observed in both eyes (more profound ipsilateral) because at the ipsilateral level of the brainstem there are axons with projections to the contralateral motor nuclei of the oculomotor (CN III), trochlear (CN IV), and abducens (CN VI) cranial nerves.[3] Observation of characteristics of nystagmus can aid in the distinction of central versus peripheral vestibular disease. These characteristics include the direction: horizontal, rotatory, or vertical; positional (change with direction of head) versus nonpositional; induced or spontaneous; and conjugate (both eyes move similar) or dysconjugate (both eyes move different). See **Table 1** with summary of signs of peripheral versus central vestibular disease.

Extensor Tone

The vestibular system provides ipsilateral facilitatory input to extensor muscles of the head, neck, trunk, and limbs and ipsilateral inhibitory input to the flexors resulting in ipsilateral increased extensor tone (see **Figs. 2** and **3**).[3] Concurrently, the VS provides

Table 1
Peripheral versus central vestibular disease

Sign	Peripheral	Central
Nystagmus	Yes	Yes
Strabismus	Yes	Yes
Head tilt	Yes	Yes
Leaning/circling	Yes	Yes
Ataxia	Yes	Yes
Nystagmus	Horizontal, rotatory	Horizontal, rotatory, vertical
Nystagmus	Does not change direction	Spontaneous change of direction
Nystagmus	Non-positional	Positional
Nystagmus	Conjugate	Conjugate, dysconjugate
Behavior/mentation	Normal	Normal or altered
Other CN	Normal (VII)	Normal or altered
Paresis/paralysis	No	Normal or altered
Proprioceptive deficits	No	Yes
Cerebellar signs	No	If yes: paradoxic

Top 5 signs are common to both components. The second tier of signs varies depending on whether peripheral or central disease. However, it should be noted that central vestibular disease can present with signs of peripheral disease. Signs such as nystagmus that are vertical, dysconjugate, positional, or change direction spontaneously always indicate central disease. Signs such as mentation alterations, multiple cranial nerves, paresis or paralysis, and proprioceptive deficits indicate central disease. If cerebellar signs are noted with concurrent vestibular disease, these indicate paradoxic vestibular disease unless 2 concurrent problems are occurring, which is uncommon.

contralateral inhibitory input to the extensor muscles. When the VS is normal, the individual can stand straight against gravity and eyes do not move spontaneously. Ipsilateral lesions will result in decreased ipsilateral input to extensor tone and lack of inhibition of flexors causing the animal to tilt, lean, flex, and move toward the side of the lesion.[1] In addition, the normal side (contralateral) has no inhibition of extensor tone contributing to leaning to the side of the lesion. In paradoxic vestibular disease, the signs are contralateral to the side of injury.[10] The cerebellum normally provides ipsilateral inhibitory input to the extensors.[10] If the cerebellum is affected, the ipsilateral inhibitory input to the extensors will be absent or decreased resulting in tilting and leaning contralateral to the side of the lesion.[3,10] These animals present signs of cerebellar and vestibular disease concurrently. Other cerebellar signs are ipsilateral, and the resulting vestibular signs are contralateral to the side of the lesion.[3] Paradoxic vestibular disease can develop if lesions occur in the rostral or medial vestibular nuclei, flocculonodular cerebellar cortex, and caudal cerebellar peduncle.[3]

Vestibular Disease

Severe signs can be seen early in vestibular disease including nystagmus, strabismus, marked head tilt, leaning, circling (tight circles), and ataxia. Ataxia can be seen with peripheral and central vestibular disease. Therefore, this sign alone does not help to distinguish between central and peripheral disease.[11] Ataxia might not always be present, specially later in the course of disease when the signs stabilize. Depending on the cause of disease signs might stabilize and the animal might appear better. During acute severe vestibular disease, the animal might collapse to one side and be unable to stand despite repeated attempts. If this is the case, obvious nystagmus is present and animals often paddle and trash in attempts to stand. This constellation of signs is often confused with seizures. When owners are questioned further, owners often claim that seizures are worse at night. A thorough discussion with the owner about history, onset of signs, and a comprehensive physical and neurologic examination should allow the clinician to determine if vestibular disease is the cause of the signs and not seizures. During neurologic examination, if vestibular disease is suspected despite lack of obvious vestibular deficits, the clinician can attempt carefully to blindfold or move the animal to a darker area to see if vestibular signs develop.[11] The author does not recommend to blindfold an animal that has obvious vestibular disease.[11] Safety must be a priority when dealing with horses with severe disease. The author recommends practicing caution when considering euthanasia based on severity of signs, because horses might improve depending on cause, anatomic region affected, treatment, and stabilization of signs over time. Some horses might fully recover. It is worthy investigating the cause, providing early supportive or specific treatment, and giving time. The author has used a large animal lift device to support the animal in the acute phase of vestibular disease. However, it might be challenging because the animal might struggle and try to roll in the lifting device. Mild intravenous (IV) sedation and keeping the lights on might aid in the management of these cases.

As mentioned earlier, signs of unilateral vestibular disease are ipsilateral to the side of the lesion and include nystagmus (usually both eyes), ventrolateral strabismus, head tilt, leaning, drifting, tight circles, and ataxia. In bilateral vestibular disease, the horse adopts a wide-based stance, no head tilt, no leaning or drifting, no circling, and lacks both physiologic and pathologic nystagmus. The head in these horses can slowly oscillate or move horizontally like in a pendular fashion from side to side. When horses get startled or try to initiate movement they might lose balance and adopt a wide-based stance. Horses might carry their neck and thorax slightly lower with thoracic limbs abducted in apparent attempts to balance themselves. Horses with bilateral THO display signs of vestibular disease in the side more severely affected. However, some cases display bilateral vestibular disease as described earlier (no nystagmus, no head tilt, no leaning or circling). These horses can look like cervical vertebral compressive myelopathy; however, a clue of having bilateral vestibular disease is the lack of physiologic nystagmus.[11] Horses with lolitrem intoxication display cerebellar signs and bilateral vestibular disease.[12–14]

In peripheral vestibular disease, usually other cranial nerves are not involved. However, due to the close proximity of facial nerve pathway to that of the vestibulocochlear nerve, injury to one might affect the other. An example of this includes THO on which the bony alterations in the stylohyoid bone and petrous part of the temporal bone affect various cranial nerves: facial, vestibular, and cochlear.[15,16] Owing to the anatomy of the temporohyoid joint, alterations in this area result in auditory loss (first alteration), then facial and vestibular deficits (see **Fig. 2**).[15] However, auditory loss might not be obvious because partial auditory loss often goes undetected unless brainstem auditory evoked responses (BAER) are done.[17] Deficits of one cranial nerve or more might be displayed in horses with THO.[15,17] Horses with THO might improve over time with medical therapy.[18,19] The best results have been reported with surgical management (ceratohyoidectomy) with some cases with complete resolution of signs and return to previous physical activity.[18,20] However, auditory loss seems to be a permanent deficit based on long-term follow up.[7,15] It is the opinion of the author that THO is the end result of various causes such as infection of the inner ear, guttural pouch infection, trauma, degenerative

Box 1
Causes of vestibular disease

Peripheral
- Infection
  - Extension from respiratory tract or guttural pouches
  - Bone infection
- Idiopathic
- Mass-occupying lesions
- Otitis media/interna
  - Bacterial, parasites (eg, ticks), fungal
- Trauma
- THO

Central
- Infection
  - Meningoencephalomyelitis[27]
    - Bacterial (several aerobic and anaerobic pathogens)
    - Parasitic
      - *Halicephalobus gingivalis*[28]
      - EPM
        - *Sarcocystis neurona, Neospora hughesi*
    - Fungal
    - Viral
- Mass-occupying lesion
  - Neoplasia
  - Granuloma
  - Abscess
- Toxicity
  - Drugs
    - Aminoglycosides (reported in other species, not reported in horses)
    - Metronidazole
  - Lolitrem B[a]
- Trauma
- Vascular
  - Air embolism/pulmonary edema//hypoxia

Central paradoxic
- Caudal cerebellar disease (eg, trauma)
- Infection
- Mass-occupying lesion
  - Neoplasia
  - Granuloma
  - Abscess
- Vascular
  - Congenital anomaly
  - Acquired
    - Vascular accident of the caudal cerebellar artery
  - Air embolism/pulmonary edema/hypoxia

Vestibulospinal tract
- Congenital anomaly
  - Other concurrent signs of spinal cord disease
- Compressive myelopathies (most common, however uncommon)
  - Only ipsilateral leaning or drifting, no head abnormalities, no nystagmus
  - Concurrent with other spinal cord sensory and motor signs
- NAD/EDM
  - Symmetric bilateral signs (no leaning or drifting)
- Trauma (other concurrent spinal cord signs)

Diseases under each component are mentioned in alphabetical order.[a] Lolitrem intoxication: horses display cerebellar signs and bilateral vestibular disease. *Abbreviations:* EPM, equine protozoal myeloencephalitis; NAD/EDM, neuroaxonal dystrophy/equine degenerative myeloencephalopathy.

joint disease, and a possible component of genetic predisposition in quarter horses (more than 50% have bilateral disease).[15] Horses with THO are on average mature adults and those with historical or recent unilateral ear infection seem to be younger. Fracture of the hyoid apparatus can predispose to THO at a later stage (suspected in racing thoroughbred horses with tongue tie, personal observation). Of interest is the finding that more than a third of the horses with THO were or are cribbers.[18] Is it possible this might predispose to THO due to repetitive mechanical stress of the hyoid apparatus? Other clinical signs can develop in horses with THO with additional fractures of the hyoid apparatus and base of the skull.[21] For further information, the reader is referred elsewhere.

Gentamicin is a widely efficacious antimicrobial used to treat gram-negative infections.[22,23] Reported toxic effects of gentamicin in humans, dogs, cats, and laboratory animals include nephrotoxicity, vestibulotoxicity, and cochleotoxicity.[24] There is 1 report of a horse with suspected vestibulotoxicity receiving gentamicin therapy.[25] Recently the author's research group investigated these effects in a small group of healthy adult horses using approved dosage of IV gentamicin for 7 consecutive days and found no nephrotoxic or vestibulotoxic effects.[26] However, auditory loss developed in 7 of 10 horses, which was irreversible in 3 horses.[26]

It is beyond the scope of this article to further describe in detail the multiple causes of vestibular disease and their specific treatments. Causes of vestibular disease in equine are listed in **Box 1**.[15,27–30] Physical, neurologic, and otoscopic examination must be part of the investigation of vestibular disease; and laboratory work and CSF analysis must be considered. Imaging diagnostic modalities for vestibular disease include skull radiographs, computed tomography, and MRI. Guttural pouch endoscopy is useful for the diagnosis of THO and BAER for the investigation of concurrent auditory loss.

DISCLOSURE

Nothing to disclose.

REFERENCES

1. Kent M, Platt SR, Schatzberg SJ. The neurology of balance: function and dysfunction of the vestibular system in dogs and cats. Vet J 2010;185:247–58.
2. De Lahunta A, Glass E, Kent M. Vestibular system: special proprioception. In: De Lahunta A, Glass E, Kent M, editors. deLahunta's veterinary neuroanatomy and clinical neurology. 3rd edition. St. Louis, MI: Saunders Elsevier; 2020. p. 319–47.
3. King AS. Special senses: Balance. In: KA S, editor. Physiological and clinical anatomy of the domestic mammals: central nervous system. Oxford, UK: Blackwell; 2008. p. 106–9.
4. Evans HE, Miller ME. The ear. In: Evans HE, Miller ME, editors. Miller's anatomy of the dog. Philadelphia, PA: W. B. Saunders; 1993. p. 988–1008.
5. Eggers SDZ. Approach to the examination and classification of nystagmus. J Neurol Phys Ther 2019;43(Suppl 2):S20–6.
6. Eggers SDZ, Bisdorff A, von Brevern M, et al. Classification of vestibular signs and examination techniques: nystagmus and nystagmus-like movements. J Vestib Res 2019;29:57–87.
7. Aleman M, Holliday TA, Nieto JE, et al. Brainstem auditory evoked responses in an equine patient population: part I--adult horses. J Vet Intern Med 2014;28: 1310–7.

8. Bentz BG, Traurig HH. Understanding and distinguishing cerebellar lesions in horses. Equine Vet Educ 2002;14:246–54.

9. Bentz BG, Traurig HH. Vestibulocerebellar deficits in a horse associated with a vascular accident of the caudal cerebellar artery. Equine Vet Educ 2002;14: 242–5.

10. King AS. Cerebellum. In: King AS, editor. Physiological and clinical anatomy of the domestic mammals: central nervous system. Oxford, UK: Blackwell; 2008. p. 171–82.

11. Aleman M. Neurologic examination in the horse. Annu Conv Am Assoc Equine Pract 2015;61:181–90.

12. Johnstone LK, Mayhew IG, Fletcher LR. Clinical expression of lolitrem B (perennial ryegrass) intoxication in horses. Equine Vet J 2012;44:304–9.

13. Johnstone LK, Mayhew IG. Flow-mediated K(+) secretion in horses intoxicated with lolitrem B (perennial ryegrass staggers). N Z Vet J 2013;61:159–64.

14. Munday BL, Monkhouse IM, Gallagher RT. Intoxication of horses by lolitrem B in ryegrass seed cleanings. Aust Vet J 1985;62:207.

15. Aleman M, Spriet M, Williams DC, et al. Neurologic deficits including auditory loss and recovery of function in horses with temporohyoid osteoarthropathy. J Vet Intern Med 2016;30:282–8.

16. Blythe LL, Watrous BJ, Schmitz JA, et al. Vestibular syndrome associated with temporohyoid joint fusion and temporal bone fracture in three horses. J Am Vet Med Assoc 1984;185:775–81.

17. Aleman M, Puchalski SM, Williams DC, et al. Brainstem auditory-evoked responses in horses with temporohyoid osteoarthropathy. J Vet Intern Med 2008; 22:1196–202.

18. Espinosa P, Nieto JE, Estell KE, et al. Outcomes after medical and surgical interventions in horses with temporohyoid osteoarthropathy. Equine Vet J 2017;49: 770–5.

19. Walker AM, Sellon DC, Cornelisse CJ, et al. Temporohyoid osteoarthropathy in 33 horses (1993-2000). J Vet Intern Med 2002;16:697–703.

20. Racine J, O'Brien T, Bladon BM, et al. Ceratohyoidectomy in standing sedated horses. Vet Surg 2019;48:1391–8.

21. Tanner J, Spriet M, Espinosa-Mur P, et al. The prevalence of temporal bone fractures is high in horses with severe temporohyoid osteoarthropathy. Vet Radiol Ultrasound 2019;60:159–66.

22. Schoster A, Amsler M, Kirchgaessner C, et al. Gentamicin plasma concentrations in hospitalized horses and retrospective minimal inhibitory concentrations of gram-negative equine pathogens. J Vet Emerg Crit Care (San Antonio) 2021; 31:323–30.

23. Bauquier JR, Boston RC, Sweeney RW, et al. Plasma peak and trough gentamicin concentrations in hospitalized horses receiving intravenously administered gentamicin. J Vet Intern Med 2015;29:1660–6.

24. Modi N, Maggs AF, Clarke C, et al. Gentamicin concentration and toxicity. Lancet 1998;352:70.

25. Dacre KJP, Pirie S, Prince DP. Choke, pleuropneumonia and suspected gentamicin vestibulotoxicity in a horse. Equine Vet Educ 2003;15:27–33.

26. Aleman MR, True A, Scalco R, et al. Gentamicin-induced sensorineural auditory loss in healthy adult horses. J Vet Intern Med 2021;35:2486–94.

27. Toth B, Aleman M, Nogradi N, et al. Meningitis and meningoencephalomyelitis in horses: 28 cases (1985-2010). J Am Vet Med Assoc 2012;240:580–7.

28. Adedeji AO, Borjesson DL, Kozikowski-Nicholas TA, et al. What is your diagnosis? cerebrospinal fluid from a horse. Vet Clin Pathol 2015;44:171–2.

29. Blythe LL. Otitis media and interna and temporohyoid osteoarthropathy. Vet Clin North Am Equine Pract 1997;13:21–42.

30. Blanke A, Fischer ML, Fuchs M, et al. Endoscopic findings of the external ear canal in a group of clinically normal horses and horses with head shaking or vestibular disease. Berl Munch Tierarztl Wochenschr 2014;127:99–107.

28. Ataoğlu AC, Boyacıoğlu O, Wierzkowska-Wcislo TA, et al. Where is your diagnosis? colon mucosal trial. Vet Clin Pathol 2015;44:171-2.

29. Dryba D. Otitis media and interna and temporomandibular osteoarthropathy. Vet Clin North Am Small Anim Pract 1997;8:31-42.

30. Bischoff, Fischer ML, Radke M, et al. Endoscopic findings of the external ear canal in a series of clinically normal horses and horses with head shaking or vestibular disease. Dtsch Tierärztl Wochenschr 2011;77:99-102.

Movement Disorders and Cerebellar Abiotrophy

Stephanie J. Valberg, DVM, PhD, DACVIM, DACVSMR

KEYWORDS

- Shivers • Stringhalt • Myoclonus • Stiff horse syndrome • Cerebellar abiotrophy

KEY POINTS

- Movement disorders in horses are enigmatic, often lack defined causes, and are currently classified by clinical signs.
- Diagnosis involves ruling out lameness and neurologic disease and characterizing the gait during walking backward and forward and trotting.
- Shivers causes abnormal hindlimb hypertonicity during walking backward and, when advanced, a few strides walking forward.
- Stringhalt causes consistent hyperflexion during walking forward and trotting and variable difficulty when walking backward.
- Other ill-defined movement disorders exist in horses whose underlying basis requires further study.

Video content accompanies this article at http://www.vetequine.theclinics.com.

INTRODUCTION

The basic neurologic circuit required for locomotion consists of (1) afferent nerves sending proprioceptive information and (2) spinal interneurons that receive afferent information and connect with (3) alpha motor neurons (lower motor neurons) that initiate muscle contraction (**Fig. 1**). An alpha motor neuron supplies a specific subset of muscle fibers, and the nerve together with its enervated muscle fibers comprises a motor unit. The overlap of numerous motor units participating in muscle contractions ensures stable force production and smooth changes from one force level to another.

A simple rhythmic locomotor pattern can be maintained at a spinal level without higher input[1]; this is due to a specific network of spinal interneurons termed central pattern generators that rhythmically transmit reciprocal excitatory and inhibitory

The author reports no conflict of interest for the information provide in this article.
Department of Large Animal Clinical Sciences, College of Veterinary Medicine, Michigan State University, 736 Wilson Road, East Lansing, MI 48824, USA
E-mail address: valbergs@msu.edu

Vet Clin Equine 38 (2022) 409–426
https://doi.org/10.1016/j.cveq.2022.05.009

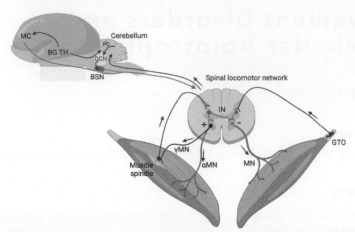

Fig. 1. Organization of neuronal control of locomotion. The selection and initiation of locomotor behavior involves various regions of the brain and brainstem. Output neurons of the basal ganglia (BG) project to the thalamus (TH), which sends projections to the motor cortex (MC) and other cortical areas as well as to areas in the brainstem. Neurons in the brainstem project to locomotor networks in the spinal cord that execute locomotion. Descending fibers from the vestibular and rubrospinal spinal pathways (brainstem nuclei [BSN]) maintain posture and modulatory signals that regulate the ongoing locomotor activity. The cerebellum receives sensory information from the spinal cord and feedback from the motor cortex, basal ganglia, and thalamus. The cerebellum coordinates locomotor behavior by integrating movement-generated feedback and internal feedback and modulating the activity in the descending pathways through Purkinje cell (PC) inhibitory connections in the deep cerebellar nuclei (DCN). Proprioceptive sensory feedback also modulates the activity of the spinal locomotor network. The spinal locomotor network consists of spinal interneurons (IN), which receive proprioceptive information from muscle spindles, and alpha motor neurons, that generate muscle contractions. A specific subset of interneurons termed *central patter generators* produce the rhythmic pattern of gaits at the spinal level. Interconnected spinal interneurons coordinate the timing of muscle contraction between agonist and antagonist muscles within a limb and between limbs. Posture and muscle length at rest are maintained by muscle spindles. Afferent impulses generated by stretch of muscle spindles stimulate alpha motor neurons (MN) to contract the muscle containing the spindle and to inhibit the antagonistic muscle. Gamma motor neurons enervate intrafusal fibers in the spindle, which maintain the shape of the spindle during contractions allowing it to maintain its exquisite sensitivity to stretch. Excessive tension at the muscle-tendon junction triggers firing of the Golgi Tendon Organ (GTO), which sends signals to the spinal cord to inhibit contraction of the muscle containing that GTO, this prevents tendon and muscle damage. (Figure created with BioRender.com.)

signals to motor units that supply ipsilateral limb muscles.[1] The importance of spinal interneurons in the process of generating rhythmic gaits is illustrated by the *DMRT3* gene mutation originally found in Icelandic horses.[2] This mutation alters specific interneurons in spinal circuits that results in the facilitation of pace, tolt, and rack gaits.

Another important component of locomotion and posture is the muscle spindle. Muscle spindles are encapsulated mechanoceptors and proprioceptors that lie in parallel with muscle fibers (see **Fig. 1**). Muscle spindles maintain their exquisite sensitivity to small changes in the length of their parent muscle through their gamma motor neurons, which constantly adjust their length and respond to stretch by signaling alpha motor neurons to initiate a contraction that prevents further stretching (the myotatic reflex).[3] During active locomotion, spindles provide proprioceptive information that allows the central nervous system to assess changes in muscle length, joint position, and velocity.[3] The Golgi tendon organ (GTO) acts to prevent excessive stretch of a muscle. The GTO is found at myotendinous junctions and senses tension, which when excessive triggers a reflex that inhibits the alpha motor neurons that supply the muscle containing the GTO (see **Fig. 1**).

Adaptation of the locomotor pattern to changes in the environment and generation of more complex motor movements requires that the brain integrate proprioceptive information and provide input to interneurons and alpha motor neurons in the spinal cord (see **Fig. 1**). The cerebellum, basal ganglia, and motor areas in the frontal cortex are the major upper motor neuron nodes that process sensory information and formulate movement patterns.[4] The cerebellum receives input from these nodes, processes a vast amount of sensory information, learns, generates feedforward movement patterns, and modulates locomotion via efferent inhibitory output that is transmitted through the deep cerebellar nuclei (see **Fig. 1**).[4]

Disruption of proprioception results in an ataxic gait, which is irregularly irregular in rhythm, whereas painful stimuli result in lameness, which produces a regularly irregular gait. Movement disorders are defined as involuntary movements that are not due to a painful stimulus and that are not associated with changes in consciousness or proprioception.[5] An important part of the diagnosis of movement disorders in horses involves ruling out lameness due to pain or mechanical restriction of gait and ruling out the presence of proprioceptive ataxia or seizure activity.

CLASSIFICATION OF MOVEMENT DISORDERS IN HORSES

The classification system in common usage for equine movement disorders is based on age-old terms stringhalt and shivers or shivering that describe a specific pattern of abnormal hindlimb movement induced by walking backward or forward (**Table 1**).[6,7] Other ill-defined movement disorders exist in horses that do not cleanly fit into these 2 categories. A more scientific classification system for horses is desirable but difficult to devise currently due to the rare nature of movement disorders, the lack of diagnostic biomarkers, clear causes, and overlap between syndromes. Attempts to apply the terminology used to classify movement disorders in other species can be problematic in horses because the triggers and pattern of abnormal limb movement are different from horse to human to small animal species.[5,8] In human and small animal medicine, the term dyskinesia is used to characterize intermittent involuntary self-limiting episodes of jerky movements that impair normal voluntary movements.[5,8] This characterization seems to fit many of the forms of stringhalt and shivers.

CLINICAL APPROACH

A diagnosis of a movement disorder in horses is made through clinical observation and characterization of the abnormal movement. There are unfortunately no hematologic or serum biochemical biomarkers that are useful for diagnosing a movement disorder. An important part of assessing a movement disorder is ruling out lameness, proprioceptive deficits, and conscious movement as the cause of the abnormal movement. The clinical approach can be assisted by using a diagnostic workflow such as the one provided in **Table 1**. This approach considers the environment because examination of the horse in a new environment can reduce signs of some movement disorders and enhance signs of movement disorders such as shivers due to the exacerbating effects of stress/excitement. Signalment including age, breed, sex, and height are important to consider because geldings, certain breeds, and taller horses are most often afflicted by movement disorders, and an early age of onset can

Table 1
A diagnostic workflow sheet that can be used to assess movement disorders in horses

Diagnostic Approach

Horse	Age:	Breed:	Sex:
	Season:	Pasture access:	Height:

Age at onset of movement disorder: Acute onset: Progressing over time:

Lameness evaluation:

Neurologic assessment:

Potential triggers: circle   Stress   Relaxed   Startling   Stall rest   Farrier   Initiating movement   Footing   Ground feeding

Movement assessment

In stall for at least 1 h before examination

Grade: 0 = absent, 1 = intermittent mild, 2 = intermittent moderate severe

	Right hind			Left hind			Forelimbs		
	HF	HE	Normal	HF	HE	Normal	HF	HE	Normal
Standing									
Lifting hoof									
Backing up 10 strides									
Walking on hard surface									
Turning at walk									
Trotting hard surface									
Canter if possible									
Score difficulty backing									
Score steepness of croup when backing									
Was facial twitching observed									
Was tail elevated, trembling									
Was symmetric muscle atrophy present									

Abbreviations: HE, hyperextension; HF, hyperflexion.

indicate a poorer prognosis for shivers.[9,10] In the history, it is important to ascertain age of onset, season of onset, and degree of progression of the movement disorder; access to pasture and presence of weeds; and drought on pastures. Any potential triggers for the movement can be identified by determining if specific gaits, handling of the limb, difficulties with the farrier, stress, excitement, startling, trailering, soft or hard surfaces, or painful conditions seem to induce or exacerbate the movement disorder. Any previous history of lameness or neurologic disease should be noted.

The order of evaluating movements is important in the clinical examination. Movement disorders are most apparent when the horse has been stall rested for several hours. The horse should be observed exiting the stall because this may be the time point when a movement disorder is most noticeable. During the physical examination, mentation and cranial nerves should be evaluated to rule out cerebral or brainstem lesions. The horse's muscle mass should be inspected for muscle development, symmetry, atrophy, and fasciculations and muscles palpated to assess tone and evidence of pain or sensitivity. Subsequently, each limb should be held in a comfortable flexed position for 10 to 15 seconds. The limb should be flexed directly upward and not drawn out behind the horse or abducted, and any excessive abduction, withdrawal reflex, or tremoring should be noted. The limb should not be abducted by the handler or flexed excessively so as not to elicit any pain at this point; this can be reserved for a lameness examination.

During the active examination, the severity of the gait abnormality should be graded as absent, intermittently present, or consistently present with the degree of abnormal movement graded mild, moderate, or severe. The first gait evaluated should be walking backward because the abnormality in this gait may abate after more exercise and it is key for the diagnosis of shivers. The horse's willingness to back up, the ability to back up in a straight line, and the timing of the foot fall (4 beat, 2 beat, pacing) should be assessed. Presence of sliding of the toe backward on the ground, abduction, adduction, hyperextension of the hock, or hyperflexion of the hock should be noted and graded. The slope of the croup, tail elevation, and trembling and facial muscle twitching should be noted during backing.

The horse should then be observed at a walk on a straight line (minimum 10 strides) and then while turning and performing a serpentine and tight circle. Evidence of proprioceptive deficits, pain, or a gait abnormality should be noted for each limb. If a gait abnormality is evident, each limb should be graded and the specific timing of an intermittent gait abnormality should be recorded (eg, on initiation of walking, when turning). The abruptness of the trajectory of the hoof arc should be noted when initiating the swing phase and when terminating the swing phase during the stride as well whether the limb was adducted or abducted during the stride. If tolerated, the horse should be observed at a trot on soft and hard surfaces as well as on the lunge line at a canter and the gait abnormality graded. Any knuckling of the fetlock should be recorded. If lameness is suspected, a thorough lameness examination can be performed at this point, and, if there is any question of foot soreness, an abaxial nerve block is performed. This is because foot soreness can produce a gait that strongly resembles stringhalt.

Unfortunately, there are no diagnostic imaging techniques or tissue biopsies that are of value for the diagnosis of movement disorders specifically; they can of course be of value in ruling out other potential diseases that alter the pattern of locomotion.

DIFFERENTIAL DIAGNOSES

Any painful orthopedic condition can cause standing hyperflexion, and lameness can often be discerned during the active lameness examination. Lameness that can be confused with a movement disorder like stringhalt or shivers includes bilateral hindlimb hoof pain, upward fixation of the patella, and fibrotic myopathy.[6] Painful hindlimb hoof conditions can produce a gait that strongly resembles stringhalt particularly when walked on hard surfaces. An abaxial nerve block helps to distinguish the 2 conditions. Upward fixation of the patella can be distinguished from shivers and stringhalt by observing that the limb is hyperextended when the patella becomes upwardly fixated and then the horse may jerk and hyperflex the stifle to release the patella. This period of hyperextension before hyperflexion is not observed with shivers or stringhalt.[7,11] Fibrotic myopathy restricts forward movement and causes protraction of the hoof before placement on the ground at the walk (Video 1). Stringhalt or shivers-forward hyperflexion have a much more pronounced degree of hyperflexion than observed with fibrotic myopathy.

Neuropathies in horses can produce a stringhalt-like gait. Causes include Scandinavian knuckling disease,[12] idiopathic polyneuropathy, equine protozoal myelitis,[13] and vitamin E deficiency.[14] These causes can be distinguished clinically by evaluating horses for evidence of muscle atrophy, proprioceptive or cranial nerve deficits, and weakness as well as by performing ancillary diagnostic tests. Lathyrism toxicity can cause a spastic gait abnormality in horses without evidence of proprioceptive deficits.[15] Unlike stringhalt or shivers, gait deficits with lathyrism tend to worsen with increased exercise duration and speed. In addition, the stride length of all limbs is short, asymmetry is particularly apparent in hindlimbs, and the coordination between limbs is inappropriate with lathyrism.

SPECIFIC MOVEMENT DISORDERS
Standing Hyperflexion

One of the most common movement disorders in horses is hyperflexion and abduction of the hindlimb that is only observed when the horse is manually asked to lift the limb (Video 2).[7,9] The term shivers has been applied by some veterinarians to this abnormal movement. However, because these horses do not show hyperflexion with forward or backward gaits and because shivers has a poorer prognosis, the term standing hyperflexion is more appropriate.[7,9] The author recommends that the term shivers be reserved for horses with abnormal hindlimb movement apparent when walking backward and lifting the limb but not consistently present when horses walk forward.

Clinical signs: Horses with standing hyperflexion are more often geldings with an average age of 12 years (range, 6–23 years).[7] When asking a horse to pick up a hindlimb, affected horses will exhibit a jerky hyperflexion of the hock and stifle often with the limb abducted, and it will remain fixed in that posture for several seconds or more (see Video 2). If the limb is picked up without exceeding a certain degree of flexion, hyperflexion may not occur. The condition is more often unilateral than bilateral.[7] The limb and muscles may tremble, and the tail may be elevated, and the horse agitated. In its most severe form, horses may lean so far toward the weight-bearing hindlimb that they almost fall over. Stress, pain, and farrier work often exacerbate standing hyperflexion.

Cause: Horses seem to have a strong withdrawal reflex when picking up the limb that in the wild may have served them well for evading predators or getting caught in impediments. Horses that are trained to have their hooves picked up seem to consciously recognize this request and will relax the withdrawal allowing the limb to be manipulated. Observation of horses suggests that this withdrawal reflex is hyperactive in standing hyperflexion and that these horses are not able to consciously relax the limb.

There seem to be 3 potential causes of standing hyperflexion.

1. Pain: Any painful condition of the hindlimb can induce a strong withdrawal response when the limb is flexed.
2. Early onset of shivers: Shivers may begin with standing hyperflexion. If this is the case the horses are usually young, predominantly geldings, and 16.3 hands or taller.
3. Hyperactive reflex arc without the ability to relax the limb consciously.

Diagnostic approach: The diagnostic approach outlined in the workflow sheet is a valuable approach to diagnose standing hyperflexion (**Table 2**). Horses with standing hyperflexion will have normal forward and backward gaits. Clinical examination to rule out behavioral issues, musculoskeletal pain, or a neuropathy is vitally important.

Treatment: If a primary neuropathy or painful condition is present then this obviously needs to be addressed. For horses with hyperactive withdrawal for unknown causes, reducing clinical signs requires a calm low-key approach to picking up the hindlimb because stress and excitement exaggerate the condition. The hoof should be raised to the least extent necessary. Some horses can be trained to flex the fetlock with the hoof on the ground so it can be cleaned without triggering the withdrawal response. For farrier work, sedation with detomidine can be helpful. Trimming hooves is usually safest performed with the weight-bearing hindlimb positioned against a wall for support. Some owners have used nippers to trim the feet by having horses stand in sand while the owner digs out an area in front of the hoof to facilitate the placement of the nippers.

Prognosis: For horses with primary standing hyperflexion, this disorder usually remains static. If an early case of shivers, horses often progress by the age of about 7 years to have difficulty walking backward.[9]

Shivers

The term *shivers* (also known as shivering) arises from the clonic-tonic muscle contractions that occur in the hindlimbs of affected horses.[6] Shivers is an age-old disease commonly seen in male horses of warmblood, thoroughbred, and draught breeds that are on average 17 hands tall and more but can affect other breeds.[9]

Clinical signs: Shivers is a remarkable movement disorder in that backward walking can be severely impaired, yet entrained forward gaits such as trotting and cantering are normal. Clinical signs of shivers are usually evident by age 7 years.[9] When manually picking up a hindlimb or when the horse is asked to walk backward, the tail may be elevated and 1 or both pelvic limbs will pause during the movement and be held abducted in hypertonic flexion with tremulous muscles.[7,11] The condition can initially be unilateral and intermittent but progresses to being bilateral. When the limb is handled, horses with shivers often jerk the limb into a hyperflexed abducted position, which may suddenly release, at which point the hoof slams to the ground. Approximately 17% of horses with shivers show signs of facial twitching while walking backward.[9] Signs are more apparent during periods of excitement or concurrent with other painful conditions and will diminish when pain or excitement diminish.[6,7,9] Trot or canter gaits are completely normal. Varying patterns of hindlimb movement during backward and forward walking has led to subdivision of shivers into 3 categories.

Shivers-hyperflexion: Shivers-hyperflexion seems to be the most common form of shivers.[7] Horses walk forward normally and show signs of hindlimb hyperflexion when walking backward and manually lifting the hindlimb (Videos 3 and 4). Signs are usually bilateral, although one hindlimb can be more severely affected than the

Table 2
The presence of hyperflexion or hyperextension in forms of shivers and stringhalt

Movement Disorder	Picking Up Hoof	Backing Up	Walking	Trotting	Cantering
Standing hyperflexion	Consistent HF	Absent	Absent	Absent	Absent
Shivers-hyperextension	Difficult-HE	Difficult-HE	Absent	Absent	Absent
Shivers-hyperflexion	Consistent HF	Consistent HF	Absent	Absent	Absent
Shivers-forward hyperflexion	Consistent HF	Consistent HF	Intermittent	Absent	Absent
Stringhalt-PSH	Consistent HF	Consistent HF	Consistent HF	Consistent HF	Variable
Stringhalt-unipedal or idiopathic	Variable	Variable	Consistent HF	Consistent HF[a]	Variable

The absence of clinical signs at gaits such as the walk and trot help to differentiate the movement disorders.
Abbreviations: HE, hyperextension; HF, hyperflexion; PSH, pasture-associated stringhalt.
[a] Some horses may warm out of hyperflexion at the trot.

other. During hyperflexion, the hindlimb is abducted and the affected limb pauses in the hyperflexed state before quickly returning to the ground (**Fig. 2**).[7] Horses with shivers are usually resistant to walking backward and have difficulty backing up in a straight line.[11] Upon backing, the tail head is elevated in most horses and muscle fasciculations may be observed. Manual lifting of a hindlimb is usually resisted and induces hyperflexion in the opposite hindlimb or eventually the hindlimb being handled. Some horses will show signs of treading in their hindlimbs or hyperflexion when drinking or feeding from buckets on the ground. Walking, trotting, and cantering are normal (see **Fig. 2**).

Shivers-FHF: Shivers-hyperflexion can progress to the point at which abnormal hyperflexion of both hindlimbs occurs in 20% or fewer strides with forward walking, as well as with backward walking, and manual lifting of the limb (Video 5).[7] Hyperflexion while walking backward occurs with the limb abducted, the hip less flexed, and the distal limb drawn farther caudally than observed in horses with stringhalt (see **Fig. 2**).[7] At the initiation of forward walking, tail head elevation and marked abduction and hyperflexion of hindlimbs occurs for the first few strides or when changes occur in surface, direction, or speed of walking. A notable pause occurs with hyperflexion before

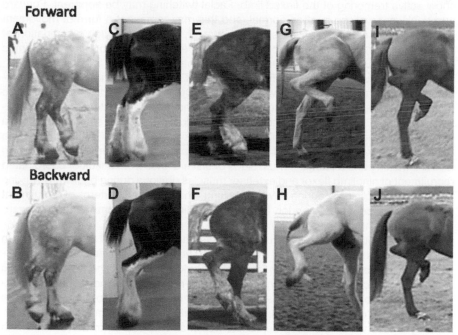

Fig. 2. Hindlimb position at peak trajectory in horses with forms of shivers and stringhalt during backward (*top row*) and forward walking (*bottom row*). Control horse (*A, B*) and horses with shivers hyper-extension (C,D), shivers-hyperflexion (*E, F*), shivers-forward hyperflexion (*G, H*), and pasture stringhalt (*I, J*). Horses with shivers-hyperextension walk forward normally but show exaggerated extension of all four limbs when asked to walk backward. Horses with shivers-hyperflexion have hyperflexion when walking backward and a normal limb trajectory when walking forward. Horses with shivers-forward hyperflexion have consistent hyperflexion and abduction walking backward and intermittent hyperflexion and abduction when walking forward. Horses with pasture-associated stringhalt have hyperflexion consistently when walking backward and forward. Traumatic and idiopathic forms of stringhalt may not show hindlimb hyperflexion when walking backward.

the limb is returned to the ground. Extreme difficulty with manual leg lifting is often present at this point such that it becomes impossible for either hindlimb to be lifted manually, or they slam the foot down rapidly. Trotting and cantering are normal; however, these horses often compete at a lower level of competition than they had before forward hyperflexion.

Shivers-hyperextension: Horses with shivers-hyperextension show reluctance to walk backward accompanied by constant or intermittent hindlimb hyperextension during backward walking (Video 6).[7] During the backward stride, both hindlimbs are placed farther caudally than normal, with a hyperextended hock and stifle. Horses may not move their forelimbs because the hindlimbs at the initiation of backward walking, which, when combined with hindlimb hyperextension, results in a stretched saw-horse appearance. A lack of coordination of forelimb and hindlimb movements is readily apparent when backing up. The tail head may be elevated, and the croup steeply sloped and muscle fasciculations apparent during backward walking. Manual lifting of the hindlimbs is often not possible due to hyperextension. Horses, however, walk forward normally and appear normal at the trot.

Forelimb shivers: Some horses have been diagnosed with "forelimb shivers" if they show signs of increased resistance to flexing the carpus, and then, when flexed, they show active tremoring of the flexed limb. Facial twitching may be apparent. Forward and backward walking is often normal, and this may represent a form of movement disorder in horses. Such cases should, however, have a thorough examination of the caudal neck and imaging of cervical facets because nerve root impingement is a more likely cause for muscle contractions and pain in this area.

Etiology of shivers: Surface electromyography (sEMG) has been used to study muscle activation patterns in horses with shivers.[16] During backward walking, hindlimb muscle activation patterns show sustained, elevated flexor and extensor muscle activation with loss of the precise agonist and antagonist firing patterns required for a normal gait. Although a movement disorder was only obvious with backward walking during sEMG studies, altered and elevated firing patterns were present even during forward walking and trotting.[16] Thus, signs of shivers arise from a lack of coordinated recruitment of hindlimb flexor and extensor muscles obvious during backward walking but present subclinically during forward walking. The disrupted patterns of recruitment seems to only be severe enough initially to be clinically apparent during backward walking and lifting of the hindlimb.

A thorough neuropathological study of the peripheral and central nervous system in a small number of warmblood and thoroughbred horses with shivers identified selective distal axonal degeneration in cerebellar Purkinje cells as the sole pathologic finding.[17] When compared with controls, calretinin-negative, calbindin-positive, glutamic acid decarboxylase-positive spheroids were increased 80-fold in Purkinje cell axons within the deep cerebellar nuclei of horses with shivers. The numbers of end terminal synapses within the deep cerebellar nuclei also appeared to be reduced with degeneration being most evident in the lateral nuclei (dentate and interpositus).[17] Axons of Purkinje cells are the sole efferent output from the cerebellum, and their pattern of connections in the deep cerebellar nuclei roughly maintains the temporal and spatial features conserved within the cerebellum itself[18]; this has led to the hypothesis that in equine shivers, the reduced or loss of regional cerebellar inhibitory output via the deep cerebellar nuclei leads to enhanced excitation of selected efferent targets that modulate hindlimb muscle tone in response to specific motor actions.[16,17]

Arguments against a cerebellar origin for shivers include the lack of ataxia that is a prominent feature of diffuse cerebellar disease like cerebellar abiotrophy[19] and the restriction of the movement disorder to backward walking. The focal lesion in the output of Purkinje cells in deep cerebellar nuclei of horses with shivers would not seem to involve sensory processing by Purkinje cell bodies as is the case in cerebellar abiotrophy. The cerebellum processes sensory information and shares this with nerve cells in the brainstem and cerebral cortical areas creating locomotor patterns via an excitatory motor drive (see **Fig. 1**).[4] Inhibitory output from Purkinje cells via the deep cerebellar nuclei restrains this excitatory drive and shapes it into specific spatiotemporal patterns of neural activity for locomotor modules.[4] It is possible that the inhibitory drive for locomotor modules important for backward walking, an unnatural gait, could be disrupted in horses with shivers. The fact that sEMG indicates abnormal muscle recruitment at a walk and trot in horses with shivers and that signs of facial twitching occur while walking backward potentially supports a cerebellar rather than a peripheral disruption of neuromuscular function; however, this requires further investigation.

Treatment: Owners of horses with shivers have tried numerous treatment regimens to improve signs of shivers without great success.[9] The author has performed a treatment trial in 3 warmbloods and 3 Clydesdales with shivers using 4 mg/kg levodopa per day for 2 weeks as well as 1 trial giving 8 mg/kg phenytoin twice daily for 2 weeks without any change in the gait pattern (personal observation). Supplementation with vitamin E is recommended if horses are deficient, because low vitamin E levels can cause gait disturbances in some horses. It was previously thought that polysaccharide storage myopathy played a role in shivers and horses have been provided a low-starch high-fat diet.[20] The role of polysaccharide storage myopathy has been ruled out; however, and there is no indication that this type of diet will modulate shivers in any way.[21] Stall rest, reduced turnout, limited exercise, lameness, and illness can temporarily precipitate more severe signs of shivers[9]; these may stabilize after removal of the precipitating factor. Some owners report that horses improve with physical therapy; however, this has yet to be documented in the literature. Regular exercise, limited time in stalls, a balanced diet, and a low-stress lifestyle seem to be sound recommendations for horses with shivers.

Prognosis: Despite the best therapeutic attempts that owners can provide, 70% of cases of shivers progressively worsen over time.[9] The rate of progression is difficult to predict, however. In the author's experience horses can be serviceable for a decade after the initial diagnosis and may show a gradual decline in their level of performance after 10 to 15 years of age. In other cases, however, horses can show a rapid progression of disease for unknown reasons.

Stringhalt

Stringhalt differs from shivers in that it produces consistent abnormal limb movement during forward gaits.[7] Stringhalt is characterized by consistent excessive and prolonged flexion of one or both hindlimbs during walking and trotting (see **Fig. 2**). The affected hindlimbs show a rapid steep ascending trajectory during the initial swing phase with the stifle and hock held in an adducted position (see **Fig. 2**).[7] Hyperflexion is inconsistent during backward walking or picking up the hindlimb. The cause for this abnormal gait has been proposed to be disruption of the afferent or efferent fibers supplying muscle spindles and GTO.[22] Disruption of these stretch or tension feedback loops could interfere with the muscle's ability to gauge the number of motor units required for a normal smooth muscle contraction resulting in hypertonicity and hyperreflexia. Stringhalt seems to have several causes, which has led to subclassifications of stringhalt.

Unipedal stringhalt

Clinical signs: Horses with unipedal stringhalt show consistent signs of hyperflexion of 1 hindlimb at a walk and trot, although the extent of hyperflexion may diminish after a period of exercise (Video 7).[23] Hindlimb hyperflexion may be present to some extent at a canter. Hyperflexion is variably present when horses are asked to back up or when manually lifting the limb. Changes in surface such as from soft to hard ground may exacerbate hyperflexion.

Diagnosis: A diagnosis of unipedal stringhalt is made by clinical observation of a unilateral hyperreflexive gait consistently present at a walk and trot and is supported by evidence of previous trauma to the metatarsus or hock. The movement disorder workflow form outlined in an earlier section may be beneficial for distinguishing unipedal stringhalt from other movement disorders, orthopedic pain, and peripheral polyneuropathies.

Cause: The cause of unipedal stringhalt is not always known, but, in many cases, there is a history of trauma to the dorsal metatarsus or hock region.[23] Other potential causes include peripheral neuropathies and disorders[12] related to vitamin E deficiencies.[14]

Treatment: The most common treatment of unipedal stringhalt is a lateral digital extensor myotenotomy, which removes the extensor tendon and 7 to 10 cm of the muscle belly.[23,24] Success rates vary with individual cases. There is a single report of improved clinical signs of stringhalt after repeated injection of botulinum toxin type A into the lateral digital extensor or long digital extensor and vastus lateralis muscles.[25]

Prognosis: Horses with stringhalt are known to function as trail horses and have been successful in jumping competitions. The prognosis for return of a normal gait after surgery is guarded because the degree of improvement noted with surgery is unpredictable and signs may recur in the future.[23,24]

Pasture-associated stringhalt

Pasture-associated stringhalt (PSH) is a form of stringhalt reported in Australia, New Zealand, Europe, South America, and the United States in horses that are grazing drought-affected, poor-quality pastures that contain the plant *Hypochaeris radicata* (commonly referred to as catsear, flatweed, and false dandelion).[10,26–29] Many but not necessarily all horses grazing an affected pasture will develop clinical signs with affected horses typically being mature and taller animals.[10]

Clinical signs: Horses with PSH show hyperflexion of both hindlimbs with some degree of asymmetry possible (see **Fig. 2**). Clinical signs vary in severity, and a grading system has been devised for PSH cases.[10]

Grade description

I Only noticeable when horse was backed, turned, or stressed.[10]

II Slight limb jerkiness when horse moves off at a walk or trot.

III Moderate hyperflexion noted when walking or trotting especially when initiating or stopping movement.

IV Severe hyperflexion with hindlimbs hitting abdomen when backing and turning. Horse is unable to trot.

V Hindlimb held hyperflexed for prolonged periods when initiating movement, which is characterized by plunging, leaping, and hopping motion.

VI Prolonged recumbency following grade IV to V stringhalt gait.

In its mildest form, horses only exhibit hyperflexion when nervous, turned sharply, or when forced to walk backward. In its most severe form both hindfeet may leave the ground simultaneously and exhibit a hopping action in which hyperflexion becomes progressively more exaggerated.[10] The trajectory of the hoof shows a rapid steep ascent during the initial swing phase with the fetlock sometimes striking the abdomen (Video 8).[7] Knuckling of the hindlimb occurs in some cases. Horses may show extreme difficulty walking backward with excessive hyperflexion (Video 9). Rarely, the forelimbs may show knuckling and hypermetria. Muscle atrophy develops in most affected horses, with the long and lateral digital extensor muscles the most severely affected.[10] Up to 20% of horses develop laryngeal hemiplegia.

Diagnosis: Diagnosis of PSH is based on the presence of characteristic bilateral hindlimb hyperflexion during backward and forward walking and trotting in horses exposed to pastures with *H radicata* and the absence of orthopedic pain or other neurologic diseases. Unlike shivers, hyperflexion is consistently present (75% of strides) at a walk and the stifle and hock are held adducted rather than abducted.[7] The distinguishing features between PSH and unipedal stringhalt are the involvement of both hindlimbs as well as exposure to *H radicata*. Low plasma vitamin E concentrations and mild increase in muscle and liver enzyme activity have occasionally been noted with PSH.[10,27,28] If performed, electromyography of hindlimb muscles reveals increased insertional activity, fibrillation potentials, and positive sharp waves, consistent with denervation.[10]

Cause: H radicata is a perennial, edible herb native to Europe but an invasive weed that has been introduced to Australia, New Zealand, the Americas, and parts of Asia.[10] A neurotoxin, potentially scyllo-inositol, is believed to be produced by *H radicata* under certain environmentally stressful conditions.[30] Outbreaks in pastured horses typically occur during drought conditions in late summer or early autumn after several weeks of grazing incriminated pastures.[28] Disease might not become evident until 1 to 3 weeks after removal from affected pastures.[31] The pathologic lesion identified in PSH horses is a Wallerian-type distal axonopathy of the tibial, deep, and superficial peroneal as well as recurrent laryngeal nerves accompanied by myofiber atrophy in the muscles supplied by affected nerves.[10,30]

Treatment: Given enough time, most horses will spontaneously recover from PSH.[10] Phenytoin at dosages of 15 mg/kg body weight orally every 12 to 24 h seems to be effective in decreasing clinical signs.[32] Given the individual variability in absorption of phenytoin, monitoring plasma concentrations has been recommended particularly for long-term administration.[10] Some horses with PSH have been reported to improve by following lateral digital extensor myotenotomy, although others only recovered after a prolonged convalescence.[28,31] Other supplements that have been given to PSH horses include thiamine, taurine, vitamin E, vitamin C, magnesium, L-tryptophan, and potassium bromide.[10] There is little theoretic basis for many of these supplements and no scientific evidence to support their use.

Prognosis: Most horses recover over a period of 6 to 18 months with milder cases recovering more quickly. Recovery can take more than 2 years for complete resolution in severe cases, and rarely, horses never recover completely.[28,31]

Idiopathic bilateral stringhalt

There seems to be other forms of bilateral stringhalt in North America not associated with ingestion of *H radicata* or trauma. These cases present with consistent bilateral hyperflexion at a walk and trot that is not as extreme as that seen with PSH, and horses will back up and lift a hindleg normally (Video 10, S.J.V., personal observation). Examination of one such case by the author did not identify degeneration or demyelination in the peroneal or tibial nerves or atrophy in the extensor or flexor muscles of the hindlimbs. The cause remains unknown.

Some movement disorders in horses do not fit into the classic forms of shivers or stringhalt. Horses may show intermittent hyperflexion when walking in pastures or treading from limb to limb when fed from the ground with no other clinical signs. Some horses may show abduction and hyperflexion of the hindlimbs with every stride at the walk. The rarity of these syndromes and the infrequency of full postmortem examination of the nervous system in cases of movement disorders makes these syndromes enigmatic.

Miscellaneous Movement Disorders

Hitch: Although hyperflexion is present in most forward strides with stringhalt, some horses will have an intermittent pause in the normal stride cycle. The cause of this "hitch" in their gait is unknown, and it has been seen most frequently in draft breeds. Rarely, Oldenburg horses have an unusual intermittent movement disorder that is only present at a walk when the horse is relaxed (Videos 11 and 12). The gait shows abduction with mild hock hyperflexion, a slight pause at the height of the stride, and then adduction of the limb when placing the limb on the ground. When the walk is more animated this gait is not apparent.

Clydesdale swing: Clydesdales can present with an unusual constellation of gait abnormalities, which may represent one breed-specific disorder or multiple movement disorders. In its simplest form the gait resembles unilateral stringhalt; however, hyperflexion may be more intermittent and most apparent after standing still for a period. In other cases, the hock may swing laterally in an abducted plane, pause with hyperflexion, and then be adducted before being placed on the ground; this usually occurs after standing still or when turning and can affect one or both hindlimbs. It can be very difficult to induce affected Clydesdales to walk backward.

Stiff horse syndrome: There are a few reports of a disorder in horses characterized by muscle rigidity and episode of severe muscle contractions and termed *stiff horse syndrome*, named after a similar human disorder stiff person syndrome.[33,34] Affected horses have been adults of a variety of breeds.[33,34] Unlike shivers or stringhalt, rather than a particular locomotor movement inducing muscle spasms, spasms are often initially induced by startling or excitement. This syndrome can resemble shivers-hyperextension, except that spasms occur with stiff horse syndrome during periods of inactivity.

Horses show an insidious onset of waxing and waning muscle stiffness progressing to acute painful muscle contractions often initially initiated by startling or touching.[33,34] Horses may spend prolonged time in recumbency showing increased muscle tone and when standing assume a stretched-out stance or camped understance with painful cramps, and lordosis lasting from seconds to minutes (**Fig. 3**).[22] Serum creatine kinase level is within the normal range. Horses can appear normal during trotting and cantering. Electromyography has shown increased motor unit firing in the absence of any limb movement, which seems to be due to a decrease in gamma-aminobutyric acid (GABA), an essential inhibitory neurotransmitter.[33] Antibodies directed against glutamic acid decarboxylase (GAD), which produces the active form of GABA in the central nervous system, have been identified in the cerebrospinal fluid of confirmed cases.[33] A definitive diagnosis is established by measuring GAD antibodies in serum and the cerebrospinal fluid using specialized human diagnostic laboratories. The reason why antibodies are produced is unknown; infection has been speculated to be a potential trigger.[22,33,34] Oral prednisolone at 2 mg/kg/d or dexamethasone decreasing from 80 mg once per day to 8 mg every other day have been used successfully to treat horses; however, recurrence can require reinstitution of treatment.[33,34] The prognosis is guarded, and cases may progress to become very painful and debilitating.[22]

Congenital myoclonus in Peruvian Paso foals: A small number of Peruvian Paso foals have been identified that show signs of hyperresponsiveness at birth to touch and

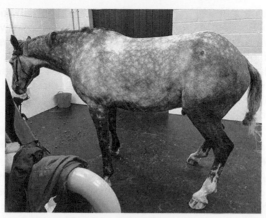

Fig. 3. The hypercontracted hindlimb musculature of a horse with stiff horse syndrome. Note the protracted hyperflexion of both hindlimbs giving a crouched appearance that persisted for several minutes following stimulation. (Photo courtesy of Dr. Federica Cantatore.)

environmental stimuli that results in prolonged myoclonic muscle contractions and stiff extended limbs.[35] Foals have difficulty rising but can stand when assisted; however, they develop a hypertonic rigid sawhorselike stance when startled that fixes them in place until the startle response fades. A 40% to 60% deficit in spinal glycine receptors has been identified in the spinal cord of affected foals.[35] The genetic basis of this disorder has yet to be identified.

CEREBELLAR ABIOTROPHY

Cerebellar abiotrophy is the most common cerebellar disease in horses reported in Arabian, Gotland pony, and Oldenburg horse breeds.[19,36–38] This condition affects foals aged less than 1 year and occurs most frequently in 1- to 6-month-old foals with 2 equine cases reported in adults.[19,36,39,40]

   Clinical signs: Many foals are born with no abnormalities and later develop disease; however, occasionally they are affected at or shortly following birth.[19,36,39] Clinical signs include intentional head tremor, hypermetric forelimb gait, symmetric ataxia, wide-based stance and gait, dysmetria, and spasticity especially when stepping over obstacles.[19] The limb may be hyperflexed when walking, resulting in slamming of the foot to the ground. A menace reflex frequently is absent or diminished; however, it is important to consider that a depressed menace reflex is present in normal foals until at least 2 weeks of age. Foals have no change in mentation and rarely show nystagmus and are not weak. Once affected Arabian foals reach maturity, the condition becomes static, although mild improvement has been observed. The cerebellar abiotrophy that occurs in Oldenburg horses is progressive and fatal with atypical histologic lesions compared with the syndrome that occurs in Arabian foals.[38]

   Diagnosis: Antemortem diagnosis of cerebellar abiotrophy is based on a typical history and the clinical signs of intention tremor, lack of menace, failure to blink to bright light, and ataxia in Arabian or part-Arabian foals or Gotland pony foals. Genetic testing is available for Arabian foals.[41] MRI of affected Arabian foals reveals a smaller cerebellum than healthy foals and a larger relative cerebellar cerebrospinal fluid space.[42] At postmortem, no gross abnormalities are notable; however, careful examination of the cerebellum may reveal an increased lobular pattern with prominent folia. The weight ratio of the cerebellum to the cerebrum may be reduced significantly in foals with cerebellar abiotrophy.[19,37] The most prominent histopathologic finding is the widespread loss of Purkinje neurons and occasional clear spaces where the Purkinje neuron should have been.[39,43] Thinning of the molecular layer occurs with gliosis of the granular layer and loss of cellularity.[43,44]

Cause: Cerebellar abiotrophy is inherited as an autosomal recessive trait in Arabians horses due to a single-nucleotide polymorphism on chromosome 2 (13074277G > A), located in the fourth exon of *TOE1* and in proximity to *MUTYH* on the antisense strand.[41,45] This mutation results in loss of Purkinje neurons with secondary loss of the granular layer of the cerebellum. Up to 20% of Arabian horses are carriers, and the mutation has been found in Bashkir curly horses, Welsh ponies, and Trakehner horses at low frequencies.[46]

Treatment and prognosis: No treatment exists for cerebellar abiotrophy. As noted previously, signs may be progressive until the foal reaches maturity. Signs may stabilize or improve slightly with time.[19,40]

ACKNOWLEDGMENTS

Shivers research was funded by Mary Anne McPhail Endowment, The University of Minnesota College of Veterinary Medicine and the United States Eventing Association.

SUPPLEMENTARY DATA

Supplementary data related to this article can be found online at https://doi.org/10.1016/j.cveq.2022.05.009.

CLINICS CARE POINTS

- Diagnosis of movement disorders in horses requires ruling out proprioceptive deficits and painful or mechanical lameness. The specific gaits affected and pattern of abnormal hindlimb movement help to distinguish shivers and stringhalt.

REFERENCES

1. Carp JSWR. Motor neurons and spinal control of movement. In: Encyclopedia of life sciences. Cichester (England): John Wiley & Sons; 2010.
2. Andersson LS, Larhammar M, Memic F, et al. Mutations in DMRT3 affect locomotion in horses and spinal circuit function in mice. Nature 2012;488:642–6.
3. Dimitriou M, Edin BB. Human muscle spindles act as forward sensory models. Curr Biol 2010;20:1763–7.
4. Caligiore D, Pezzulo G, Baldassarre G, et al. Consensus Paper: Towards a Systems-Level View of Cerebellar Function: the Interplay Between Cerebellum, Basal Ganglia, and Cortex. Cerebellum 2017;16:203–29.
5. Cerda-Gonzalez S, Packer RA, Garosi L, et al. International veterinary canine dyskinesia task force ECVN consensus statement: Terminology and classification. J Vet Intern Med 2021;35:1218–30.
6. Baird JD, Firshman AM, Valberg SJ. Shivers (shivering) in the horse: A review. In: American association of equine. practitioners 2006;359–64.
7. Draper AC, Trumble TN, Firshman AM, et al. Posture and movement characteristics of forward and backward walking in horses with shivering and acquired bilateral stringhalt. Equine Vet J 2015;47:175–81.

8. Garone G, Capuano A, Travaglini L, et al. Clinical and genetic overview of paroxysmal movement disorders and episodic ataxias. Int J Mol Sci 2020;21: 3603.
9. Draper AC, Bender JB, Firshman AM, et al. Epidemiology of shivering (shivers) in horses. Equine Vet J 2015;47:182–7.
10. El-Hage CM, Huntington PJM IG, Slocombe RF, et al. Pasture-associated string-halt: contemporary appraisal of an enigmatic syndrome. Equine Vet Educ 2019; 31:154–62.
11. Seino KKS T, Vig M, Kyllonen S, et al. Three-dimensional kinematic motion analysis of shivers in horses: a pilot study. J Equine Vet Sci 2019;79:13–22.
12. Grondahl G, Hanche-Olsen S, Brojer J, et al. Acquired equine polyneuropathy in Norway and Sweden: a clinical and epidemiological study. Equine Vet J Suppl 2012;(43):36–44.
13. Dubey JP, Lindsay DS, Saville WJ, et al. A review of Sarcocystis neurona and equine protozoal myeloencephalitis (EPM). Vet Parasitol 2001;95:89–131.
14. Finno CJ, Valberg SJ. A comparative review of vitamin E and associated equine disorders. J Vet Intern Med 2012;26:1251–66.
15. Holbrook TC, Gilliam LL, Stein FP, et al. Lathyrus hirsutus (Caley Pea) intoxication in a herd of horses. J Vet Intern Med 2015;29:294–8.
16. Aman JE, Valberg SJ, Elangovan N, et al. Abnormal locomotor muscle recruitment activity is present in horses with shivering and Purkinje cell distal axonopathy. Equine Vet J 2018;50:636–43.
17. Valberg SJ, Lewis SS, Shivers JL, et al. The Equine Movement Disorder "Shivers" Is Associated With Selective Cerebellar Purkinje Cell Axonal Degeneration. Vet Pathol 2015;52:1087–98.
18. Grimaldi G, Manto M. Topography of cerebellar deficits in humans. Cerebellum 2012;11:336–51.
19. Mayhew IG. Congenital, genetic and familial disorders. In: Large animal neurology. Chichester (England): Willey-Blackwell; 2009. p. 185–6.
20. Valentine BA, de Lahunta A, Divers TJ, et al. Clinical and pathologic findings in two draft horses with progressive muscle atrophy, neuromuscular weakness, and abnormal gait characteristic of shivers syndrome. J Am Vet Med Assoc 1999;215:1661–5, 1621.
21. Firshman AM, Baird JD, Valberg SJ. Prevalences and clinical signs of polysaccharide storage myopathy and shivers in Belgian draft horses. J Am Vet Med Assoc 2005;227:1958–64.
22. Mayhew IG. Disorders of posture and movement. In: Mayhew IG, editor. Large animal neurology. 2nd edition. Chichester, West Sussex: Willey-Blackwell; 2009. p. 133–42.
23. Crabill MR, Honnas CM, Taylor DS, et al. Stringhalt secondary to trauma to the dorsoproximal region of the metatarsus in horses: 10 cases (1986-1991). J Am Vet Med Assoc 1994;205:867–9.
24. Baxter GMS TS. Lameness in the extremities. In: Baxter GM, editor. Lameness in horses. 6th edition. Chichester: Willey Blackwell; 2011. p. 767 769.
25. Wijnberg ID, Schrama SE, Elgersma AE, et al. Quantification of surface EMG signals to monitor the effect of a Botox treatment in six healthy ponies and two horses with stringhalt: preliminary study. Equine Vet J 2009;41:313–8.
26. Araujo JA, Curcio B, Alda J, et al. Stringhalt in Brazilian horses caused by Hypochaeris radicata. Toxicon 2008;52:190–3.
27. Araya O, Krause A, Solis de Ovando M. Outbreaks of stringhalt in southern Chile. Vet Rec 1998;142:462–3.

28. Domange C, Casteignau A, Collignon G, et al. Longitudinal study of Australian stringhalt cases in France. J Anim Physiol Anim Nutr (Berl) 2010;94:712–20.
29. Gay CC, Fransen S, Richards J, et al. Hypochoeris-associated stringhalt in North America. Equine Vet J 1993;25:456–7.
30. Domange C, Canlet C, Traore A, et al. Orthologous metabonomic qualification of a rodent model combined with magnetic resonance imaging for an integrated evaluation of the toxicity of Hypochoeris radicata. Chem Res Toxicol 2008;21: 2082–96.
31. Huntington PJ, Jeffcott LB, Friend SC, et al. Australian Stringhalt–epidemiological, clinical and neurological investigations. Equine Vet J 1989;21:266–73.
32. Huntington PJ, Seneque S, Slocombe RF, et al. Use of phenytoin to treat horses with Australian stringhalt. Aust Vet J 1991;68:221–4.
33. Nollet H, Vanderstraeten G, Sustronck B, et al. Suspected case of stiff-horse syndrome. Vet Rec 2000;146:282–4.
34. Purcell TB, Sellers AD, Goehring LS. Presumed case of "stiff-horse syndrome" caused by decreased gamma-aminobutyric acid (GABA) production in an American Paint mare. Can Vet J 2012;53:75–8.
35. Gundlach AL, Kortz G, Burazin TC, et al. Deficit of inhibitory glycine receptors in spinal cord from Peruvian Pasos: evidence for an equine form of inherited myoclonus. Brain Res 1993;628:263–70.
36. Baird JD, Mackenzie CD. Cerebellar hypoplasia and degeneration in part-Arab horses. Aust Vet J 1974;50:25–8.
37. Bjorck G, Everz KE, Hansen HJ, et al. Congenital cerebellar ataxia in the gotland pony breed. Zentralbl Veterinarmed A 1973;20:341–54.
38. Koch PF H. Die Oldenberger Fohlenataxie als Erbkrankheit. Tierarztl Umsch 1950;5:317–20.
39. Palmer AC, Blakemore WF, Cook WR, et al. Cerebellar hypoplasia and degeneration in the young Arab horse: clinical and neuropathological features. Vet Rec 1973;93:62–6.
40. Foley AG,J, Almes K, Patton K, et al. Cerebellar abiotrophy in a 6-year-old Arabian mare. Equine Vet Educ 2011;23:130–4.
41. Brault LS, Cooper CA, Famula TR, et al. Mapping of equine cerebellar abiotrophy to ECA2 and identification of a potential causative mutation affecting expression of MUTYH. Genomics 2011;97:121–9.
42. Cavalleri JM, Metzger J, Hellige M, et al. Morphometric magnetic resonance imaging and genetic testing in cerebellar abiotrophy in Arabian horses. BMC Vet Res 2013;9:105.
43. Scott EY, Woolard KD, Finno CJ, et al. Cerebellar abiotrophy across domestic species. Cerebellum 2018;17:372–9.
44. Blanco A, Moyano R, Vivo J, et al. Purkinje cell apoptosis in arabian horses with cerebellar abiotrophy. J Vet Med A Physiol Pathol Clin Med 2006;53:286–7.
45. Scott EY, Woolard KD, Finno CJ, et al. Variation in MUTYH expression in Arabian horses with Cerebellar Abiotrophy. Brain Res 2018;1678:330–6.
46. Brault LS, Penedo MC. The frequency of the equine cerebellar abiotrophy mutation in non-Arabian horse breeds. Equine Vet J 2011;43:727–31.

Pathologic Conditions of the Nervous System in Horses

Rebecca E. Ruby, MSc, BVSc, Jennifer G. Janes, DVM, PhD*

KEYWORDS

- Equine • Neuropathology • Postmortem examination • Disease

KEY POINTS

- Horses are susceptible to a variety of processes that can impact neurologic function.
- Antemortem neuroanatomic localization is important to confirm the underlying disease process.
- Complete histories, clinical examinations, and ancillary diagnostic testing in conjunction with postmortem examination are often needed for a definitive diagnosis.
- Not all equine neurologic diseases have macroscopic or microscopic lesions.

INTRODUCTION

Pathologic examination of the equine central and peripheral nervous system (PNS) requires an understanding of equine macroscopic and microscopic anatomy, anatomic neurolocalization, and common causes of neurologic dysfunction. Additionally, the physical ability and tools to remove the brain, spinal cord, and peripheral nerves of interest are needed. Often to reach a diagnosis a complete history, summary of the clinical physical and neurologic examination, appropriate ancillary diagnostics in conjunction with a postmortem examination is needed for a definitive diagnosis. The definition of a "neurologic necropsy" will vary between institutions and laboratories. The focus of this article is to provide the reader with an understanding of pathologic findings which correlate to more common equine neurologic diseases.

DISCUSSION
Neuroanatomy Overview

The central and peripheral nervous systems are composed of a highly intricate network of specialized cells and supportive structures that facilitate a variety of sensory and motor functions. The central nervous system (CNS) is composed of the brain and spinal cord. Primary cellular components of the CNS include neurons, macroglial

Department of Veterinary Science, University of Kentucky Veterinary Diagnostic Laboratory, 1490 Bull Lea Road, Lexington, KY 40511, USA
* Corresponding author.
E-mail address: jennifer.janes@uky.edu

Vet Clin Equine 38 (2022) 427–443
https://doi.org/10.1016/j.cveq.2022.04.006
0749-0739/22/© 2022 Elsevier Inc. All rights reserved.

cells (astrocytes and oligodendrocytes), and microglial cells embedded in the neuropil. Other important cellular components include ependymal cells, choroid plexus epithelia, and a dense vascular network. A combination of tight junctions between blood vessels, pericytes, and foot processes of astrocytes covered by a basement membrane comprises the blood–brain barrier. Axons are projections from the neurons that function to conduct nerve impulses to the appropriate synapses to other neurons or effector cells. Axons are located in the CNS and PNS. The sensory and motor components of the cranial and spinal nerves which innervate skeletal muscle, as well as the nerves and ganglia of the enteric and autonomic systems, comprise the PNS.[1]

Macroscopically the brain is made up of the cerebral hemispheres, cerebellum, and brain stem covered by meninges (dura mater, arachnoid and pia mater) which thereby create the epidural, subdural, and subarachnoid spaces. Each cerebral hemisphere is composed of a superficial layer of gray matter which contains neurons and subjacent white matter that contains the nerve fibers. The junction of the gray and white matter is distinct on macroscopic examination. In contrast, the spinal cord is composed of superficial white matter that borders central gray matter composed of dorsal and ventral horns. Sensory pathways are located in the dorsal horn and motor pathways in the ventral horn. The spinal cord is also covered by the meninges.

Injury or infection to the nervous system can occur via the hematogenous route, direct extension due to trauma or compromise of surrounding structures (ie, cribriform plate), or retrograde axonal transport (ie, Rabies). The cells of the nervous system undergo stereotypical changes in response to various types of injury or infection. Axons exhibit Wallerian degeneration which is characterized by focal swelling of the axons, termed spheroids. Other changes seen with Wallerian degeneration include digestion chambers that contain fragmented axons or gitter cells (a type of macrophage). Wallerian degeneration is seen with acute focal injury to an axon, typically due to trauma. Depending on the inciting cause, neuronal changes range from neuronal loss, chromatolysis (swelling of the cell body and dispersion of Nissl substance), apoptosis, necrosis, intracytoplasmic or intranuclear inclusions or vacuolations seen with storage diseases. Areas of softening or necrosis of the neural tissue are termed malacia. Compromise to the vascular support can result in hemorrhages or infarction. Inflammation in response to infectious agents is characterized by inflammatory cell populations which vary in composition based on infectious agent and chronicity. Bacterial infections are often highly neutrophilic while parasitic or protozoal infections may have a significant eosinophilic component. In general, macroscopic and microscopic lesion patterns can often provide insight into potential disease differentials.[2]

Inflammatory/Infectious Diseases

Equine protozoal myeloencephalitis

Equine protozoal myeloencephalitis (EPM) is most commonly caused by infection with *Sarcocystis neurona*, less commonly *Neospora hughesi* and rarely other protozoan organisms.[3] Postmortem examination is considered the gold standard for a diagnosis of EPM and is achieved by demonstrating the appropriate inflammatory lesions within the brain and spinal cord with the visualization of protozoa. Macroscopic lesions are less common than microscopic but do occur and include hemorrhage and malacia (**Fig. 1**). Histologic lesions include necrosis, malacia, mixed inflammation with lymphocytes, histiocytes, plasma cells, eosinophils, and neutrophils infiltrating the meninges, surrounding blood vessels, and scattered within the neural parenchyma. Protozoal agents may be difficult to visualize, especially in cases treated before euthanasia. Detection of protozoa in tissues examined with hematoxylin and eosin staining ranges from 20% to 36%.[4] This percentage can be increased with immunohistochemistry

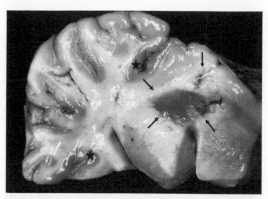

Fig. 1. A focal region of yellow discoloration and malacia with scattered hemorrhage is evident in the white matter (*black arrows*). Malacia or softening is also observed in the gray matter of the cerebral cortex (*asterisk*). Microscopic examination and PCR confirmed EPM.

(IHC) and/or polymerase chain reaction (PCR). As chronicity of the disease increases, the inflammatory cell population becomes predominantly histiocytic and eosinophilic and with treatment may become sparser and be replaced with glial scarring. The protozoan organism may affect any portion of the spinal cord or brain and antemortem localization is likely to increase the likelihood of finding areas of inflammation at postmortem.[5]

Rare cases of other CNS protozoan infections have been reported including *Trypanosoma cruzi*.[6] In these cases, diagnosis is confirmed at postmortem based on the morphologic appearance of the protozoa and PCR of formalin fixed or fresh tissues. *Toxoplasma gondii* can infect most warm-blooded mammals and seroprevalence studies show a seroprevalence ranging from 8.9% to 16.4%.[7] Initial evaluation of protozoal encephalomyelitis in horses implicated *T. gondii* but the organism was later identified as *S. neurona*. To date, no cases of neurologic disease in horses caused by *T. gondii* have been confirmed. Systemic toxoplasmosis has been reported in a horse, raising the possibility that the involvement of the neurologic system could occur.[8] Any need to reference any of the information about toxoplasmosis.

Viral encephalomyelitis

In general, there is an overlap in pathologic findings in cases of viral encephalitis. Diagnosis of viral encephalitis is most commonly achieved by using fluorescent antibody tests (FAT), PCR, or IHC. PCR is readily available for the most common equine viruses with neurotropism and combining this modality with histologic examination is the simplest method of achieving a diagnosis. Viral encephalitis is typically characterized by perivascular cuffs, inflammation within the neuropil, neuronal degeneration, and neuronophagia. Inflammation may range from neutrophilic to lymphocytic with histiocytes present in some cases.

West Nile Virus infection may result in grossly evident areas of hemorrhage or malacia within the thoracic and/or lumbar spinal cord (**Fig. 2**). Histologic findings are most prevalent in the brainstem and thoracolumbar spinal cord and are characterized by a nonsuppurative encephalomyelitis with gliosis and neuronal degeneration.[9,10] The severity of changes is variable between cases and outbreaks.

The alphaviruses, (Eastern, Western and Venezuelan encephalitis) rarely result in gross lesions. These viruses infect neurons resulting in microscopically evident neuronal necrosis, neuronophagia, and gliosis.[11] Microscopic changes predominate

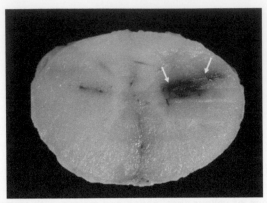

Fig. 2. Section of equine thoracic spinal cord. Focal hemorrhage is encompassing the gray and white matter (yellow *arrows*). Microscopic examination and PCR confirmed nonsuppurative myelitis due to West Nile Virus.

within the gray matter and necrotizing vasculitis, thrombosis, and malacia may be seen in severe cases. Perivascular cuffs of lymphocytes and neutrophils with microglial proliferation are seen. The cerebral cortex is the anatomic region most severely affected with histologic lesions decreasing in frequency and severity moving caudally.[12]

In the case of equine herpesvirus 1 (EHV-1) and rarely EHV-4, hemorrhage and vasculitis are observed, most commonly within the spinal cord, but also in some cases within the brain. Gross lesions include hemorrhage and in severe cases malacia of the nervous tissue. The characteristic lesions are a nonsuppurative necrotizing vasculitis with thrombosis most marked within the brainstem and spinal cord.[13] PCR of the spinal cord, respiratory tract or EDTA blood collected antemortem will all confirm the presence of this virus.[14]

Due to the zoonotic and fatal nature of rabies infection, accurate and rapid postmortem diagnostics are imperative. The preferred test for rapid diagnosis is fluorescent antibody testing on fresh or frozen brains. A section of cerebellum and brainstem, regions that have been shown to have the highest viral antigen load, are submitted to state laboratories for FAT on fresh tissue. When fresh tissue is not available, then histologic examination and IHC are indicated. Histologic findings are variable in distribution and severity and include nonsuppurative inflammation within the brain, meninges, and/or spinal cord and parotid adenitis. Identification of acidophilic intracytoplasmic inclusions is pathognomonic for rabies but an inconsistent finding and an absence of these inclusions do not rule out a diagnosis of rabies.[15] Lesion distribution includes the brainstem, cerebellum, spinal cord, hippocampus, trigeminal ganglion. Lesions are more commonly observed within the spinal cord when compared with the brain. Gross lesions are often absent but may include hemorrhage within the spinal cord.

General bacterial or mycotic pathogens
Bacterial and mycotic infections are generally rare and may be due to bacteremia following a primary infection at another organ site. Typically, a random, multifocal inflammatory pattern is observed within the brain and/or spinal cord. Inflammation may be sporadic or large abscesses or granulomas may occur.[16,17] Appropriate culture methods, visualization of infectious organisms in tissue section, PCR or IHC will also aid in a diagnosis.

Neuroborreliosis

Neuroborreliosis occurs due to transmission of the spirochete bacterium *Borrelia burgdorferi* via the *Ixodes* spp. tick. From a pathologic perspective, diagnosis requires the demonstration of appropriate inflammatory lesions and a confirmatory test that demonstrates the presence of *B burgdorferi*. Many types of inflammation including lymphohistiocytic, neutrophilic, eosinophilic, and plasmacytic have been reported. The histologic findings reported include leptomeningitis, encephalomyelitis, vasculitis, ganglionitis, radiculoneuritis, and neuritis.[18–20] Neuritis of cranial nerves and peripheral nerves has been reported, but the collection of most of these nerves is not routinely conducted at necropsy; therefore, neurolocalization and/or a complete history will aid in the collection of the appropriate samples. Inflammation in a variety of other organ systems has also been reported. Confirmatory testing requires the demonstration of the spirochete via argyrophilic stains, IHC, or PCR. In the authors' opinion, a definitive diagnosis is often difficult to reach in some cases even with these additional test modalities.

Botulism

Horses are highly susceptible to botulism as compared with other species.[21] The causative agent of botulism is *Clostridium botulinum*. It is capable of producing 8 toxins (A,B,C_1,C_2,D,E,F) with B and C_1 neurotoxins reported to cause disease in horses.[22] Common routes of exposure in horses include ingestion via contamination of feed material with preformed toxin either by forage degradation or degrading small animal or rodent carcasses.[23–25] Occasional cases of botulism due to wound contamination have been reported in horses. In foals, ingestion of contaminated soil allowing for sporulation in the gastrointestinal tract (toxoinfectious botulism) has been reported.[22] Mechanistically, the neurotoxin acts by binding receptors at peripheral neuromuscular junctions and interferes with acetylcholine release. Thereby lower motor neuron function is impacted. Clinical signs include weakness, poor muscle tone, dysphagia, muscle fasciculations, and recumbency to name a few.

From a postmortem standpoint, gross and microscopic lesions are not observed. However, submitted feed samples and/or gastrointestinal contents obtained during the postmortem examination can be tested for the toxin at laboratories that offer botulinum testing.

Tetanus

Clostridium tetani, the causative agent of tetanus, is a common inhabitant of soil throughout the world. Two toxins, tetanospasmin and tetanolysin are produced by the bacteria. Tetanospasmin is produced in anaerobic environments (ie, wounds). It travels retrograde along axons to access the CNS. It then binds to inhibitory motor neurons. Thereby inhibitory neurotransmitters such as glycine and GABA are unable to balance excitatory nerve actions from upper motor neurons resulting in the clinically observed muscle spasms. Other clinical signs include hyperesthesia and third eyelid prolapse.

Similar to other diseases, gross and microscopic lesions are not observed outside of the potential identification of the wound that allowed entry. Diagnosis is typically presumptive based on the history of a wound, inadequate vaccination, and development of clinical signs as bacterial isolation is difficult.[26,27]

Aberrant parasite migration

Multiple case reports of aberrant parasite migration exist. Two have characteristic pathologic findings and are discussed here. *Halicephalobus gingivalis* is a free-living nematode that invades multiple tissues, including the oral and nasal cavities, adrenal glands, kidney, lymph nodes, brain, and spinal cord. Tissue invasion results in granulomatous and eosinophilic inflammation centered on nematode larvae. Horses with neurologic signs often have inflammation within both the brain and other organs.[28] *Parelaphostrongylus tenuis*, while more frequently observed in camelids and ruminants, has been demonstrated in cases of acquired cervical scoliosis and results in histologic findings of inflammation and necrosis of the dorsal gray column, dorsal nerve roots and adjacent white matter. In some cases, nematode larvae are observed.[29,30] Migration of other nematodes will typically result in inflammation centered on migratory tracks within variable sections of the nervous system.

Noninflammatory Diseases

Cervical vertebral stenotic myelopathy

Cervical vertebral stenotic myelopathy (CVSM) occurs when malformations within the vertebral column cause vertebral canal narrowing and subsequent spinal cord compression.[31,32] Currently, the literature has identified 2 categories of affected horses: (1) young, growing horses typically onset under 5–6 years of age and (2) older horses often associated with significant osteoarthritis.[33,34] Macroscopic pathology associated with CVSM presents as various abnormalities involving the cervical vertebrae and/or associated soft tissue (ie, ligamentum flavum, articular process joint capsule, or intervertebral disk material) in the cervical column.[35–38] The vertebral body can subluxate dorsally into the vertebral canal (**Fig. 3**) or flaring of the caudal epiphysis can reduce vertebral canal height. Articular processes joints exhibit a variety of changes that can lead to vertebral canal narrowing including osteoarthritis, osteochondrosis, subchondral sclerosis, bone cysts, articular process spatial asymmetry that can cause encroachment of the spinal cord, synovial cysts, and thickened joint capsules. Regarding the spinal cord, in some cases, a palpable depression is evident at the site of compression.

In cases of CVSM submitted for necropsy, the inclusion of the results of imaging studies (radiographs, myelogram, and/or computed tomography) aids the pathologist in targeting regions of interest. Preservation of both sides of the bony portion of the cervical column and intact cord is difficult. If lesions are anticipated to be lateralized based on imaging then noting this on the submission form ensures the preservation of the side of the column for examination. When performing a complete examination of the cervical spinal column, the column should be examined in neutral and flexed positions with attention to areas of suspected compression or abnormal motion. The spinal cord is then removed and examined for macroscopic areas of distortion or hemorrhage. The cord may be fixed whole in 10% neutral buffered formalin. To facilitate adequate fixation the dura should be opened along the length of the spinal cord and small incisions can be made into the cord approximately every 2 to 3 cm. After the

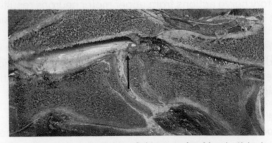

Fig. 3. Dorsal deviation of the cranial aspect of the vertebral body (*black arrow*) into the cervical vertebral canal causing spinal cord compression.

cord is removed, individual vertebrae of interest should be disarticulated to examine the articular processes.

Characteristic histologic lesions that indicate compressive injury to the spinal cord are observed in CVSM cases. In the white matter, Wallerian degeneration characterized by varying degrees of demyelination, presence of gitter cells, dilated myelin sheaths, and spheroids (swollen axons) are consistent with sites of compression. In chronic cases, perivascular fibrosis, motor neuron loss, astrocytosis, and microglial scars are observed.[39] Distribution of the lesions within the funiculi of the white matter aids in lesion localization. Pathologic changes are typically visualized in the dorsal, lateral, and superficial funiculi at the compression site. The dorsal and superficial lateral funiculi, which contain the ascending nerve tracts, are affected cranial to the site of compression, whereas the descending nerve tracts in the ventral and the deep portion of the lateral funiculi are affected caudal to the site of compression.

Neonatal encephalopathy
Neonatal encephalopathy (NE) is a common neurological disease of neonatal foals with variable clinical signs which range from dissociation with the mare to recumbency, seizures, and irregular respiratory patterns. Despite the high prevalence of this condition, the pathophysiology, pattern of neurologic injury, and mechanisms of disease are still poorly understood. Pathologic descriptions of the CNS in foals with NE describe variable pathology which includes laminar necrosis, neuronal necrosis, perineuronal edema, perivascular hemorrhage and vascular hyperplasia.[40] A more recent description of postmortem examination in foals with NE observed neuronal necrosis and/or degeneration within the CNS considered consistent with ischemia.[41] At the University of Kentucky Diagnostic Laboratory, identification of significant microscopic abnormalities within the brain of foals with NE are infrequent, and when identified often consist of scattered neuronal necrosis or cerebral hemorrhage. Despite overt neurologic deficits, it is common to have no significant macroscopic or microscopic changes identified at postmortem examination in foals with NE.

Degenerative/Nutritional

Neuronal axonal dystrophy/equine degenerative myeloencephalopathy
Clinically neuronal axonal dystrophy (NAD) and equine degenerative myeloencephalopathy (EDM) manifest as progressive, symmetric ataxia in young horses typically within the first year of life. Genetic predisposition, alpha-tocopherol deficiency, and diets low in vitamin E are proposed predisposing factors to disease development.[42–44] The pathogenesis is still being investigated, however, oxidative stress on the CNS, either from lack of antioxidants or exposure to environmental oxidants, is the current premise. EDM is considered to be a more advanced form of NAD. Young age is not a prerequisite as similar neurologic signs and microscopic findings have been recognized in older horses.

Macroscopic examination of the brain and spinal cord is typically unremarkable in these cases. Broadly, axonal loss and secondary demyelination comprise the lesions. For NAD, dystrophic axons are localized to the cuneate and gracile nuclei in the medulla oblongata, whereas in EMD, the spinal cord is also affected.[45] Axonal loss throughout all spinal cord funiculi is observed with the cranial cervical and midthoracic spinal cord affected and typically more severe lesions in the thoracic cord. The spinocerebellar tracts in the dorsolateral funiculi and motor tracts in the ventromedial funiculi are more heavily impacted. Other histologic lesions include axonal spheroids, gliosis, lipofuscin accumulation within macrophages, neurons, and endothelium, neuronal degeneration in the dorsal root ganglia, or pigment retinopathy.[46,47]

Equine motor neuron disease

Equine motor neuron disease (EMND) is an acquired neurodegenerative disease that clinically presents as muscle wasting, weakness, weight loss and shifting of weight between the limbs.[48] Pigmentary retinopathy has also been reported in affected horses.[47,49] Risk factors include limited access to pasture, alpha-tocopherol deficiency, vitamin E deficient diets and predominate high grain diets with minimal hay leading to increased susceptibility of the nervous system to oxidative stress.[50,51] Biopsy of the ventral branch of the spinal accessory nerve has been found to be a reliable antemortem test for diagnosis of chronic cases.[52]

Postmortem macroscopic findings include varying degrees and location of skeletal muscle atrophy with typically the medial heads of the triceps vastus intermedius along the femur most severely affected. Lesions are not observed grossly with the brain, spinal cord, or peripheral nerves. Histologically, as the disease name indicates, one of the primary observed lesions is degeneration and loss of motor neurons in the brain stem (cranial nerve nuclei V (facial), VII (trigeminal), XII (hypoglossal), and nucleus ambiguus), and ventral horn of the spinal cord. Neuronal changes include chromatolysis, pyknotic nuclei, neuronophagia, neuronal loss, and accumulation of lipofuscin. Wallerian degeneration is observed in the downstream spinal and peripheral nerves due to impaired motor neuron function. Lesions in the affected skeletal muscle are compatible with denervation atrophy including angular atrophic fibers, with type 1 fibers preferentially affected, and degeneration of intramuscular nerves.[53]

Polyneuritis equi

Polyneuritis equi (PNE), previously known as cauda equina syndrome, is a rare, slowly progressive idiopathic polyneuritis involving the peripheral nerves along the sacrococcygeal region.[54] Studies have focused on the components of the observed granulomatous inflammation suggestive of a potential immune-mediated process.[55] Affected horses can exhibit ataxia, rear limb weakness and decreased tail, anal, perianal, urinary tone and in some cases cranial nerve involvement. Regarding antemortem diagnostics, biopsy of the sacrocaudalis dorsalis lateralis muscle was found to be supportive of a clinical diagnosis of PNE in a case report.[56]

On postmortem examination, macroscopic lesions include thickening and discoloration of the extradural segments of the sacral and coccygeal nerves. Foci of hemorrhage may be interspersed. Microscopically, the thickened nerve segments are due to granulomatous inflammation with extensive fibrosis. IHC studies have identified CD8+ T cells, CD20+ B cells, and plasma cells among the macrophages.[55] Nerve segments distal to the grossly enlarged portions can exhibit both degeneration and regeneration of axons. Cranial nerves may also be affected and these nerves should be collected and examined if a history of nerve deficits is reported.

Congenital

Some structural abnormalities, such as meningoencephalocele/meningocele, are easily identified at birth (**Fig. 4**) However, internal abnormalities such as hydrocephalus, dysplasias, hypoplasia may manifest with nonspecific neurologic abnormalities. A complicating factor in the early identification of congenital diseases affecting the nervous system is the overlap of clinical signs caused by a portion of these conditions and the clinical signs observed in cases of NE. In some cases, such as occipitoatlantoaxial malformations and abnormalities of the structure of the CNS, computed tomography or magnetic resonance imaging allows for antemortem diagnosis. In other conditions, progression of disease and signalment will strongly support a diagnosis that is confirmed with postmortem findings.

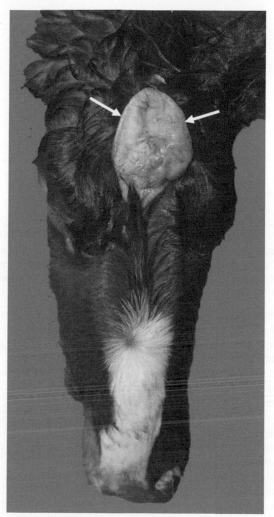

Fig. 4. Protrusion of white-pink tissue (*white arrows*) along the symphysis of the frontal bones. Histopathology confirmed a meningocele.

Cerebellar abiotrophy occurs in Arabians, Swedish Gotland ponies, and the American Miniature Horse. Cerebellar disease is noted between birth to 6 months of age. Histologically, a loss of Purkinje cells and granule cells is observed in the cerebellar folia.[57]

Toxic/Metabolic

Nigropallidal encephalomalacia

Chronic ingestion, typically over 1 month or more, of *Centraurea spp.* plants (ie, yellow star thistle, Russian knapweed) can cause depression, abnormal prehension, salivation, recumbency.[58] Death often occurs due to emaciation and starvation due to impaired oral function. Intoxication is most common in late summer or fall when other pasture forages have come depleted. Repin is suspected to be the neurotoxic component of the plant. The proposed pathogenesis is that repin causes glutathione depletion leading to oxidative damage and neuronal cell death. Lesions are localized to the

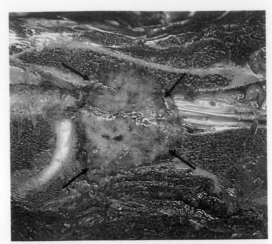

Fig. 5. A parasagittal view of the third cervical vertebra identified a focal, well-demarcated tan-red soft mass encompassing the dorsal lamina and vertebral body with spinal cord compression (*white arrows*). Histology confirmed multicentric lymphosarcoma involving the spleen and cervical vertebra.

globus pallidus and substantia nigra. Both structures are components of the basal ganglia and are involved in voluntary movement.[59]

Foci of malacia are localized to the substantia nigra and globus pallidus. Typically these foci are bilateral but can be unilateral. Malacic areas are soft, yellow, and often gelatinous. Histologically, these foci are composed of well-demarcated regions of liquefactive necrosis typically with loss of neurons, necrotic blood vessels, infiltrates of gitter cells, and regions of edema.

Equine leukoencephalomalacia

Equine leukoencephalomalacia, commonly known as "moldy corn poisoning" occurs when horses ingest moldy feed over a period of 1 month or more. Corn or corn by-products in the feed are contaminated with a saprophytic fungus, *Fusarium verticil-lioides,* or *proliferatum* which produces multiple mycotoxins, both toxic and nontoxic. Fumonisin B1 is considered to be the most significant mycotoxin related to the development of clinical signs and disease.[60] Fumonisin B1 disrupts sphingolipid metabolism which is important for various cellular and metabolic functions in the brain.

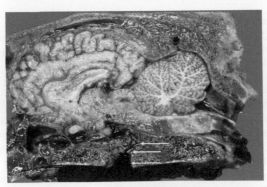

Fig. 6. Parasagittal section of the head identified an acute fracture of the basosphenoid bone (*white arrows*) with associated hemorrhage.

Other processes impacted by fumonisin B1 production include damage to the microvasculature and cardiovascular function. Clinical signs include weakness, circling, ataxia and pharyngeal paralysis to name a few. In horses, whereby there is liver involvement icterus and elevated total bilirubin can be observed.[61]

As the disease name implies, macroscopic lesions are largely localized to the cerebral white matter. Extensive, irregular regions of malacia and hemorrhage are scattered throughout the subcortical white matter on the cut section. Gyri may be flattened but cerebral edema is not observed. If malacia extends to the brain stem and spinal cord, then gray matter involvement can be appreciated. Microscopically, edema, hemorrhage, and necrosis comprise the grossly observed malacic areas. Blood vessels in the area are often infiltrated by eosinophils and plasma cells and variably contain thrombi.

Lead
While lead poisoning is more commonly reported in food animals, it is reported in horses as well. In contrast to food animals, disease in horses is more often due to chronic exposure. The source of exposures in horses is reported to be the inhalation of fumes next to lead smelters, exposure to lead-based materials (ie, paint, caulk, gasoline), or grazing on contaminated pasture. Clinically horses present with depression, cranial nerve deficits leading to laryngeal/pharyngeal paralysis, general paralysis due to peripheral nerve dysfunction or convulsions. In general, lead has limited absorption and is largely excreted over time through bile, feces, milk or urine. Tissue deposition is observed in the liver, kidney and bones.[62,63]

Macroscopic lesions within the central or PNS are typically none. Microscopically, axonal degeneration distal to motor neurons correlates to the clinical peripheral neuropathy. Evaluation of lead in the tissues (liver, kidney, or bone) in conjunction with clinical signs and postmortem findings are confirmatory for lead poisoning.[64]

Swainsonine toxicosis
Swainsonine toxicosis, commonly referred to as locism in North America, is due to the ingestion of locoweeds (*Astragalus* sp., *Oxytropis* sp.) over a period of time. The plants contain indolizidine alkaloid swainsonine. This alkaloid is absorbed and inhibits lysosomal alpha-mannosidase and Golgi mannosidase II ultimately resulting in neuronal swelling and vacuolation due to accumulations of mannose in the lysosomes. Swainsonine toxicosis is an induced storage disease. Clinical signs include ataxia, behavioral changes, and loss of condition. Younger animals are more likely to have irreversible damage as compared with adults due to maturing neurons.[65,66]

Pathognomonic macroscopic lesions are not observed. Microscopically, neurons in the central and peripheral nerves have a foamy appearance due to the microvacuolization of the cytoplasm. Axonal spheroids can be seen in the cerebellum and brainstem. Cytoplasmic vacuolations have also been reported in renal, thyroid, and pancreatic epithelial cells.

Metabolic encephalopathy
In the horse, massive insults to the liver, kidney, or gastrointestinal tract impacting overall organ function can lead to increases in ammonia and other metabolites causing metabolic impairment of cerebral function. Of these hepatic encephalopathy is the most common. A variety of conditions have reported to cause hepatic encephalopathy including but not limited to equine serum hepatitis, cholangitis, choliathiasis, portosystemic shunts in foals, or toxic plant ingestion (ie, pyrrolizidine alkaloid containing plants).[67–74]

Macroscopic lesions are specific to the primary insult. For example, horses with serum hepatitis have shrunken, flaccid, "dish rag livers" due to hepatocyte loss.

Microscopic lesions in cases of metabolic encephalopathy are represented by the proliferation of Alzheimer's type II astroglial cells typically arranged in pairs and clusters throughout the cerebral cortex.[71] Myelin vacuolation that is observed in other species with metabolic encephalopathy is not typically observed in affected horses. Colitis may cause similar neurologic disease and microscopic findings within the brain.

Neoplasia

Primary neoplasia, with the exception of pituitary adenomas, of the CNS is rare in horses. Lymphosarcoma may arise within only the CNS neoplasia or as part of multicentric lymphoma with neoplastic cells present in other organs in addition to the CNS. Clinical signs will depend on the location of the neoplasm which may occur in the brain or spinal cord. In some cases, neoplastic cells may be observed in a cerebral spinal fluid sample or a mass effect may be identified with imaging.[75] A variety of neoplasms have been described and typically result in clinical signs related to what area of the nervous system they arise. Metastatic spread or direct invasion of the nervous system occurs with neoplasia from other organs and may result in compression of the nervous tissue (**Fig. 5**) or pathologic fracture of the vertebral bodies.[75]

Cholesterol granulomas are most frequent within the fourth ventricle but have more clinical significance when formed within the lateral ventricle. They are easily identified at postmortem examination. These nodules are found in 15% to 20% of horses, most commonly with no associated neurologic dysfunction. In a small number of cases the mass becomes large enough to obstruct the interventricular foramen and lead to hydrocephalus and secondary pressure atrophy.[76,77] can we add lymphoma?

Trauma

Trauma to the neurologic system may result in a range of findings at postmortem examination. In acute cases, lesions may be limited to hemorrhage or fractures with the distortion of the nervous tissue. If there is time for damage to the neurologic system to manifest microscopically then areas of hemorrhage or malacia may be observed macroscopically. Axonal, myelin, or neuronal degeneration may be observed microscopically. If the animal survives for several days, then reparative attempts are observed. These include the presence of hemosiderophages, gitter cells, gliosis, and glial scarring. In a small number of cases, minimal gross or histologic findings are observed despite a traumatic episode being observed immediately before death. Common sites of fracture which result in neurologic dysfunction or death include the basosphenoid bone, frontal skull, and spinal column (**Fig. 6**).

Anesthesia

Cases of post anesthetic neurologic dysfunction include mentation changes, blindness, myelopathy, and peripheral neuropathies. Postanesthetic cerebral necrosis was described in 5 horses. All horses developed signs of prosencephalic disease between 5 hours and 7 days of anesthesia. Grossly, areas of malacia were observed within the brain and microscopic findings included laminar neuronal necrosis to diffuse necrosis of the gray and white matter.[78]

Post anesthetic myelopathy or myelomalacia occurs infrequently in horses undergoing general anesthesia. These cases may show the weakness of the hind limbs following recovery, progressing to recumbency. Reported lesions include symmetric necrosis of the gray matter, hemorrhage within the gray matter of the thoracic and spinal cord.[79] Clinically lesions are typically localized to L4-S3. The cause is unknown with spinal cord ischemia proposed as a primary mechanism.[80]

Neuropathies are reported and commonly include the femoral nerve, peroneal nerve, radial nerve, and facial nerve.[81,82] Pathologic findings often include perineural hemorrhage, edema, and findings of nerve degeneration.

Field Necropsy

The authors recognize that they have access to an unparalleled team of necropsy technicians and necropsy suite. In general removal of the entire spinal cord and brain takes 30 to 45 minutes. In a field setting it is unlikely that all instrumentation needed for spinal cord removal will be available. If the entire animal cannot be transported to a diagnostic laboratory, then several options exist to increase the chances of a diagnosis.

Option 1- Removal of the head at the atlanto-occipital (AO) joint. This procedure only requires a sharp knife. CSF can be collected sterilely immediately postmortem from the dorsal or ventral approach to the AO space. Following the disarticulation of the head the cranial aspect of the cervical spinal cord can be extended by gripping the dura and a long scalpel blade will allow for several inches of cord to be collected. The head and spinal cord can be submitted for testing. Most laboratories that perform necropsies will receive heads for processing.

Option 2- Neurolocalized to cervical spine-following removal of the head, the cervical spinal column can be removed with a knife and pressure. The neck is skinned and muscle removed. Disarticulation is performed at C7-T1 with subsequent cuts at this location intermixed with strong upwards or downward manipulation of the cervical column resulting in tearing of the intervertebral disc and freeing of the cervical column. This portion may also be sent to a diagnostic laboratory, particularly useful in suspected cases of cervical compressive lesions.

Option 3- Shipment of small samples only. Collect EDTA blood, whole blood in a red top tube, respiratory swabs, ocular fluid, and CSF. If the horse is seen before death then collection/and submission of a complete blood count, blood chemistry panel as well as CSF analysis may help to determine the cause of disease. Postmortem radiographs may also help to identify sites of fracture. If possible, remove the head and obtain samples of the brainstem and cervical spinal cord. While this will not allow for the diagnosis of several degenerative conditions, many infectious diseases can be identified with this sample set.

SUMMARY

The variety of neurologic diseases which affect horses makes pathologic examination of the nervous system a complex and lengthy process. An understanding of the common causes of neurologic disease, antemortem neurolocalization, and supplementation of the necropsy examination with ancillary testing will help to diagnose a large number of causes of neurologic disease. In cases of infectious disease, the infectious agent will either be visible microscopically or PCR or IHC will be used for confirmatory testing. In cases of degenerative and noninflammatory disease, a stereotypical reaction pattern within the CNS is expected to correlate with a clinical history or macroscopic evidence of nervous system distortion. Metabolic disease and intoxications will require additional testing to confirm an underlying cause of neurologic dysfunction. A general understanding of neuropathology and collaborative relationship with your local pathologists will aid in definitive diagnosis of neurologic diseases.

DISCLOSURE

The authors have nothing to disclose.

REFERENCES

1. Cantile Carlo YS. Nervous system - cytopathology of nervous tissue. In: Maxie MG, editor. Jubb, Kennedy, and Palmer's pathology of domestic animals1, Sixth edition. St. Louis: Elseiver; 2016. p. 251–64.
2. Miller AD, Zachary JF. Nervous system - dysfunction/responses to injury. In: Zachary JF, editor. Pathologic basis of veterinary disease. St. Louis: Elseiver; 2017. p. 815–30.
3. Dubey J, Lindsay D, Saville W, et al. A review of Sarcocystis neurona and equine protozoal myeloencephalitis (EPM). Vet Parasitol 2001;95(2–4):89–131.
4. Hamir A, Moser G, Galligan D, et al. Immunohistochemical study to demonstrate Sarcocystis neurona in equine protozoal myeloencephalitis. J Vet Diagn Invest 1993;5(3):418–22.
5. Henker LC, Bandinelli MB, de Andrade CP, et al. Pathological, immunohistochemical, and molecular findings of equine protozoal myeloencephalitis due to Sarcocystis neurona infection in Brazilian horses. Trop Anim Health Prod 2020;52(6): 3809–17.
6. Bryan LK, Hamer SA, Shaw S, et al. Chagas disease in a Texan horse with neurologic deficits. Vet Parasitol 2016;216:13–7.
7. Li X, Ni HB, Ren WX, et al. Seroprevalence of Toxoplasma gondii in horses: a global systematic review and meta-analysis. Acta Trop 2020;201:105222.
8. Kimble KM, Gomez G, Szule JA, et al. Systemic toxoplasmosis in a horse. J Comp Pathol 2021;182:27–31.
9. Snook CS, Hyman SS, Piero FD, et al. West Nile virus encephalomyelitis in eight horses. J Am Vet Med Assoc 2001;218(10):1576–9.
10. Cantile C, Del Piero F, Di Guardo G, et al. Pathologic and immunohistochemical findings in naturally occurring West Nile virus infection in horses. Vet Pathol 2001; 38(4):414–31.
11. Del Piero F, Wilkins PA, Dubovi EJ, et al. Clinical, pathologic, immunohistochemical, and virologic findings of eastern equine encephalomyelitis in two horses. Vet Pathol 2001;38(4):451–6.
12. Steele K, Twenhafel N. Pathology of animal models of alphavirus encephalitis. Vet Pathol 2010;47(5):790–805.
13. WHITWELL KE, Blunden A. Pathological findings in horses dying during an outbreak of the paralytic form of Equid herpesvirus type 1 (EHV-1) infection. Equine Vet J 1992;24(1):13–9.
14. Pusterla N, Hussey GS. Equine herpesvirus 1 myeloencephalopathy. Vet Clin North Am Equine Pract 2014;30(3):489–506.
15. Bassuino DM, Konradt G, Cruz RA, et al. Characterization of spinal cord lesions in cattle and horses with rabies: the importance of correct sampling. J Vet Diagn Invest 2016;28(4):455–60.
16. Toth B, Aleman M, Nogradi N, et al. Meningitis and meningoencephalomyelitis in horses: 28 cases (1985-2010). J Am Vet Med Assoc 2012;240(5):580–7.
17. Raphel C. Brain abscess in three horses. J Am Vet Med Assoc 1982;180(8): 874–7.
18. Imai D, Barr B, Daft B, et al. Lyme neuroborreliosis in 2 horses. Vet Pathol 2011; 48(6):1151–7.
19. Johnstone L, Engiles J, Aceto H, et al. Retrospective evaluation of horses diagnosed with neuroborreliosis on postmortem examination: 16 cases (2004–2015). J Vet Intern Med 2016;30(4):1305–12.

20. Divers T, Gardner R, Madigan JE, et al. Borrelia burgdorferi infection and Lyme disease in North American horses: a consensus statement. J Vet Intern Med 2018;32(2):617–32.
21. Critchley E. A comparison of human and animal botulism: a review. J R Soc Med 1991;84(5):295–8.
22. Whitlock RH, Buckley C. Botulism. Vet Clin North Am Equine Pract 1997;13(1): 107–28.
23. Broughton J, Parsons L. Botulism in horses fed big bale silage. Vet Rec 1985; 117(25–26):674.
24. Ostrowski SR, Kubiski SV, Palmero J, et al. An outbreak of equine botulism type A associated with feeding grass clippings. J Vet Diagn Invest 2012;24(3):601–3.
25. Wichtel J, Whitlock R. Botulism associated with feeding alfalfa hay to horses. J Am Vet Med Assoc 1991;199(4):471–2.
26. Green SL, Little CB, Baird JD, et al. Tetanus in the horse: a review of 20 cases (1970 to 1990). J Vet Intern Med 1994;8(2):128–32.
27. Van Galen G, Delguste C, Sandersen C, et al. Tetanus in the equine species: a retrospective study of 31 cases. Tijdschr Diergeneeskd 2008;133(12):512–7.
28. Kinde H, Mathews M, Ash L, et al. Leger J. Halicephalobus gingivalis (H. deletrix) infection in two horses in southern California. J Vet Diagn Invest 2000;12(2): 162–5.
29. Johnson AL, De Lahunta A, Divers TJ. Acquired scoliosis in equids: case series and proposed pathogenesis. Paper presented at. AAEP Proceedings 2008.
30. Mittelman NS, Divers TJ, Engiles JB, et al. Parelaphostrongylus tenuis cerebro-spinal nematodiasis in a horse with cervical scoliosis and meningomyelitis. J Vet Intern Med 2017;31(3):890–3.
31. Mayhew IG, delahunta A. A.spinal cord disease in the horse. Cornell Vet 1978; 68(Suppl 6):1–207.
32. Dimock WW, Errington B. J. Incoordination of Equidae: Wobblers. J Am Vet Med Assoc 1939;XCV(750):261–7.
33. Levine JM, Adam E, MacKay RJ, et al. Confirmed and presumptive cervical verte-bral compressive myelopathy in older horses: a retrospective study (1992–2004). J Vet Intern Med 2007;21(4):812–9.
34. Levine JM, Ngheim PP, Levine GJ, et al. Associations of sex, breed, and age with cervical vertebral compressive myelopathy in horses: 811 cases (1974-2007). J Am Vet Med Assoc 2008;233(9):1453–8.
35. Nout Y, Reed S. Cervical vertebral stenotic myelopathy. Equine Vet Education 2003;15(4):212–23.
36. Powers B, Stashak T, Nixon A, et al. Pathology of the vertebral column of horses with cervical static stenosis. Vet Pathol 1986;23(4):392–9.
37. Stewart RH, Reed SM, Weisbrode SE. Frequency and severity of osteochondrosis in horses with cervical stenotic myelopathy. Am J Vet Res 1991;52(6):873–9.
38. Janes JG, Garrett KS, McQuerry KJ, et al. Cervical vertebral lesions in equine ste-notic myelopathy. Vet Pathol 2015;52(5):919–27.
39. Summers BACJ, de Lahunta A. Injuries to the central nervous system. veterinary neuropathology. St. Louis, MO: Mosby; 1995. p. 193–8.
40. Palmer A, Rossdale P. Neuropathological changes associated with the neonatal maladjustment syndrome in the Thoroughbred foal. Res Vet Sci 1976;20(3): 267–75.
41. Lyle-Dugas J, Giguere S, Mallicote MF, et al. Factors associated with outcome in 94 hospitalised foals diagnosed with neonatal encephalopathy. Equine Vet J 2017;49(2):207–10.

42. Aleman M, Finno CJ, Higgins RJ, et al. Evaluation of epidemiological, clinical, and pathological features of neuroaxonal dystrophy in Quarter Horses. J Am Vet Med Assoc 2011;239(6):823–33.

43. Burns EN, Finno CJ. Equine degenerative myeloencephalopathy: prevalence, impact, and management. Vet Med (Auckl) 2018;9:63–7.

44. Finno CJ, Miller AD, Sisó S, et al. Concurrent equine degenerative myeloencephalopathy and equine motor neuron disease in three young horses. J Vet Intern Med 2016;30(4):1344–50.

45. Beech J. Neuroaxonal dystrophy of the accessory cuneate nucleus in horses. Vet Pathol 1984;21(4):384–93.

46. Finno CJ, Valberg SJ, Shivers J, et al. Evidence of the primary afferent tracts undergoing neurodegeneration in horses with equine degenerative myeloencephalopathy based on calretinin immunohistochemical localization. Vet Pathol 2016; 53(1):77–86.

47. Finno CJ, Kaese HJ, Miller AD, et al. Pigment retinopathy in warmblood horses with equine degenerative myeloencephalopathy and equine motor neuron disease. Vet Ophthalmol 2017;20(4):304–9.

48. Divers TJ, Mohammed HO, Cummings JF. Equine motor neuron disease. Vet Clin North Am Equine Pract 1997;13(1):97–105.

49. Riis RC, Jackson C, Rebhun W, et al. Ocular manifestations of equine motor neuron disease. Equine Vet J 1999;31(2):99–110.

50. Cummings JF, de Lahunta A, Mohammed HO, et al. Endothelial lipopigment as an indicator of α-tocopherol deficiency in two equine neurodegenerative diseases. Acta Neuropathol 1995;90(3):266–72.

51. Divers TJ, Mohammed HO, Cummings JF, et al. Equine motor neuron disease: findings in 28 horses and proposal of a pathophysiological mechanism for the disease. Equine Vet J 1994;26(5):409–15.

52. Jackson CA, De Lahunta A, Cummings JF, et al. Spinal accessory nerve biopsy as an ante mortem diagnostic test for equine motor neuron disease. Equine Vet J 1996;28(3):215–9.

53. Cantile Carlo YS. Nervous system - progressive motor neuron diseases. In: Maxie MG, editor. Jubb, Kennedy and Palmer's pathology of domestic animals1, 6th edition. St. Louis: Elsevier; 2016. p. 330–1.

54. Milne F, Carbonell P. Neuritis of the cauda equina of horses: a case report. Equine Vet J 1970;2(4):179–82.

55. Van Galen G, Cassart D, Sandersen C, et al. The composition of the inflammatory infiltrate in three cases of polyneuritis equi. Equine Vet J 2008;40(2):185–8.

56. Aleman M, Katzman SA, Vaughan B, et al. Antemortem diagnosis of polyneuritis equi. J Vet Intern Med 2009;23(3):665–8.

57. Blanco A, Moyano R, Vivo J, et al. Purkinje cell apoptosis in arabian horses with cerebellar abiotrophy. J Vet Med A Physiol Pathol Clin Med 2006;53(6):286–7.

58. Cordy D. Nigropallidal encephalomalacia in horses associated with ingestion of yellow star thistle. J Neuropathol Exp Neurol 1954;13:330–42.

59. Chang H, Rumbeiha W, Patterson J, et al. Toxic equine parkinsonism: an immunohistochemical study of 10 horses with nigropallidal encephalomalacia. Vet Pathol 2012;49(2):398–402.

60. Marasas WFO, Kellerman TS, Gelderblom WC, et al. Leukoencephalomalacia in a horse induced by fumonisin B₁isolated from Fusarium moniliforme. Onderstepoort J Vet Res 1988;55(4):197–203.

61. Uhlinger C. Leukoencephalomalacia. Vet Clin North Am Equine Pract 1997;13(1): 13–20.

62. Dollahite J, Younger R, Crookshank H, et al. Chronic lead poisoning in horses. Am J Vet Res 1978;39(6):961–4.
63. Schmitt N, Brown G, Devlin EL, et al. Lead poisoning in horses. Arch Environ Health An Int J 1971;23(3):185–95.
64. Cantile CYS. Nervous system-lead poisoning. In: Maxie MG, editor. Jubb, Kennedy and Palmer's pathology of domestic animals1, 6th edition. St Louis, Missouri: Elsevier; 2016. p. 316–7.
65. James LF, Van Kampen KR, Staker GR. Locoweed (Astragalus lentiginosus) poisoning in cattle and horses. J Am Vet Med Assoc 1969;155:525–30.
66. Pfister J, Stegelmeier B, Gardner D, et al. Grazing of spotted locoweed (Astragalus lentiginosus) by cattle and horses in Arizona. J Anim Sci 2003;81(9):2285–93.
67. Peek S, Divers T. Medical treatment of cholangiohepatitis and cholelithiasis in mature horses: 9 cases (1991–1998). Equine Vet J 2000;32(4):301–6.
68. Peek SF, Divers TJ, Jackson CJ. Hyperammonaemia associated with encephalopathy and abdominal pain without evidence of liver disease in four mature horses. Equine Vet J 1997;29(1):70–4.
69. Bouchard P, Weldon A, Lewis R, et al. Uremic encephalopathy in a horse. Vet Pathol 1994;31(1):111–5.
70. Frye MA, Johnson JS, Traub-Dargatz JL, et al. Putative uremic encephalopathy in horses: five cases (1978–1998). J Am Vet Med Assoc 2001;218(4):560–6.
71. Hasel KM, Summers B, De Lahunta A. Encephalopathy with idiopathic hyperammonaemia and Alzheimer type II astrocytes in Equidae. Equine Vet J 1999;31(6):478–82.
72. Aleman M, Nieto JE, Carr EA, et al. Serum hepatitis associated with commercial plasma transfusion in horses. J Vet Intern Med 2005;19(1):120 2.
73. Pearson EG. Liver failure attributable to pyrrolizidine alkaloid toxicosis and associated with inspiratory dyspnea in ponies: three cases (1982-1988). J Am Vet Med Assoc 1991;198(9):1651–4.
74. Stegelmeier BL. Pyrrolizidine alkaloid-containing toxic plants (Senecio, Crotalaria, Cynoglossum, Amsinckia, Heliotropium, and Echium spp.). Vet Clin North Am Food Anim Pract 2011;27(2):419–28.
75. Paradis MR. Tumors of the central nervous system. Vet Clin North Am Equine Pract 1998;14(3):543–61.
76. Maulet B, Bestbier M, Jose-Cunilleras E, et al. Magnetic resonance imaging of a cholesterol granuloma and hydrocephalus in a horse. Equine Vet Education 2008; 20(2):74–9.
77. Lloyd-Edwards RA, Willems DS, Beukers M, et al. Presumed cholesterinic granulomas detected on CT in horses are associated with increased lateral ventricle height and age. Vet Radiol Ultrasound 2020;61(3):269–78.
78. McKay J, Kelly D, Senior M, et al. Postanaesthetic cerebral necrosis in five horses. Vet Rec 2002;150(3):70–4.
79. Zink MC. Postanesthetic poliomyelomalacia in a horse. Can Vet J 1985;26(9):275.
80. Trim CM. Postanesthetic hemorrhagic myelopathy or myelomalacia. Vet Clin North Am Equine Pract 1997;13(1):73–7.
81. Wagner AE. Complications in equine anesthesia. Vet Clin North Am Equine Pract 2008;24(3):735–52, x.
82. Moreno KL, Scallan EM, Friedeck WO, et al. Transient pelvic limb neuropathy following proximal metatarsal and tarsal magnetic resonance imaging in seven horses. Equine Vet J 2020;52(3):359–63.

Printed and bound by CPI Group (UK) Ltd, Croydon, CR0 4YY

03/10/2024

01040482-0009